Devices for Blood Analysis: Hematology Essentials

Devices for Blood Analysis: Hematology Essentials

Editor: Marko Emanuel

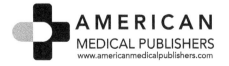

AMERICAN
MEDICAL PUBLISHERS
www.americanmedicalpublishers.com

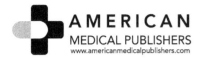

Cataloging-in-Publication Data

Devices for blood analysis : hematology essentials / edited by Marko Emanuel.
       p. cm.
Includes bibliographical references and index.
ISBN 978-1-63927-655-4
1. Blood--Analysis. 2. Blood--Analysis--Equipment and supplies. 3. Hematology.
4. Blood--Diseases. 5. Diagnosis, Laboratory. 6. Hemodynamic monitoring.
I. Emanuel, Marko.
RB45 .D48 2023
616.075 61--dc23

American Medical Publishers,
41 Flatbush Avenue,
1st Floor, New York,
NY 11217, USA

ISBN 978-1-63927-655-4 (Hardback)

Contents

Preface

Blood is a type of body fluid found in the circulatory system of human beings and other vertebrates. It carries essential substances including oxygen and nutrients to the cells. It also carries-back the metabolic waste products and carbon dioxide from the cells to lungs, kidneys and digestive system to be removed by the body. Blood analysis refers to the laboratory investigation of a blood sample that helps to gather information about its chemical and physical properties. For carrying out blood analysis, blood sample is drawn from the veins of fingers, arms or earlobes. In certain cases, the blood cells of the bone marrow might also be examined. Micro devices have great potential for the growth of portable and point-of-care diagnostic devices, specifically for blood analysis. The development of micro and nano devices for the analysis of blood, integrates numerous research fields including electronics, micro or nanotechnologies, medicine, informatics, mechanics, biotechnology, chemistry and optics. This book explores all the important aspects of blood analysis devices in the present day. It is a valuable compilation of topics, ranging from the basic to the most complex advancements in the field of hematology. The readers would gain knowledge that would broaden their perspective in this area.

This book is the end result of constructive efforts and intensive research done by experts in this field. The aim of this book is to enlighten the readers with recent information in this area of research. The information provided in this profound book would serve as a valuable reference to students and researchers in this field.

At the end, I would like to thank all the authors for devoting their precious time and providing their valuable contribution to this book. I would also like to express my gratitude to my fellow colleagues who encouraged me throughout the process.

Editor

Dielectric Characterization and Separation Optimization of Infiltrating Ductal Adenocarcinoma via Insulator-Dielectrophoresis

Ezekiel O. Adekanmbi, Anthony T. Giduthuri and Soumya K. Srivastava *

Department of Chemical and Materials Engineering, University of Idaho, Moscow, ID 83844-1021, USA; adek5632@vandals.uidaho.edu (E.O.A.); gidu3424@vandals.uidaho.edu (A.T.G.)
* Correspondence: srivastavask@uidaho.edu

Abstract: The dielectrophoretic separation of infiltrating ductal adenocarcinoma cells (ADCs) from isolated peripheral blood mononuclear cells (PBMCs) in a ~1.4 mm long Y-shaped microfluidic channel with semi-circular insulating constrictions is numerically investigated. In this work, ADCs (breast cancer cells) and PBMCs' electrophysiological properties were iteratively extracted through the fitting of a single-shell model with the frequency-conductivity data obtained from AC microwell experiments. In the numerical computation, the gradient of the electric field required to generate the necessary dielectrophoretic force within the constriction zone was provided through the application of electric potential across the whole fluidic channel. By adjusting the difference in potentials between the global inlet and outlet of the fluidic device, the minimum (effective) potential difference with the optimum particle transmission probability for ADCs was found. The radius of the semi-circular constrictions at which the effective potential difference was swept to obtain the optimum constriction size was also obtained. Independent particle discretization analysis was also conducted to underscore the accuracy of the numerical solution. The numerical results, which were obtained by the integration of fluid flow, electric current, and particle tracing module in COMSOL v5.3, reveal that PBMCs can be maximally separated from ADCs using a DC power source of 50 V. The article also discusses recirculation or wake formation behavior at high DC voltages (>100 V) even when sorting of cells are achieved. This result is the first step towards the production of a supplementary or confirmatory test device to detect early breast cancer non-invasively.

Keywords: dielectrophoresis; electrophysiological properties; crossover frequency; wake or recirculation formation; dielectric spectra

1. Introduction

Noncommunicable diseases (NCDs) kill more than 36 million people annually representing 63% of global deaths [1]. Breast cancer, a subset of NCDs, accounts for over 500,000 of these deaths [2] with an incidence of about 1.1 million new cases being reported per year [3]. In the United States, as of March 2017, more than 3.1 million women with a history of breast cancer has been reported [4]. About 85% of these breast cancers occur in women who have no family history of breast cancer [4] and one in eight women develop breast cancer in her lifetime. As of now, the main cause of breast cancer cannot be pinned down exactly, but scientists have hypothesized where breast cancer originates. Our bodies consist of many cells, which can be replaced as they age. Old cells tend to copy their DNA before splitting into new ones. However, the copying process could cause mutation which may result in cellular abnormalities called tumors. When tumor cells grow and invade neighboring tissues, they are termed cancerous [5,6]. Breast cancer that starts in the cells of the glands are termed adenocarcinoma

(ADCs), which can be invasive ductal (indicates that the cancer cells present in the milk ducts (Ductal Carcinoma in-situ)) and can begin to infiltrate and replace the normal surrounding tissues of the duct walls (accounts for 80% of breast cancer), also known as invasive lobular. According to the National Cancer Institute, around 90% of breast cancers are adenocarcinomas. If untreated, breast cancers can grow bigger, taking over more surrounding breast tissue. When breast cancer cells break away from the original cancer, they can enter the blood or lymph vessels. Traveling through these vessels, cancer cells may settle in other areas of the breast or in the lymph nodes of the breast tissue, forming new tumors. This is called metastasis. These adenocarcinomas are the most difficult tumor to accurately identify the primary site [7].

Diagnosis of adenocarcinoma is achieved by examining features such as tubular myelin, intranuclear surface apoprotein tubular inclusions, Langerhans cells associated with neoplastic cells, cytoplasmic hyaline globules, glycogen, lipid droplets, and cytoplasmic crystals. The diagnostic is painful since a tissue biopsy is utilized to extract the different types of cells mentioned above making it a cumbersome, time consuming, and costly process since they are ultrastructural features that are needed to be observed through electron microscopes. Another technique to diagnose adenocarcinoma is through the application of immunohistochemistry that has also been explored using estrogen and progesterone receptor proteins, thyroid transcription factor-I and surfactant apoproteins [7]. However, specificity and sensitivity are the main issues associated with this method. An alternative technique including a less invasive route is desirable to address some of the drawbacks of the current diagnostic tools used such that it is rapid, easy-to-use, economical, and sensitive. The combination of peripheral blood mononuclear cells (PBMCs) and microfluidics makes an excellent alternative that is explored through this article.

In this article, we explore the use of PBMCs to detect these cancerous cells since they are known to circulate in the peripheral blood of patients, especially when breast cancer is spread beyond the ducts into other parts of the breast tissues or other organs through blood [8]. PBMCs are typically isolated from whole blood using density gradient centrifugation commonly in Ficoll-Pacque PLUS and the Histopaque 1077 media [9]. To discriminate and subsequently separate ADCs from PBMCs, increased interests have been rooted in exploring the utilization of the cell physical properties in lieu of other methods including antibody-conjugation, which is time consuming and can impact ADCs' properties and viability [10]. Leveraging physical characteristics in the form of size-based filtration [11–13], density-gradient separation [14–16], and inertial-hydrodynamic discrimination [17–19] has been explored in the past until Shim et al. reported that size and density distributions of ADCs tend to overlap with those of PBMCs, leading to occasional inefficiency in the separation of ADCs based on size and density. An alternative technique is to utilize the electrophysiological property differences between PBMCs and ADCs in a microfluidic device, termed as dielectrophoresis (DEP).

Dielectrophoresis (DEP), a microfluidic and an electrokinetic technique that could be utilized to detect ADCs from a heterogenous population of PBMCs, utilizes electric signatures like cell capacitance and conductance in a non-uniform electric gradient, and seems to be a novel alternative [20–25]. DEP is a promising technique that is utilized to characterize and manipulate different types of cells like red blood cells, bacteria, virus, yeast, and proteins. It also is capable of detecting subtle changes on the cells based on their state, i.e., alive and dead, healthy and infected. In this article we choose to characterize PBMCs and ADCs utilizing DEP as a detection tool via quantifying the unhealthy or diseased cells, i.e., cancer cells because it employs no moving parts, it is non-destructive for the bioparticles, and utilizes low electric current on a micro-chip without the need of antibody tagging or fluorescent labels making it a portable system. Reduced response time and higher throughput and accuracy makes DEP a promising technique for cancer cell detection.

When a bioparticle is subjected to a non-uniform electric field, the dielectrophoretic forces and the dipole-dipole forces between the particles (dipole moments) are generated based on the differences between the electrical properties (capacitance and conductance) of cells and the surrounding fluid [23]. Traditionally, DEP based cancer cell separations employ metallic electrodes to capture infected cells, by creating non-uniform electric fields using AC voltage [16,25]. AC DEP device offers a major disadvantage in the form of decreased metal electrode functionality due to fouling when biological samples are manipulated [24,26]. Also, these devices often have high cost associated with the fabrication containing metal parts [24,27]. To address the challenges posed by AC DEP device, we chose to explore DC electric current (insulator-based DEP (iDEP)) as an alternative to electrode-based DEP. iDEP employs insulating objects or structures created by microfabrication embedded in the channel to generate spatial non-uniformities in the field [28,29]. With the electrodes placed in the inlet and outlets, here electroosmotic forces can be utilized for inducing flows, eliminating the need for the pumps for continuous operation [30]. The aim of this work, therefore, is to determine experimentally if there are differences in the electrophysiological properties of normal PBMCs and ADCs and to use these differences, if they exist, to numerically attempt their detection (using DC signals) on a microchip—an important step towards the development of a supplementary diagnostic device for ADCs.

In this article, we develop an in silico based COMSOL Multiphysics model for continuously detecting ADCs from a heterogenous population of PBMCs in a microchannel with modified geometry. To create non-uniformity in the electric field, an array of semi-circular insulating obstacles are embedded in the microchannel. First, a PDMS-based microwell was constructed to house a horizontally arranged 100 μm apart platinum electrode (Figure 1) to obtain the characteristic membrane properties of both ADCs and PBMCs. The properties, validated against the available data in the literature, are then utilized to in conjunction with Finite Element Method (FEM) to model and simulate the trajectory of both cells (ADCs and PBMCs) in a semicircular-insulator-based 2D microfluidic channel. While the characterization of the ADCs gives the innate electrical signatures that is characteristic of moderately differentiated infiltrating ductal adenocarcinoma, the utilization of FEM sets a workable model that could serve as a platform for fabricating a novel diagnostic device for ADCs.

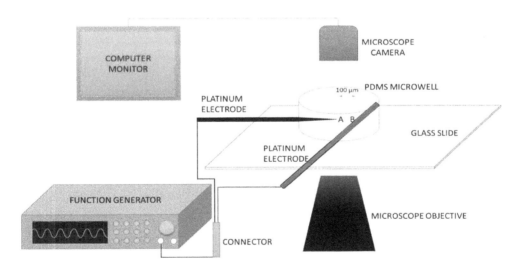

Figure 1. The experimental set-up for the measurement of dielectrophoresis (DEP) crossover frequency using a novel microwell platform to obtain electrophysiological properties, i.e., conductivity and permittivity of peripheral blood mononuclear cell (PBMCs) and adenocarcinoma cells (ADCs) that will aid in designing an early detection platform for breast cancer.

2. Theory of Dielectrophoresis

Crossover frequency measurement is a novel dielectrophoretic-based method of characterizing the dielectric properties of many biological particles. By crossover frequency, we mean the frequency at which cells suspended in a microwell in an osmotic concentration medium, change their direction of motion towards or away from the high field region in an electric-field-gradient-based system. When a bioparticle (i.e., cell) is placed between the two electrodes as shown in Figure 1, the cell can either move to A or B depending on its polarizability relative to the medium in which it is suspended. Cells move to A (pDEP) if they are more polarizable than the medium and to B (nDEP) if the reverse occurs. At varying conductivity of the suspending medium, various crossover frequency data (f_{xo}) can be generated. In this current work, these data are generated, plotted and fitted with a model (Equation (1)) using least square regression and the confidence of the fit was found through the coefficient of regression analysis. A voltage drop at the electrode boundary is considered to be significant at frequencies below 15 kHz [30]. Also, because the reservoirs of microdevice are typically considered as an enormous source of ions compared with the microchannels themselves, any voltage drop can be neglected between the electrode and the inlet or outlet to the microchannel. In this study, the operating conditions for the crossover frequency quantification are maintained above the reported threshold and thus can neglect the voltage drop at the boundary of the electrodes that are placed in the inlet and outlet reservoirs. According to Pethig [31] or a biological cell whose interfacial polarization between the plasma membrane and the cytoplasm results in a dispersion frequency far below 1 MHz for the cell effective dielectric permittivity and conductivity, the first crossover frequency, f_{xo1}, of the cell membrane is given by:

$$f_{xo1} = f_{xo1}(C_{mem}, G_{mem}, \sigma_m):$$
$$f_{xo1} = \frac{1}{\sqrt{2}} \frac{\sigma_m}{\pi R C_{mem}} \sqrt{1 - \frac{RG_{mem}}{2\sigma_m} - 2\left(\frac{RG_{mem}}{2\sigma_m}\right)^2} \tag{1}$$

$$\forall C_{mem} = \varepsilon_{mem}/d \tag{2}$$

$$G_{mem} = \sigma_{mem}/d \tag{3}$$

In terms of total particles and medium properties, f_{xo1} can also be represented as

$$f_{xo1} = \frac{1}{2\pi} \left\{ \frac{(\sigma_m - \sigma_p)(\sigma_p + 2\sigma_m)}{(\varepsilon_p - \varepsilon_m)(\varepsilon_p + \varepsilon_m)} \right\}^{1/2} \tag{4}$$

where, C_{mem} is the specific membrane capacitance, G_{mem} the membrane conductance, σ_m the conductivity of the suspending medium, ε_{mem} the permittivity of the membrane, σ_{mem} the conductivity of the membrane, d is the characteristic dimension of the cell membrane and R, the radius of the particle. In an iDEP system, the DEP force, $\vec{F}_{DEP}$, acting on the particles due to the field gradient is a function of the particle and medium characteristics and is given as:

$$\vec{F}_{DEP} = 2\pi\varepsilon_m r^3 \left(\frac{\sigma_p - \sigma_m}{\sigma_p + 2\sigma_m}\right) \nabla \left|\vec{E}_{DC}\right|^2 \tag{5}$$

where the quantity $\left(\frac{\sigma_p - \sigma_m}{\sigma_p + 2\sigma_m}\right)$ is the Clausius-Mossotti factor (CM), which is the parameter that determines whether $\vec{F}_{DEP}$ will be positive (as in pDEP) or negative (as in nDEP) and $\nabla \left|\vec{E}_{DC}\right|^2$ is the field distribution parameter that enhances particle polarization and dielectrophoretic separation effect.

This force is usually balanced with the viscous drag within the fluid system. Prior to the utilization of DEP-viscous force balance for particle separation, electrokinetic forces (electroosmotic and electrophoretic forces) would have been utilized to pump the particles to the separation region through the electroosmotic channel wall condition and the electrostatic interaction of the electric field with the particles.

Electroosmotic flow is generated due to the action of the electric field on charged interior surfaces having electrical double-layer (EDL). For the microscale flow, surface charge generated at the solid wall-ionic liquid interface is a significant interfacial property to affect the flow. This is because the surface charge at the solid–liquid interface can redistribute the charged ions in the ionic liquid and forms the electrical double layer (EDL) with local net charge density. However, because of the characteristic length of the EDL known as Debye length is small and has the typical values from several nanometers to one micrometer (significantly small compared to the dimensions of the channel), thus the effect of EDL on the microscale flow is usually neglectable and it can only produce obvious effect on the nanoscale fluid flow. When an external electric field is applied on the ionic liquid with EDL within a microchannel, the liquid will be driven by the electric field and form the electroosmotic flow (EOF), which is a typical fluidic transport phenomenon over the microscale [32,33]. The nature and magnitude of the charge in EDL is characterized by the Zeta potential [34]. Electroosmotic mobility of fluid is a function of the Zeta potential of the microdevice, i.e., microchannel construction material and is given by [35]:

$$\mu_{EO} = \frac{-\xi\varepsilon_m}{\eta} \tag{6}$$

where, μ_{EO} is the electroosmotic mobility, ε_m is the permittivity of medium, ξ is the Zeta potential of the material and η is the viscosity of suspending medium (buffer). The electrophoretic mobility unlike the electroosmotic mobility that depends on the material, depends on the Zeta potential of the particle itself and is given by [36]:

$$\mu_{EO} = \frac{\xi_p\varepsilon_m}{\eta} \tag{7}$$

where, ξ_p is the Zeta potential of the particle. At the separation region, the particle experiences a dielectrophoretic force that is impacted by the particle mobility. The DEP mobility is a function of CM factor and for a spherical particle it is expressed as [37]:

$$\mu_{DEP} = \frac{\pi d_p^2 \varepsilon_m}{12\eta}CM \tag{8}$$

where, d_p is the particle diameter and η is the medium viscosity.

3. Materials and Methods

3.1. Microwell Fabrication

Silicone elastomer mixed with its curing agent in 10:1 ratio (Sylgard 184, Dow Corning, Midland, MI, USA) was placed in a desiccator chamber under 0.27-mTorr vacuum in order to remove the bubbles formed during the mixing process. After three successive degassing operations lasting for 15 min, at an interval of 5 min between each run, the clear PDMS was poured into a clean petri dish and cured in the oven at 70 °C for 1 h. This step was followed by dicing the PDMS into 1″ × 1″ squares. A 3-mm hole was punched into each of the diced PDMS to create a well onto which the cell suspension was pipetted. Scotch tape was used to remove any dirt/dust from the PDMS after which it is was irreversibly sealed to a borosilicate glass slide through plasma oxidation of 50 W RF power for 1 min. High purity platinum wire was connected to the microwell as shown in Figure 1. With the aid of an Olympus IX71 inverted microscope (Olympus, Tokyo, Japan), the distance (100 μm) between the electrode tips was set. Loctite's self-mix epoxy was used to keep the electrode spacing intact. The epoxy also prevented any leakage of liquid when the microwell was filled with cell suspension. This was evident when anhydrous copper sulfate was dispensed around the filled microwell, in a regulated environment, did not cause any change in color, i.e., from its natural white to blue color.

3.2. Cell Pretreatment

The DEP suspending medium (dextrose solution) was prepared and characterized as described in our previous article [38]. The prepared 100 mL suspending medium was divided into five separate beakers. Into each beaker, except the first, calculated volume of phosphate buffer saline (PBS) was added to successively change the conductivity of the DEP suspending medium to obtain the following conductivities (in mS/m): 50, 60, 74, 88 and 97. Female normal peripheral mononuclear cells (PBMCs) and infiltrating ductal adenocarcinoma cells (ADCs) with no identifiable angiolymphatic invasion were obtained from Conversant Bio, Huntsville, AL, USA. Also, the cells obtained did not have any identifiable information about the patient itself except their gender and age (Institutional Review Board - IRB exempt). The cells were prepared for experiment according to the supplier's instructions. Thereafter, a known number of cells were transferred into each of the five DEP suspending medium solution where they were washed twice and diluted in 1:400 cell: suspending medium ratio before being pipetted into the DEP microwell for experiment.

3.3. Measurement of Crossover Frequency

After the assurance that the microwell was leakage-free, the platinum electrodes were connected to the two terminals of an 80 MHz Siglent SDG 2082X Arbitrary Waveform Generator (Siglent Technologies, Solon, OH, USA), which supplied an 8 V peak-to-peak sinusoidal AC signal of shifting frequencies. 5 µL of the PBMCs suspension prepared as discussed in Section 3.2 was transferred into the microwell and allowed to equilibrate. Then, about 4 µL was carefully siphoned from the well so that fewer cells (between 4–7 cells) were present in the field-of-view for the experiment. Having fewer cells does not only reduce the influence of particle-particle interaction, but also enhances clarity in visualizing cells for crossover frequency determination. The waveform generator was then switched on to generate electric field gradient around the electrodes. Movement of cells was monitored and captured with a high-speed camera at 30 fps as a function of the changing field frequency until the crossover frequency was found. There was no movement of cells or flow when the waveform generator was turned off. The experiment was repeated four times (technical replicates) and there were two set of biological replicates obtained for the experiments and the crossover frequency was found in each case. More experiments were run using the other modified medium at varying conductivities thus obtaining crossover frequency spectra. The PBMCs are majorly lymphocytes (>80%) ~10 µm in diameter while ADCs are ~20 µm in diameter. Measurements were made at room temperature conditions, i.e., $T = 24 \pm 1\,°C$.

4. Finite Element Modeling and Simulation

In this section, attention was given to the numerical modelling and simulation performed using the dielectric properties obtained from the crossover frequency measurements in Section 3.3. COMSOL Multiphysics 5.3a (Comsol Inc., Stockholm, Sweden) was used to solve fluid flow, electrostatics, and particle tracing modules in an integrated stationary and time-dependent fashion. The architecture of the separation device (Figure 2) was arrived at after a series of parameter modification that ensured a complete separation of ADCs from its mixture with PBMCs. The design was made in 2D because the width to depth ratio was more than 5:1.

Electric current mode was used to solve, in steady states, the current conservation equation based on Ohms law and electric displacement relations using the electric potential as the dependent variable. This was solved in steady state because the charge relaxation time for the conducting media (water, in this case 3.6×10^{-6} s) is less than the external time scale for device operation (10 s). Solving this Ohm's law with the charge conservation and electric displacement equations gives the electric field, E, which was used to compute the electroosmotic boundary condition used in the creeping flow analysis according to $u_{EO} = \mu_{EO}E$, where u_{EO} is the electroosmotic velocity- the velocity of the bulk of the fluid flowing in the channel due to electric field effects. In the incompressible creeping flow analysis (as is the usual case in microfluidic channel where the Reynolds number is significantly less than unity and viscous force is dominant), the steady state form Stokes equation together with the continuity equation was solved as the synergistic conservation of momentum and mass, which account for the velocity profile within the fluidic channel. The magnitude of this velocity as a function of the position within the channel was then used to solve the drag force (Table 1) acting on the particles flowing within the channel through numerical coupling. The drag force is then counterbalanced by the dielectrophoretic force, Equation (5), at the region where the magnitude of electric field norm was modified as a result of the constrictions placed between the inlet and the outlet channels. Each particle moving through the microdevice was tracked using the particle tracing module solved in time-dependent mode. Tracking the particles enabled the statistics through which the device parameters (like voltage, device dimensions, etc.) that generated the desired separation of the particles were noted. Using a free triangular customized mesh, with different sizes, growth rate, and curvature factor for both constrictions and the remaining regions within the channel, the geometry was discretized and made ready for finite element analysis. Multifrontal massively parallel (MUMPS) solver, which performs Gaussian factorization, was used in the stationary mode to obtain the velocity profile and the electric field norms. MUMPS solved for the velocity profile and the electric field norms these values with a relative tolerance of 0.001 and without any recourse to lumping while computing the fluxes. GMRES (generalized minimal residual solver), a solver that approximates solutions by the vector in a Krylov subspace with minimal residual, was used in the transient domain to track the particles with respect to their position in space and velocity magnitude as a function of time. The final geometry of the device where complete separation occurs was 1.4 mm in length with 5 semi-circular constriction of radius 0.1 mm and inter-structural constriction spacing of 85 µm. The distance D (Figure 2) between the constriction end and the upper channel wall was fixed to be 35 µm. This distance forbids two cancer cells to pass through the separation region at any given time. This design was made to prevent any form of shielding that may eventually result in incomplete separation. Table 1 provides a list of parameters, variables, boundary conditions in each type of study utilized in COMSOL, and equations associated with the modeling and simulation. Zeta potential for PDMS was assumed to be −0.1 V and a relative permittivity of 80 was used in the simulation. The flow velocity at the inlet was assumed to be 0.001 m/s.

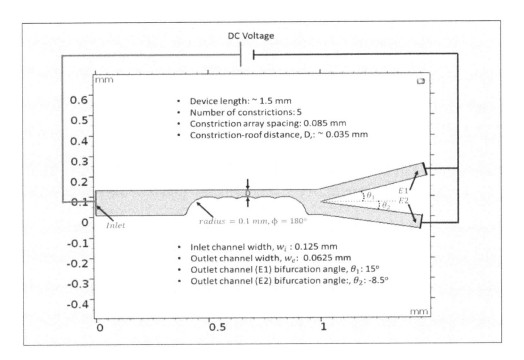

Figure 2. Optimal device design geometry obtained by COMSOL modeling and simulation utilizing the electrophysiological properties of PBMCs and ADCs from the PDMS microwell. Entire microfluidic platform is ~1.5 mm with semi-circular constrictions embedded in the channel. Inlet channel is 125 µm wide and the two outlet channel widths are ~62.5 µm. Pt electrodes in the inlet and outlet ports is connected to a DC power supply to further sort ADCs from healthy PBMCs.

Table 1. List of parameters, variables, discretization, type of study utilized, and the equations associated that was incorporated into COMSOL package for optimizing the device geometry and sorting of adenocarcinoma (ADCs) from healthy peripheral blood mononuclear cells (PBMCs).

Physics/Parameters	Tag	Dependent Variable	Discretization	Study	Equation
Electric current	ec	V	Lagrange Quadratic	Stationary	$\nabla \cdot J = Q_{j \cdot v}$ $J = \sigma E + J_e$ $E = -\nabla V$ Wall boundary- insulated $(\boldsymbol{n} \cdot \boldsymbol{J} = 0)$
Fluid Flow	spf	u	P2 + P1	Stationary	$\nabla \cdot \left[-p\boldsymbol{I} + \mu(\nabla \boldsymbol{u} + (\nabla \boldsymbol{u})^T \right] +$ $\boldsymbol{F} = 0$ $\rho \nabla \cdot (u) = 0$ Wall boundary- electroosmosis $u = \mu_{eo} E_t$ $\forall \; \mu_{eo} = \frac{\epsilon_r \epsilon_0}{\mu} \xi ; E_t = E - (E \cdot n)n$
Particle tracing	ptf	q, v	Formulation	Transient	$\frac{d(m_p v)}{dt} = \boldsymbol{F}_t$ $\boldsymbol{F}_D = \frac{1}{\tau_p} m_p (\mathbf{u} - \mathbf{v})$ $\tau_p = \frac{\rho_p d_p^2}{18\mu}$ $\boldsymbol{F}_{DEP} =$ $2\pi r_p^3 \epsilon_0 real(\epsilon_r^*) real(K) \nabla |E|^2$ $K = \frac{\epsilon_{r,p}^* - \epsilon_r^*}{\epsilon_{r,p}^* + 2\epsilon_r^*} \forall \epsilon_r^* = \epsilon_r$ in stationary field Wall boundary- particles bounce-off walls
			Newtonian		
			Drag law		
			Stokes		

Meshing	Calibration	Mesh Type	Max size	Boundary layer transition
	Fluid dynamics	Free triangular	0.001 mm	Smooth transition to interior mesh

Stationary solver	MUMPS
Transient Solver	GMRES

5. Results and Discussion

In this section, we finally discuss and present the important results to prove that breast cancer can be detected early enough using whole blood. This simulation study demonstrating sorting of ADCs from PBMCs will further be validated experimentally (beyond the scope of this article). Our results are categorized into sections demonstrating: (1) experimental evidence of electrophysiological characterization of both healthy PBMCs and breast cancer ADCs, (2) validation of our microwell technique by comparing with studies from literature and (3) modeling and simulation parameters like meshing, stationary analysis, transient analysis.

5.1. Electrophysiological Characterization of PBMCs and ADCs Experimentally

In estimating the properties of both PBMCs and ADCs movement of cells toward or away from high field region was tracked until the crossover frequencies were found in case at changing properties of the suspending medium. Figure 3A,B shows an ADC cell experiencing positive and negative DEP force (pDEP and nDEP) respectively. In Figure 3C,D, we manually tracked the movement of the target cell as previously demonstrated for prostate cancer in Hele-Shaw flow cell by Huang et al. [39]. Figure 3E shows the first crossover frequency behavior when cells experience a switch from nDEP to pDEP. This first crossover frequency, usually in Hz–kHz range is mainly due to the membrane associated proteins, shape, and size of the cell. The first crossover frequency is often enough to study the phenotype of the cells; however, to characterize their genotype, the 2nd crossover frequency value has to be obtained, often in MHz range.

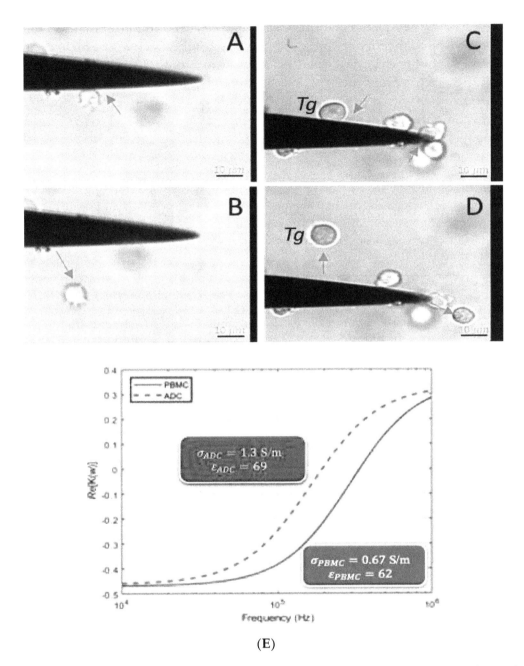

Figure 3. ADC cells experiencing DEP in the microwell at varying AC frequencies- (**A**) shows the ADC cells experiencing positive DEP (pDEP) wherein the cells move towards the high-field region or the triangular electrode in here and (**B**) shows the ADC cells experiencing nDEP behavior wherein the cells move away from the high field region. (**C,D**) are the images resulting from manual tracking of the target cell (labeled Tg) as demonstrated in [39]. (**E**) shows a plot of real part of Clausius-Mossotti factor varying with frequency (Hz). Here the cells initially experience nDEP (negative DEP) and as the frequency increases, they switch to pDEP (positive DEP) where the switch is termed as first crossover frequency.

The crossover frequency data for PBMCs and ADCs were fitted using Equation (1). This equation is an ideal model owing to the spherical nature of lymphocytes. Equation (1) is also suitable for ADCs even though they are a little distorted. Kirby and Huang et al. had reported that an isotopically inhomogeneous non-spherical cell can still be analyzed, to a good approximation, with single shell model since the spherical harmonic solutions used in the eigenfunction expansion approximations for DEP force can help define the effective particle properties [39,40]. Since the second crossover frequencies could not be obtained due to the limitation of the measuring equipment, often obtained at high frequency range (>50 MHz), the cytoplasmic properties used in the simulation were as reported by Qiao et al. using impedance measurement [41]. The total (effective) particle conductivity, σ_p, and permittivity was obtained as described by Adekanmbi et al. [3] and Pethig [31] respectively. Table 2 provides the dielectric properties obtained from our experiments that are compared to the other published literature values in case of PBMCs. It should be noted that the conductivity of the infected ADCs rise sharply compared to the healthy PBMCs that may be attributed to the introduction of new membrane permeation pathways, to membrane peroxidation damage, and to changes in membrane fluidity following infection [42].

Table 2. Dielectric properties, i.e., conductivity and permittivity obtained from our novel electrokinetic technique based on cell response obtained at crossover frequency for ADCs and healthy PBMCs using an osmotic concentration suspending medium maintained at osmotic conductivity and permittivity. Literature reported values has been compared with our novel technique for PBMCs only as a measure of validation [43].

Property	ADCs (Infiltrating Ductal Adenocarcinoma Cells)	PBMCs (Lymphocytes)		Suspending Medium
	Crossover Freq. Technique	Crossover Freq. Technique	Literature Reported [43]	
Conductivity (S/m)	1.3	0.67	0.66	0.055
Permittivity	69	62	59.62	80

The data fitted using MATLAB in Figure 3E were analyzed using chi-square test. The expected value of the crossover frequency is determined from the curves in Figure 3E at $Re\ (K(w)) = 0$ to prove that the fitting is reasonable. The χ^2 critical value at 0.05 significance value is obtained to be 11.07. The χ^2 test statistic value for ADCs and PBMCs are found to be 1.1804 and 2.413 respectively. Since, the calculated test statistic is less than the critical χ^2 value, it signifies a reasonably good fit, i.e., there is no significant difference between the observed (curve) and expected (experimental) values.

However, the authors believe that this is the first time that ADCs were characterized using a novel electrokinetic technique to obtain their dielectric properties i.e., permittivity and conductivity as shown in Table 2.

5.2. Parameters Affecting COMSOL Modeling and Simulation to Obtain High Sorting Efficiencies

In this section, we discuss the factors that affect the optimization of the device geometry to achieve high sorting efficiencies that further influence early breast cancer detection obtained through sorting ADCs from healthy PBMCs.

5.2.1. Meshing of the Device Design in COMSOL

Meshing is one of the factors that strongly affect modelling requirements. Choosing the right mesh element types and sizes is highly pivotal to the accuracy of the simulation results in any finite element problem. Under-meshing can result in solutions that are far less than accurate while over meshing can result in large amount of computational time due to the mesh using too many unnecessary elements. To prevent under meshing, we used mesh elements greater than 40,000. Over meshing was, however, checked and prevented by using meshing sequence with local and global attributes. The local mesh density at the constrictions was sufficiently increased by reducing mesh size while the remaining part of the geometry (where dielectrophoretic force would not have significant effects) was meshed at increased mesh size. This meshing sequence, which was based on Lagrange quadratic representation, reduced the total number of mesh element by 45.17% and computation period by 51.06%. Since the dielectrophoretic force, which causes cells to separate based on their movement away or towards the high field region, acts significantly at the channel constriction zone, it was necessary to verify if the maximum element size (MES) at the constriction would affect the transmission probability of ADCs and to what extent would that effect be. As shown in Figure 4, the accuracy of the solution (which is a function of the transmission probability) depends on the choice of mesh size. The mesh characteristics that was found to be optimum at the applied effective potential difference is as given in Table 1.

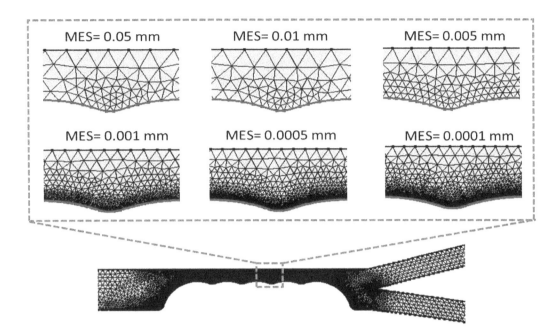

Figure 4. The discretization of the separation region, i.e., along the semicircular constrictions where maximum DEP effect is observed that causes the cells to move into categorized streamlines by adopting variable mesh element size (MES).

Figure 4 demonstrates the gradation of the discretization regime of the constriction zone as the maximum element size (MES) is progressively reduced. At MES = 0.05 mm the density of the triangular mesh is very low indicating that the inter-nodal distance within the discretized zone is large. This large distance depicts an inefficient solution capacity for the gradient of the electric field, which is evident in the low transmission probability (TP) for the ADCs (Figure 5). Transmission Probability, TP, is referred to as the ratio of the number of particles at a specified exit to the total number of the particles at the inlet. In other words, large mesh size at the constriction zone was not able to correctly solve for the electric field gradient which is necessary for dielectrophoretic influence on the particles. When the mesh size was progressively reduced, the number of elements increased correspondingly. This in turn increased the separation efficiency at the constriction zone, hence the dramatic ramping up of the percentage of ADCs that were sorted from healthy PBMCs. It is important to note that the progressive reduction in MES increases the computation time, i.e., with MES at 0.0005 mm and 0.0001 mm requiring 800% and 960% more time than at 0.001 mm. Since the TP value for MES = 0.001 mm, 0.0005 mm and 0.0001 mm are comparatively similar and >97%, the computation was carried out at 0.001 mm with an error margin of ~<0.00020%. At these values (0.001, 0.0005 and 0.0001 mm), it is safe to conclude that the stationary and transient solutions (within the margin of error) of the coupled physics do not vary with mesh condition as the TP values tend to be approximately constant. MES value beyond 0.0001 mm showed critical error warning sign in COMSOL and was computationally very expensive.

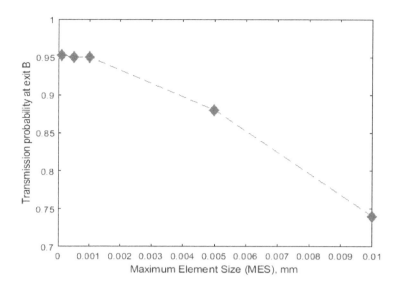

Figure 5. Transmission probability of ADCs as a function of the maximum element size at the separation zone, i.e., around the semicircular constriction region. Since MES at 0.001 mm, 0.0005 mm, and 0.0001 mm are almost similar, the simulation was completed fixing MES at 0.001 mm.

5.2.2. Stationary Field Analysis

The numerical computation comprises of two stationary fields: (a) creeping (fluid) flow and (b) electric current (ec). The electric current was solved in the stationary mode to generate the electric field that not only generated the electro-osmotic effects at the channel wall but also provided the distribution of field strength, E, whose gradient provided the necessary dielectrophoretic force at the constrictions.

As shown in Figure 6A, when DC potential difference was applied across the channel (from the inlet to outlet) and there was a distribution of the electric field as governed by the Laplace equation. The tips of the constrictions within the channel, generated the highest field strength region that was important for dielectrophoretic separation. In Figure 6, the effect of the field gradient is visually more pronounced when the flow field lines were plotted together with the electric field norm. Glaringly, the gradient of the field which was utilized by the dielectrophoretic force acting at the constrictions interfere with the velocity field. The dielectrophoretic velocity introduced at the constrictions added to the already existing electrophoretic and electroosmotic velocities apart from the increase in velocity that was introduced by the continuity equation owing to the reduction in flow area. Figure 6C shows the ripple effects generated from the surface of the constrictions outwards. The resultant effects of this streamline interference could be seen in Figure 6D–F at varying DC voltage, i.e., 10 V, 110 V, and 60 V respectively. The number of constrictions were fixed at 5 and diameter of the constriction was considered to be 100 μm.

Effects of applied potentials and constriction radius on transmission probability: It is important to verify the effects of the electric field strength at various applied potentials and constrictions on the separation efficiency of the microdevice platform. As a result, the radius of the constrictions was varied keeping the number (#) of constrictions fixed at 5 at a given time thus resolving the Laplace equation each time using different applied potential without varying the mesh conditions (Figure 7). The number of constrictions was fixed as an optimization test constraint with respect to the length of the device as well as the exploration of the possibility of initiating cellular separation with minimal insulating constrictions as previously demonstrated by Adekanmbi et al. [38].

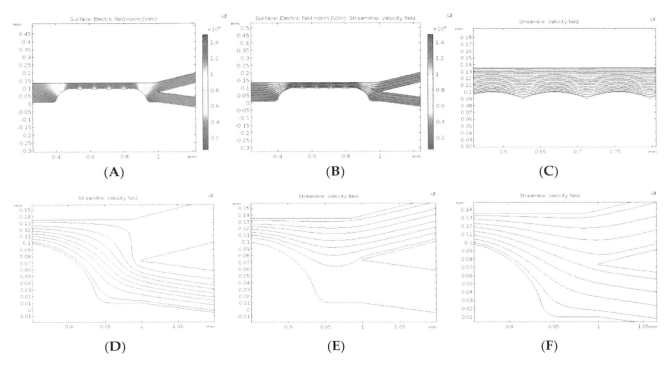

Figure 6. Field and velocity profiles obtained from solving the electrostatics and stokes equations in stationary mode. (**A**) is the electric field norm, (**B**) is the combination of the field norm with velocity streamlines, (**C**) is the zoomed image showing the effect of the constriction zone on velocity streamlines. (**D–F**) show streamlines based on changing DC voltage at 10 V, 110 V and 60 V respectively. The constriction diameter and number were fixed to be 100 μm and 5 respectively.

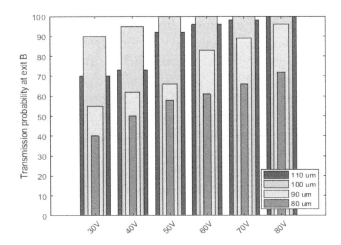

Figure 7. Effects of constriction clearance / size, i.e., diameter and DC voltage on the transmission probability of ADCs. Diameter of the constrictions were varied—80, 90, 100, and 110 μm keeping the number (#) of constrictions fixed, i.e., 5 at a given time. Perfect sorting was observed for constriction diameter of 100 μm at voltages >50 V_{DC}.

Transmission probability of the total number of PBMCs (from inlet to outlet) as a function of the constriction gap, i.e., D in Figure 2 and applied voltage using a fixed number of constriction entities, i.e., 5 was calculated and plotted as shown in Figure 7. Transmission probability (TP) is congruent to normalizing the amount of PBMCs recovered by the initial amount of PBMCs in the inlet mixture. This means, a TP value of 1 represents 100% separation of the PBMCs from its mixture with ADCs. The essence of calculating the transmission probability was to verify the selectivity of the device and to track operating parameters that would be optimal for the operability of the device. Figure 7 demonstrates the effect of varying the constriction diameter and the applied voltage on the transmission probability of PBMCs. The TP value for each of the constriction diameter was progressively increased with the changing potential. At a given DC voltage, the recovery of PBMCs was highest when the constriction diameter was 100 μm. More so, from 50 V to 80 V, 100 μm constriction diameter gave a perfect separation of the PBMCs. None of the constriction diameters gave 100% separation except 110 μm at 80 V. These variations in transmission probability could be attributed to the changing electric field strengths as the applied voltage and constriction diameter change. Changing the applied DC potential affected the electrokinetic and dielectrophoretic forces operating within the channel. Electrokinetic contributions within the channel affects the particle velocity and hence the resident time within which the particles are expected to experience strongest DEP force at the constriction zone. At <50 V, the electro-osmotic velocity of the bulk fluid medium was low enough to move the particles slowly to the constriction zone where there is ample residence time for the cells to experience sufficient induced dielectrophoretic force that would cause them to be separated adequately. However, since DEP force depends on square of the field gradient, the low DC potential (<50 V) could not generate the required electric field gradient that is sufficient to induce strong negative dielectrophoretic force necessary for sorting the cells into their respective differential outlets.

Since increasing electric potential could result in increased Joule heating of the microdevice leading to unwholesome modification of the electrokinetic and dielectrophoretic effects, 100 μm constriction diameter was considered to be the ideal dimension for the separation device platform. Furthermore, operating at a lower voltage, i.e., ~60 V_{DC} seems to reduce the risk of Joule heating within the insulator-based dielectrophoretic device.

5.2.3. Transient Analysis

Particle tracking analysis was used to trace the movement of both ADCs and PBMCs along the whole microdevice platform. There is no change observed in the particles' trajectory when the particle position is placed either at the center or the edge of the inlet, since a uniform particle distribution is selected in COMSOL within the channel. There is no surface interaction with the particles due to the "bounce-off" condition selected in COMSOL. Particles were seen moving through the channel inlet until they were acted upon by the dielectrophoretic force at the constriction which tend to move the particles either towards or away from the constriction surface depending on the properties of the medium, ADCs, PBMCs, and the generated electric field gradient. From the equation of the dielectrophoretic force (Equation (5)), the force experienced by both PBMCs and ADCs at the constriction depends on the square of the electric field gradient as well as the radius of the particle to the third power. The membrane conductivity of both ADCs and PBMCs are both less than that of the medium. Therefore, it is expected that both of them would experience negative DEP.

Figure 8 demonstrates the scenario where ACDs and PBMCs were partially and completely separated while shifting the applied voltage for a constriction number of 5 and diameter of 100 μm at fixed medium properties. Figure 8A depicts incomplete separation at DC voltage below 50 V. At this applied voltage the strength of the applied electric field was not sufficient enough to push away the PBMCs. At 50 V, the generated field gradient had made the DEP force more negative such that the PBMCs were pushed away enough from the high field region to cause their separation from ADCs (Figure 8B). No separation was observed at higher DC voltages, i.e., >100 V (Figure 8C). However, there was separation at ~100 V but with some interesting modification to the flow streamlines as shown in Figure 9.

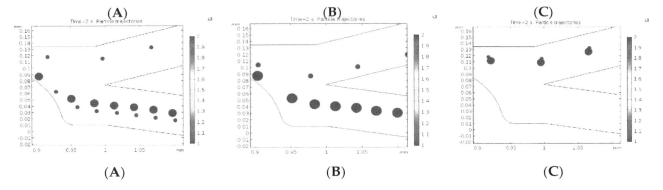

Figure 8. Particle trajectories showing partial (**A**,**C**) and complete separation (**B**) at various voltage conditions. The constriction diameter was fixed at 100 µm along with number of constrictions at 5. **A**) shows incomplete separation at <50 V$_{DC}$, (**B**) complete separation at 50 V$_{DC}$, (**C**) no separation at V100 V$_{DC}$.

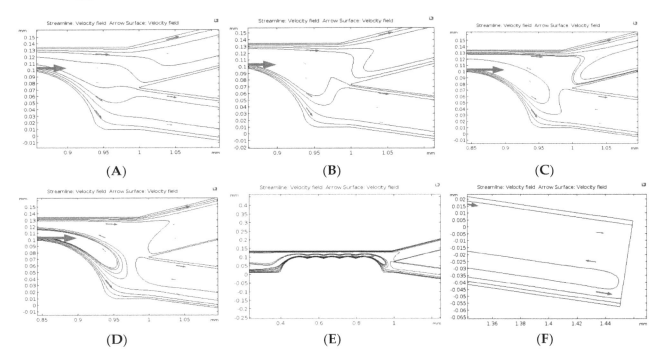

Figure 9. Velocity streamlines at various applied DC voltage conditions at fixed number of constrictions (5) and constriction size (100 µm); (**A**) and (**B**) shows streamlines at 60 V$_{DC}$ and 100 V$_{DC}$ respectively; (**C**) partial recirculation observed at 120 V$_{DC}$; (**D**) increasing recirculation at 200 V$_{DC}$; (**E**) shows the recirculation effects that caused non-compliant behavior of cells to the DEP force; and (**F**) close-up of some cells that tend to reach the exit showing recirculation as well.

In Figure 9A, the operating DC voltage is 60 V while Figure 9B is at 100 V. At 120 V (Figure 9C), some streamlines are being recirculated and this recirculation became more and more pronounced as the applied voltage increased to 200 V (Figure 9D–F). Figure 9D shows the close-up section of the bifurcation zone at 200 V, where in more recirculation of streamlines are being observed. Figure 9E is a close-up representation of the streamline recirculation showing some of the cells that were forced to move in a circular reverse direction to the DEP force. As shown in Figure 9F, some of the cells that were heading towards the exit ports are also forced to move towards the inlet, i.e., recirculated back into the main channel.

This interesting development may be associated with the inter-relation of the high potentials with the electric current within the channel, which, could generate a substantial amount of temperature rise that interferes with the conductivity of the fluid-particle system. Since dielectrophoretic force is a function of conductivity of the fluid-particle system, DEP is hampered as Joule heating becomes more predominant due to the increased temperature. This simulation neglected particle-particle interaction on the basis of experiments since the cell suspension were to be diluted to an extent where in the cells will substantial be far apart that their interaction can be considered inconsequential.

5.3. Validation of the DEP Microwell Technique

The electrophysiological properties for PBMCs obtained data through our novel microwell platform via DEP crossover frequency measurement were validated by comparing the reported data in literature obtained through DEP electro-rotation measurement as reported by Chan et al. [43]. The samples used in this research and the reported literature values were from non-pregnant young female (<50 years of age) since pregnancy tends to substantially lower the specific membrane conductance of PBMCs [43]. The electrophysiological properties for PBMCs obtained from our experiments and the literature reported values were used to run the simulation independently under the same operating conditions. Figure 10 shows the results of the comparative simulation where a log-log plot of transmission probability (TP) and the progression time were plotted. Statistically, the p-value obtained for this comparison was 0.1 (at 0.01 significance level) implying that we do not have sufficient evidence to reject the null hypothesis of "no significant difference" between the two outcomes.

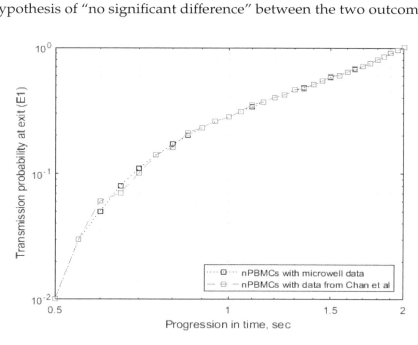

Figure 10. Validation of the electrophysiological properties of healthy PBMCs obtained from the DEP microwell platform using crossover frequency measurement and the literature reported values based on electro-rotation experiments [43]. Both the samples were derived from non-pregnant young women (<50 years of age).

6. Conclusions

Continuous dielectrophoretic separation of infiltrating ductal adenocarcinoma cells (ADCs) from isolated peripheral blood mononuclear cells (PBMCs) using direct current in a semi-circular insulator-based microchannel has been numerically studied. The electrophysiological properties for PBMCs used in simulations were obtained in a novel DEP microwell platform that characterized the behavior of the cells under varying AC frequency by measuring the DEP crossover of the cells. The first and second crossover frequency obtained were curve-fitted using a single shell model to obtain the conductivity and permittivity of the PBMCs. PBMCs vary in size and the sample used in this experiment was majorly small size lymphocytes, i.e., ~10 μm in diameter.

Dielectrophoretic force is a function of the gradient of the electric field-a factor that also depend on the applied voltage as well as the constriction radius. In order to induce sufficient field gradient for the dielectrophoretic separation of ADCs from PBMCs, the applied DC potential and the constriction diameter were dynamically varied until a regime of perfect simulation was obtained at constriction diameter of 100 μm and applied DC potential of ~50 V. The number of constrictions in the channel also affects separation efficiency and 5 semi-circular constrictions lead to optimal sorting of ADCs from PBMCs. This insulator-DEP based method of separating infiltrating ductal adenocarcinoma cells (ADCs) from isolated peripheral blood mononuclear cells (PBMCs) using direct current provided a cheaper, less cumbersome, easier-to-use, and yet efficient approach when compare with previous methods that used deformability, magnetism, or dielectric affinity column. Discretization of domain (meshing) in numerical analysis is an important factor that affect the accuracy of the solution obtained from solving any associated physics within a microchannel. In this paper, effort was made to strike a balance between the computational requirements of the mesh size and the desired transmission probability. Mesh size (local and global) was carefully chosen such that the resultant solution of the simulation did not vary with meshing. To aid our understanding of the choice of applied potential and how it relates with the separation efficiency, we found out that increasing the voltage beyond 100 V DC would lead to no separation, i.e., both PBMCs and ADCs moved into one exit channel.

Another interesting phenomenon was observed at higher voltages (>100 V) along with separation was recirculation behavior of cells. Some of the cells that were moving towards the exit channels were forced to change their direction back to the inlet. Recirculation increased especially between the constriction region and the bifurcation into exit channels with increasing DC potential. This behavior or wake formation is due to increased Joule heating as the temperature rises in the microfluidic platform with increasing DC potential since DEP is a function of the conductivity of the medium.

This DEP spectroscopy technique based on crossover measurement allows characterizing the intracellular differences and physical properties of cells, without any labeling, without affecting cell integrity and viability. Finally, this method confirms a high potential of emerging lab-on-chip (LOC) platforms in the early diagnosis and the treatment of breast cancer especially in young women where mammography is ineffective and/or painful.

Author Contributions: Conceptualization, S.K.S.; methodology, E.O.A.; software, E.O.A. and A.T.G.; validation, E.O.A., A.T.G. and S.K.S.; formal analysis, E.O.A. and A.T.G.; investigation, E.O.A.; resources, S.K.S.; data curation, E.O.A.; writing—original draft preparation, E.O.A.; writing—review and editing, S.K.S.; visualization, S.K.S.; supervision, S.K.S.; project administration, S.K.S.; funding acquisition, S.K.S. All authors have read and agreed to the published version of the manuscript.

Acknowledgments: We would also like to acknowledge the past undergraduate researchers Amanda Vu and Sheila Briggs for their help in DEP microwell experiments.

References

1. Cao, B.; Bray, F.; Ilbawi, A.; Soerjomataram, I. Effect on longevity of one-third reduction in premature mortality from non-communicable diseases by 2030: A global analysis of the sustainable development goal health target. *Lancet Glob. Health* **2018**, *6*, e1288–e1296. [CrossRef]
2. Konigsberg, R.; Obermayr, E.; Bises, G.; Pfeiler, G.; Gneist, M.; Wrba, F.; de Santis, M.; Zeillinger, R.; Hudec, M.; Dittrich, C. Detection of epcam positive and negative circulating tumor cells in metastatic breast cancer patients. *Acta. Oncol.* **2011**, *50*, 700–710. [CrossRef] [PubMed]
3. Adekanmbi, E.; Srivastava, S. Dielectrophoretic applications for disease diagnostics using lab-on-a-chip platform. *Lab Chip* **2016**, *16*, 2148–2167. [CrossRef] [PubMed]
4. Breast Cancer Statistics. Available online: https://www.breastcancer.org/symptoms/understand_bc/statistics. (accessed on 24 March 2020).
5. den Toonder, J. Circulating tumor cells: The grand challenge. *Lab Chip* **2011**, *11*, 375–377. [CrossRef]
6. Karabacak, N.M.; Spuhler, P.S.; Fachin, F.; Lim, E.J.; Pai, V.; Ozkumur, E.; Martel, J.M.; Kojic, N.; Smith, K.; Chen, P.I.; et al. Microfluidic, marker-free isolation of circulating tumor cells from blood samples. *Nat. Protoc.* **2014**, *9*, 694–710. [CrossRef]
7. Hammar, S.P. Metastatic adenocarcinoma of unknown primary origin. *Hum. Pathol.* **1998**, *29*, 1393–1402. [CrossRef]

8.   Mego, M. Emerging role of circulating tumor cells in cancer management. *Indian J. Med. Paediatr. Oncol.* **2014**, *35*, 237–238. [CrossRef]

9.   Whole Blood is the Best Biospecimen for Isolating Peripheral Blood Mononuclear Cells. Available online: https://www.dls.com/biopharma/blog/3-reasons-whole-blood-is-necessary-for-pbmc-isolation (accessed on 5 February 2020).

10.   Gascoyne, P.R.; Shim, S. Isolation of circulating tumor cells by dielectrophoresis. *Cancers* **2014**, *6*, 545–579. [CrossRef]

11.   Nagrath, S.; Sequist, L.V.; Maheswaran, S.; Bell, D.W.; Irimia, D.; Ulkus, L.; Smith, M.R.; Kwak, E.L.; Digumarthy, S.; Muzikansky, A. Isolation of rare circulating tumour cells in cancer patients by microchip technology. *Nature* **2007**, *450*, 1235–1239. [CrossRef]

12.   Deng, G.; Herrler, M.; Burgess, D.; Manna, E.; Krag, D.; Burke, J.F. Enrichment with anti-cytokeratin alone or combined with anti-epcam antibodies significantly increases the sensitivity for circulating tumor cell detection in metastatic breast cancer patients. *Breast Cancer Res.* **2008**, *10*, R69. [CrossRef]

13.   Wlodkowic, D.; Cooper, J.M. Tumors on chips: Oncology meets microfluidics. *Curr. Opin. Chem. Biol.* **2010**, *14*, 556–567. [CrossRef]

14.   Plouffe, B.D.; Lewis, L.H.; Murthy, S.K. Computational design optimization for microfluidic magnetophoresis. *Biomicrofluidics* **2011**, *5*, 13413. [CrossRef] [PubMed]

15.   Liu, Y.; Hartono, D.; Lim, K.M. Cell separation and transportation between two miscible fluid streams using ultrasound. *Biomicrofluidics* **2012**, *6*, 012802. [CrossRef] [PubMed]

16.   Gascoyne, P.R.; Wang, X.B.; Huang, Y.; Becker, F.F. Dielectrophoretic separation of cancer cells from blood. *IEEE Trans. Ind. Appl.* **1997**, *33*, 670–678. [CrossRef]

17.   Becker, F.F.; Wang, X.B.; Huang, Y.; Pethig, R.; Vykoukal, J.; Gascoyne, P.R. Separation of human breast cancer cells from blood by differential dielectric affinity. *Proc. Natl. Acad. Sci. USA* **1995**, *92*, 860–864. [CrossRef] [PubMed]

18.   Moon, H.-S.; Kwon, K.; Kim, S.-I.; Han, H.; Sohn, J.; Lee, S.; Jung, H.-I. Continuous separation of breast cancer cells from blood samples using multi-orifice flow fractionation (MOFF) and dielectrophoresis (DEP). *Lab Chip* **2011**, *11*, 1118–1125. [CrossRef] [PubMed]

19.   Yang, F.; Yang, X.; Jiang, H.; Butler, W.M.; Wang, G. Dielectrophoretic separation of prostate cancer cells. *Technol. Cancer Reserach Treat.* **2013**, *12*, 61–70. [CrossRef]

20.   Zerbino, D.D. Biopsy: Its history, current and future outlook. *Likars'ka sprava* **1994**, *3–4*, 1–9.

21.   An, J.; Lee, J.; Lee, S.H.; Park, J.; Kim, B. Separation of malignant human breast cancer epithelial cells from healthy epithelial cells using an advanced dielectrophoresis-activated cell sorter (DACS). *Anal. Bioanal. Chem.* **2009**, *394*, 801–809. [CrossRef]

22.   Alshareef, M.; Metrakos, N.; Juarez Perez, E.; Azer, F.; Yang, F.; Yang, X.; Wang, G. Separation of tumor cells with dielectrophoresis-based microfluidic chip. *Biomicrofluidics* **2013**, *7*, 11803. [CrossRef] [PubMed]

23.   Srivastava, S.K.; Daggolu, P.R.; Burgess, S.C.; Minerick, A.R. Dielectrophoretic characterization of erythrocytes: Positive abo blood types. *Electrophoresis* **2008**, *29*, 5033–5046. [CrossRef]

24.   Srivastava, S.K.; Gencoglu, A.; Minerick, A.R. Dc insulator dielectrophoretic applications in microdevice technology: A review. *Anal. Bioanal. Chem.* **2011**, *399*, 301–321. [CrossRef]

25.   Pethig, R. Review article-dielectrophoresis: Status of the theory, technology, and applications. *Biomicrofluidics* **2010**, *4*, 022811. [CrossRef] [PubMed]

26.   Gencoglu, A.; Minerick, A. Chemical and morphological changes on platinum microelectrode surfaces in ac and dc fields with biological buffer solutions. *Lab Chip* **2009**, *9*, 1866–1873. [CrossRef] [PubMed]

27.   Ozuna-Chacon, S.; Lapizco-Encinas, B.H.; Rito-Palomares, M.; Martinez-Chapa, S.O.; Reyes-Betanzo, C. Performance characterization of an insulator-based dielectrophoretic microdevice. *Electrophoresis* **2008**, *29*, 3115–3122. [CrossRef] [PubMed]

28.   Chou, C.F.; Tegenfeldt, J.O.; Bakajin, O.; Chan, S.S.; Cox, E.C.; Darnton, N.; Duke, T.; Austin, R.H. Electrodeless dielectrophoresis of single- and double-stranded DNA. *Biophys. J.* **2002**, *83*, 2170–2179. [CrossRef]

29.   Cummings, E.B.; Singh, A.K. Dielectrophoresis in microchips containing arrays of insulating posts: Theoretical and experimental results. *Anal. Chem.* **2003**, *75*, 4724–4731. [CrossRef]

30.   Moncada-Hernandez, H.; Lapizco-Encinas, B.H. Simultaneous concentration and separation of microorganisms: Insulator-based dielectrophoretic approach. *Anal. Bioanal. Chem.* **2010**, *396*, 1805–1816. [CrossRef]

31. Pethig, R.R. *Dielectrophoresis: Theory, Methodology and Biological Applications*; Wiley; Hoboken, NY, USA, 2017.

32. Jing, D.; Zhan, X. Cross-Sectional Dimension Dependence of Electroosmotic Flow in Fractal Treelike Rectangular Microchannel Network. *Micromachines* **2020**, *11*, 266. [CrossRef]

33. Bhattacharyya, S.; Bera, S. Combined electroosmosis-pressure driven flow and mixing in a microchannel with surface heterogeneity. *Appl. Math. Modell.* **2015**, *39*, 4337–4350. [CrossRef]

34. Ghosal, S. Fluid mechanics of electroosmotic flow and its effect on band broadening in capillary electrophoresis. *Electrophoresis* **2004**, *25*, 214–228. [CrossRef] [PubMed]

35. Tandon, V.; Bhagavatula, S.K.; Nelson, W.C.; Kirby, B.J. Zeta potential and electroosmotic mobility in microfluidic devices fabricated from hydrophobic polymers: 1. The origins of charge. *Electrophoresis* **2008**, *29*, 1092–1101. [CrossRef] [PubMed]

36. O'Brien, R.W.; White, L.R. Electrophoretic mobility of a spherical colloidal particle. *J. Chem. Soc. Faraday Trans.* **1978**, *74*, 1607–1626. [CrossRef]

37. Srivastava, S.K.; Baylon-Cardiel, J.L.; Lapizco-Encinas, B.H.; Minerick, A.R. A continuous dc-insulator dielectrophoretic sorter of microparticles. *J. Chromatogr. A* **2011**, *1218*, 1780–1789. [CrossRef]

38. Adekanmbi, E.O.; Ueti, M.W.; Rinaldi, B.; Suarez, C.E.; Srivastava, S.K. Insulator-based dielectrophoretic diagnostic tool for babesiosis. *Biomicrofluidics* **2016**, *10*, 033108. [CrossRef]

39. Huang, C.; Liu, H.; Bander, N.H.; Kirby, B.J. Enrichment of prostate cancer cells from blood cells with a hybrid dielectrophoresis and immunocapture microfluidic system. *Biomed. Microdevices* **2013**, *15*, 941–948. [CrossRef]

40. Kirby, B.J. *Micro- and Nanoscale Fluid Mechanics: Transport in Microfluidic Devices*; Cambridge University Press: Cambridge, UK, 2010.

41. Qiao, G.; Duan, W.; Chatwin, C.; Sinclair, A.; Wang, W. Electrical properties of breast cancer cells from impedance measurement of cell suspensions. *J. Phys. Conf. Ser.* **2010**, *224*, 012081. [CrossRef]

42. Gascoyne, P.; Mahidol, C.; Ruchirawat, M.; Satayavivad, J.; Watcharasit, P.; Becker, F.F. Microsample preparation by dielectrophoresis: Isolation of malaria. *Lab Chip* **2002**, *2*, 70–75. [CrossRef]

43. Chan, K.L.; Morgan, H.; Morgan, E.; Cameron, I.T.; Thomas, M.R. Measurements of the dielectric properties of peripheral blood mononuclear cells and trophoblast cells using ac electrokinetic techniques. *Biochim. Biophys. Acta (BBA) Mol. Basis Disease* **2000**, *1500*, 313–322. [CrossRef]

2

Multinucleation of Incubated Cells and their Morphological Differences Compared to Mononuclear Cells

Shukei Sugita *, Risa Munechika and Masanori Nakamura

Department of Engineering, Nagoya Institute of Technology, Nagoya 466-8555, Japan;
mmm5ar07dd@gmail.com (R.M.); nakamura.masanori@nitech.ac.jp (M.N.)
* Correspondence: sugita.shukei@nitech.ac.jp

Abstract: Some cells cultured in vitro have multiple nuclei. Since cultured cells are used in various fields of science, including tissue engineering, the nature of the multinucleated cells must be determined. However, multinucleated cells are not frequently observed. In this study, a method to efficiently obtain multinucleated cells was established and their morphological properties were investigated. Initially, we established conditions to quickly and easily generate multinucleated cells by seeding a *Xenopus* tadpole epithelium tissue-derived cell line (XTC-YF) on less and more hydrophilic dishes, and incubating the cultures with medium supplemented with or without Y-27632—a ROCK inhibitor—to reduce cell contractility. Notably, 88% of the cells cultured on a less hydrophilic dish in medium supplemented with Y-27632 became multinucleate 48 h after seeding, whereas less than 5% of cells cultured under other conditions exhibited this morphology. Some cells showed an odd number (three and five) of cell nuclei 72 h after seeding. Multinucleated cells displayed a significantly smaller nuclear area, larger cell area, and smaller nuclear circularity. As changes in the morphology of the cells correlated with their functions, the proposed method would help researchers understand the functions of multinucleated cells.

Keywords: multinucleated cells; XTC-YF cells; morphological analysis; Y-27632; hydrophobic dish

1. Introduction

Most cell types normally have a single nucleus, whereas some types of cells contain multiple nuclei. Nuclear division without cytokinesis occurs in some types of mammalian cells, including megakaryocytes, which produce blood platelets, and some hepatocytes and heart muscle cells [1]. Cells of the monocyte/macrophage lineage can fuse and form large multinucleated giant cells that have long been recognized as a histopathological hallmark of tuberculosis, schistosomiasis and other granulomatous diseases [2]. Even mononuclear cells sometimes become multinucleated cells in culture [3].

Some studies indicate concerns of multinucleated cells to pathophysiological events. When endothelial cells obtained from sites of arteriosclerosis are cultured, they exhibit a multinucleated morphology [4]. Multinucleated cells are frequently seen in malignant neoplasms [5]. Multinucleated giant cells are found in epulis, during unusual patterns of chronic inflammation, and are responsible for eliminating foreign bodies and cell debris by phagocytosis [6].

The mechanism by which the properties of mononuclear cells are altered to a multinucleated morphology is not completely understood. Since researchers have attempted to use cells cultured in vitro for tissue engineering [7], understanding of the properties of multinucleated cells is important to produce risk-free tissues.

The ultimate goal of the present study is to investigate the properties of multinucleated cells. For the purpose, we initially established a method to efficiently obtain multinucleated cells because people still struggle with harvesting multinucleated cells. The existence of multinucleated cells of NMFH-2 and NMFH-1 cells were 10.2% and 5.00%, respectively [5]. If experimental systems to collect many multinucleated cells are established, various biochemical, molecular and immunological assays can be made. Although a method designed to incubate multinucleated cells by exclusively selecting and sub-culturing these cells has been reported, the procedure took 10 months [3]. Zang et al. observed multinucleated cells after culture on a hydrophobic substrate in the absence of myosin [8]. In this study, we tested the administration of Y-27632, a ROCK inhibitor that decreases myosin activity and cell contractility, to efficiently obtain any type of cell without gene transfer. The cells were incubated on a less hydrophilic dish and cultured with Y-27632. After establishing the method for generating multinucleated cells, the nature of the multinucleated cells was evaluated based on the morphology of the cells and cell nuclei. This experiment is based on reports that alterations in the nuclear size and shape are associated with and diagnostic markers of human diseases, including cancer and other pathologies [9,10].

2. Materials and Methods

2.1. Contact Angle of Dishes

Reportedly, multinuclear cells are more frequently observed after culture on a hydrophobic surface [8]. Thus, we initially assessed the hydrophobicity of a dish. The contact angle θ of the dish surface was measured to evaluate its hydrophobicity. A 5 μL water drop was placed on φ 35 mm plastic dish (430165, CORNING, Corning, NY, USA) and φ 35 mm glass bottom dish from Fine Plus International (FC27-10N, FPI, Kyoto, Japan) and Matsunami Glass Industry (D11140H, Matsunami, Kishiwada, Japan). After imaging the droplet from the lateral side of the dish with a digital camera (CX3, Ricoh Imaging, Tokyo, Japan), the radius r of the contact area and height h of the droplet was measured using image analysis software (ImageJ 1.48v, National Institutes of Health, Bethesda, MD, USA) as follows. First, ten points on the edge of the droplet were spotted manually and their coordinates (x_i, y_i) $(i = 1, 2, 3, \ldots, 10)$ were measured. Then, a circle that fits the measured points was calculated using the least squared method:

$$\begin{pmatrix} A \\ B \\ C \end{pmatrix} = \begin{pmatrix} \sum x_i^2 & \sum x_i y_i & \sum x_i \\ \sum x_i y_i & \sum x_i^2 & \sum y_i \\ \sum x_i & \sum y_i & \sum 1 \end{pmatrix}^{-1} \begin{pmatrix} -\sum(x_i^3 + x_i y_i^2) \\ -\sum(x_i^2 y_i + y_i^3) \\ -\sum(x_i^2 + y_i^2) \end{pmatrix} \tag{1}$$

where A, B, and C are parameters of the circle. The equation of the circle is given by:

$$x^2 + y^2 + Ax + By + C = 0. \tag{2}$$

Finally, the radius r of the circle was determined as:

$$r = \sqrt{\frac{A^2}{4} + \frac{B^2}{4} - C}. \tag{3}$$

The height of the droplet h was directly measured from lateral images of the droplet. The contact angle was calculated with the equation:

$$\theta = 2\arctan\frac{h}{r} \tag{4}$$

using the half angle method [11].

2.2. Cells

Xenopus laevis cells derived from tadpoles (XTC-YF, RCB0771, RIKEN BioResource Center, Tsukuba, Japan) were used for ease of handling. The cells were cultured at 25 °C in culture medium (Leibovitz's L-15 Medium, Wako Pure Chemical Industries, Osaka, Japan) that had been diluted two-fold with sterilized distilled water. The medium included 10% fetal bovine serum (S1820, Biowest, Nuaillé, France) and a 1% antibiotic solution (P4333, Sigma-Aldrich, St. Louis, MO, USA).

2.3. Conditions Used to Prepare Multinucleated Cells

XTC-YF cells were seeded on the FPI and Matsunami glass bottom dishes to investigate the conditions required to generate multinucleated cells. Y-27632 (257-00511, Wako Pure Chemical Industries) was added to the culture medium at a concentration of 100 μM to suppress myosin-induced contraction.

The cultured cells were fixed with 10% neutral buffered formalin for 10 min followed by washes with phosphate-buffered saline (PBS(-)) to confirm the multinucleated phenotype. The cells were immersed in 32 μM Hoechst 33342 (Molecular Probes, Thermo Fisher Scientific, Tokyo, Japan) for 20 min to fluorescently stain the cell nuclei and washed with PBS(-). Phase contrast images of the cells and fluorescently stained cell nuclei were captured using an inverted fluorescence microscope (IX-71, Olympus, Tokyo, Japan) equipped with an EM-CCD camera (iXon Ultra 888, Andor Technology, Belfast, UK) through a 20× (UPLFLN20X, Olympus) or 40× (LUCPLFLN40X, Olympus) objective lens.

For image analysis, 680 μm × 680 μm images at 20× magnification and 340 μm × 340 μm images at 40× magnification were captured. The image analysis software (ImageJ 1.48v) was used to create a superimposition of the phase contrast and fluorescence images. The total numbers of cells, N_{all}, and multinucleated cells, N_{multi}, in the images were counted. The percentage of multinucleated cells R_{multi} was defined as follows:

$$R_{multi} = \frac{N_{multi}}{N_{all}} \times 100 \ [\%].$$

(5)

2.4. Time-Lapse Imaging

Time-lapse images were captured to directly observe cell division. The XTC-YF cells were seeded on the FPI glass bottom dish, as described in Section 2.3, and observed under an inverted microscope (IX-73, Olympus) equipped with a CCD camera (DP73, Olympus). The phase contrast images of the cells were captured through the 20× objective lens at 5 min intervals from 3 to 72 h after seeding.

2.5. Morphometry of the Cells and Cell Nuclei

The XTC-YF cells were seeded on FPI glass bottom dishes, and half of the cultures were treated with 100 μM Y-27632. After a 48 h incubation, cells were fixed and stained as described in Section 2.3. The phase contrast images and images of the fluorescently labeled nuclei were captured using the setup described in Section 2.3. The images of the fluorescently labeled cell nuclei were binarized to obtain nuclear outlines. The cell shapes were manually outlined in the phase contrast image. From the outlines of the cells and nuclei, the cellular area S_{cell} and nuclear area $S_{nucleus}$ were measured. In the case of multinucleated cells, the areas of individual nuclei were measured. The cellular (α_{cell}) and nuclear ($\alpha_{nucleus}$) circularity values were measured using the following equations:

$$\alpha_{cell} = \frac{S_{cell}}{M_{cell}{}^2} \times \frac{4}{\pi}$$

(6)

$$\alpha_{nucleus} = \frac{S_{nucleus}}{M_{nucleus}{}^2} \times \frac{4}{\pi}$$

(7)

where M_{cell} and $M_{nucleus}$ represent the major axis of the best fit ellipse of the cellular and nuclear areas, respectively. A circularity value of 1 represents a perfect circle and a value of 0 indicates a (segmented) line.

2.6. Statistical Analysis

The difference in contact angle between the dishes was determined using the Tukey method. The differences in morphological data between mononuclear and multinucleated cells were determined using unpaired t-tests. The data are presented as the means $\pm$ standard deviations (SD), and the significance level was set to $p = 0.05$.

3. Results and Discussion

3.1. Contact Angle of Glass Bottom Dishes

Images of droplets on dishes are shown in Figure 1. The glass bottom dish manufactured by FPI had a significantly larger contact angle ($93 \pm 2°$, $n = 10$; Figure 1a) than the glass bottom dish from Matsunami Glass Industry ($71 \pm 4°$, $n = 10$; Figure 1b) and plastic dishes ($66 \pm 3°$, $n = 10$; Figure 1c). All groups had a significant difference in the contact angle. Based on these results, the dish manufactured by FPI is less hydrophilic than the dish manufactured by Matsunami Glass Industry and plastic dishes. Thus, in the following experiments, we used the glass bottom dish manufactured by FPI as a less hydrophilic dish and the dish from Matsunami Glass Industry as a more hydrophilic dish.

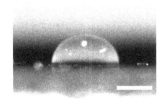 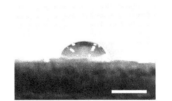 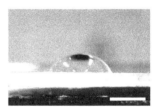

(**a**) Glass bottom dish (FPI)   (**b**) Glass bottom dish (Matsunami)   (**c**) Plastic dish (Corning)

Figure 1. Typical images of droplets plated on (**a**) glass bottom dishes manufactured by Fine Plus International (FPI) and (**b**) Matsunami and (**c**) a plastic dish. Image contrast was enhanced for visibility. Bars correspond to 2 mm calibrated at the surface of the dish.

3.2. Comparison of Multinucleated Cells Plated on Different Dishes

Figure 2 shows typical images of XTC-YF cells after the administration 100 μM Y-27632 at 48 h after seeding. Many multinucleated cells were observed after seeding on a less hydrophilic glass bottom dish (manufactured by FPI) and an incubation in medium containing Y-27632 (Figure 2a). On the other hand, when cells were seeded on a more hydrophilic dish (manufactured by Matsunami) or seeded on a less hydrophilic dish but incubated in normal medium, few multinucleated cells were observed (Figure 2b–d). Figure 3 plots the percentage of multinucleated XTC-YF cells (R_{multi}) as a function of time after seeding. On the less hydrophilic glass bottom dishes, the R_{multi} gradually increased, reaching 88% after 48 h. When the cells were seeded on the less hydrophilic dish without Y-27632 or on a more hydrophilic dish, the R_{multi} was $\leq 5\%$, even after 48 h. Therefore, the condition required to produce multinucleated XTC-YF cells was incubation on a less hydrophilic dish in media containing 100 μM Y-27632. These results were in good agreement with a previous report showing that cells exhibited a multinucleated morphology after culture on a hydrophobic surface under conditions that inhibited myosin shrinkage [8]. Since Y-27632 is a Rho-kinase inhibitor that suppresses cellular contraction, the reagent is considered to inhibit cytokinesis.

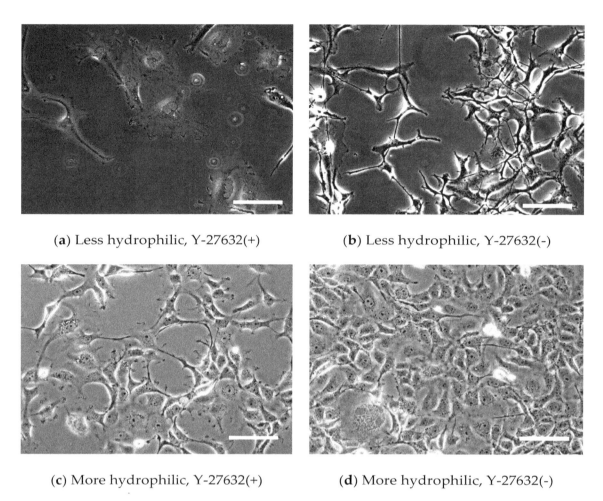

(**a**) Less hydrophilic, Y-27632(+)   (**b**) Less hydrophilic, Y-27632(-)

(**c**) More hydrophilic, Y-27632(+)   (**d**) More hydrophilic, Y-27632(-)

Figure 2. Typical images of XTC-YF cells seeded on (**a,b**) less hydrophilic (FPI) and (**c,d**) more hydrophilic (Matsunami) glass bottom dishes. Cells were incubated with (**a,c**) normal medium containing 100 μM Y-27632 and (**b,d**) normal medium alone. Multinucleate cells are shown in red and their nuclei are shown in blue. Scale bars represent 100 μm.

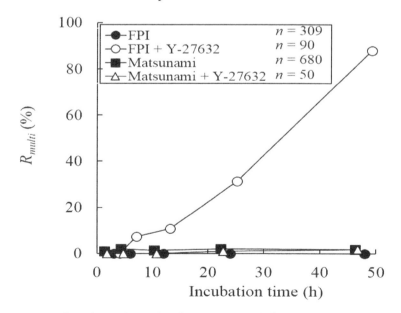

Figure 3. The percentage of multinucleated cells (R_{multi}, as defined in Equation (5)) of XTC-YF cells after seeding on less (FPI) and more hydrophilic (Matsunami) dishes and culture in the presence or absence of Y-27632. n, Number of cells.

Multinucleated cells are produced at a high rate when the contractile force of myosin is inhibited and after culture on a relatively less hydrophilic dish. Unlike the long-term culture method [3], the present method yields multinucleated cells in the usual culture period. Additionally, unlike the gene transfer method [8], the present method is designed to study multinucleated cells in situ since the modification of gene expression is not required. The present method is thus beneficial for studying effects of multinucleation on cellular functions.

The surface hydrophobicity can be controlled by coating octadecyltriethoxysilane or fluorine resin-coating. The tuning of hydrophobicity for efficient production of multinuclear cells remain as future tasks.

3.3. Changes in the Number of Nuclei during the Incubation

Time-lapse images were captured to confirm that the multinucleated cells were not generated by fusion but instead through inefficient division. The time-lapse images of XTC-YF cells seeded on the less hydrophilic dish and cultured with medium containing 100 μM Y-27632 are shown in Figure 4 and Video S1. Over time, the projected area of the cells gradually increased (Figure 4b), and cells exhibiting a mononuclear morphology at the time of adhesion developed multiple nuclei following a subsequent cell division without cytokinesis (Figure 4c–e). Thus, the XTC-YF cells became multinucleated through inefficient division. The time of the first cell division after seeding was 21.5 ± 11.5 h. Some multinuclear cells divided again and the number of nuclei increased over time (Figure 4e–h). When multinucleated cells divided, all nuclei divided at the same time (Figure 4f). However, multinucleate cells with two nuclei sometimes divided into odd numbers of nuclei, such as three or five cell nuclei (Figure 4h). As shown in Figure 4 and Video 1, cells underwent multipolar mitosis and two clusters of chromosomes segregated into a single nucleus. This chromosomal mis-segregation is likely to produce aneuploid progeny [12], which is a condition associated with cancer [13,14].

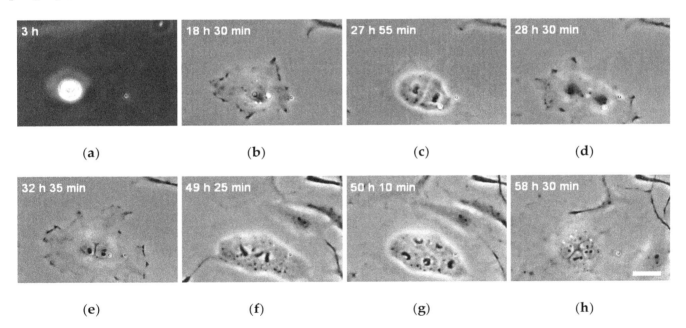

(a)   (b)   (c)   (d)

(e)   (f)   (g)   (h)

Figure 4. Typical time-lapse images of the XTC-YF cells incubated in medium containing 100 μM Y-27632 and seeded on a less hydrophilic glass bottom dish. Bars in (h) = 30 μm and are applicable to all images. The numbers in the upper left of the panels indicate the time after seeding.

Figure 5 shows the relationship between the elapsed time and the number of nuclei per cell. Forty-eight hours after seeding, many cells contained two nuclei. As shown in Figure 4 and Video 1, multinucleated cells further divided at later time points. This division increased the number of cells with more than two nuclei and decreased the number of cells with two nuclei at 72 h after seeding.

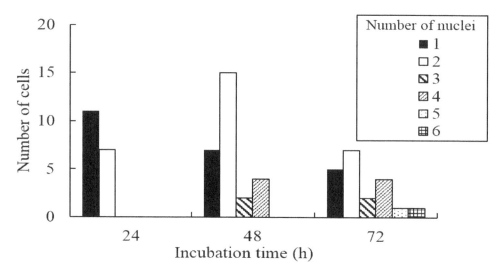

Figure 5. The number of nuclei in XTC-YF cells incubated with medium containing 100 μM Y-27632 and seeded on less hydrophilic glass bottom dishes.

3.4. Morphology of the Cells and Cell Nuclei of Multinucleated and Mononuclear Cells

Figure 6a shows the nuclear area ($S_{nucleus}$) of multinucleated and mononuclear cells. The $S_{nucleus}$ of the multinucleated cells was significantly smaller than mononuclear cells. As confirmed in Video 1, chromosome division definitely occurred, and thus the smaller nuclei observed in multinuclear cells indicated chromosomal condensation. Since the nuclear size positively correlates with nuclear import rates and the concentrations of two transport factors, importin α and Ntf2 [15], the concentrations of these factors might be reduced in multicellular cells compared with mononuclear cells. Importin α and Ntf2 modulate the import of lamin B3 [15], a major component of the nuclear lamina that supports the nuclear envelope and is involved in DNA replication [16], suggesting a possible difference in DNA replication between multinucleated and mononuclear cells.

A cell nucleus divided, as confirmed in the time-lapse movie (Video S1). Thus, normal numbers of chromosomes would be present in a single nucleus, even in the multinucleated cells. As shown in the results presented in Figure 6a, the $S_{nucleus}$ of the multinucleated cells was much smaller than mononuclear cells. Since the nuclear volume in cancer cells influences the proliferative activity [17], multinucleated cells might display differences in cell proliferation.

Figure 6b shows the cellular area (S_{cell}) of multinucleated and mononuclear cells. The S_{cell} of the multinucleated cells was significantly larger than mononuclear cells. In this study, Y-27632 was administered to obtain multinucleated cells. Since Y-27632 interferes with myosin II activity and reduces the tension of stress fibers, a cell treated with Y-27632 spreads and exhibits an increased cellular area [18]. Thus, the significant increase in the cell area of multinucleated cells might be due to the effect of Y-27632. Further experiments will be needed to determine whether Y-27632 or multinucleation increased the cell area.

According to Wilson, the ratio of the area of the cell nucleus to the area of the cell is a constant value [19]. If the ratio in multinucleated cells is defined for each nucleus within a cell, the ratio observed for multinucleated cells at 48 h after seeding (2.4 ± 0.6%) was smaller than mononuclear cells (5.9 ± 2.1%). However, multinuclear cells contain at least two nuclei. Thus, if the sum of the nuclear area in a single multinucleated cell is considered, the ratio is comparable to the nuclear area of mononuclear cells (5.0 ± 1.3%). In this sense, the ratio proposed by Wilson [19] is applicable to multinuclear cells.

Figure 6c shows the nuclear circularity ($\alpha_{nucleus}$) of multinucleated and mononuclear cells. The nuclear circularity of the multinucleated cells was significantly smaller than mononuclear cells. The circularity of the nucleus tends to decrease in the presence of an abnormal number of chromosomes in cancer cells [20]. Thus, we speculated that the nuclei of multinucleated cells contain an abnormal number of chromosomes.

Figure 6d shows the cellular circularity (α_{cell}) of the multinucleated and mononuclear cells. There were no significant differences in the cellular circularity between the multinucleated and mononuclear cells, and the cellular circularity appeared to be lower in the multinuclear cells. The cells treated with Y-27632 exhibited an increased degree of polarization and decreased circularity [21–24], or no change in cellular circularity [25]. Since Y-27632 was administered to obtain multinucleated cells in this study, the multinucleation of cells appears to decrease their circularity.

As shown in Figure 6, the morphology of the cell and cell nucleus of the multinucleated cells was completely different from the mononuclear cells. Since defects in nuclear size and shape are associated with and diagnostic markers of human disease, including cancer and other pathologies [9,10], further investigations focusing on cellular functions and their mechanisms will be required.

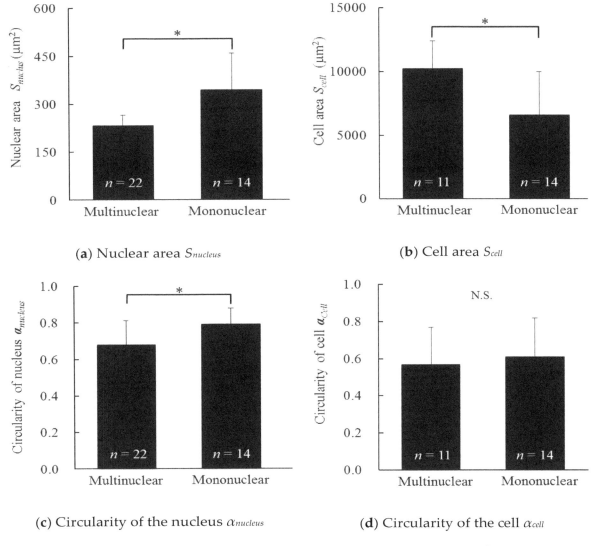

(a) Nuclear area $S_{nucleus}$

(b) Cell area S_{cell}

(c) Circularity of the nucleus $\alpha_{nucleus}$

(d) Circularity of the cell α_{cell}

Figure 6. Morphology of multinucleated and mononuclear XTC-YF cells 48 h after seeding on the less hydrophilic glass bottom dish. Morphological data, such as (a) the nuclear area, (b) cell area, (c) circularity of the nucleus, and (d) circularity of the cell, are shown. n, Number of nuclei; *, $p < 0.05$.

4. Conclusions

In summary, the present study established conditions to generate multinucleated XTC-YF cells, by seeding the cells on a less hydrophilic dish in a medium containing Y-27632. The present method quickly and easily produced multinucleated cells compared to pioneering methods [3,8]. Some cells divided to produce cells with an odd number of nuclei. The multinucleated cells had a significantly smaller nuclear area, larger cell area, and smaller nuclear circularity. The present method could contribute to improving our understanding of the nature of multinuclear cells.

Video S1: Time-lapse images of cell division.

Author Contributions: Conceptualization, S.S.; methodology, R.M.; formal analysis, R.M.; resources, S.S.; writing—original draft preparation, R.M.; writing—review and editing, S.S. and M.N.; supervision, S.S.; project administration, S.S.; funding acquisition, S.S.

References

1. Alberts, B.; Wilson, J.H.; Johnson, A.; Hunt, T.; Lewis, J.; Raff, M.; Roberts, K.; Walter, P. *Molecular Biology of the Cell: Reference edition*, 5th ed.; John, H., Wilson, T.H., Eds.; Garland Science: New York, NY, USA, 2008; p. 1099.
2. Helming, L.; Gordon, S. Macrophage fusion induced by IL-4 alternative activation is a multistage process involving multiple target molecules. *Eur. J. Immunol.* **2007**, *37*, 33–42. [CrossRef] [PubMed]
3. Sedlak, B.J.; Booyse, F.M.; Bell, S.; Rafelson Jr., M.E. Comparison of two types of endothelial cells in long term culture. *Thromb. Haemost.* **1976**, *35*, 167–177. [CrossRef] [PubMed]
4. Tokunaga, O.; Fan, J.L.; Watanabe, T. Atherosclerosis- and age-related multinucleated variant endothelial cells in primary culture from human aorta. *Am. J. Pathol.* **1989**, *135*, 967–976. [PubMed]
5. Ariizumi, T.; Ogose, A.; Kawashima, H.; Hotta, T.; Umezu, H.; Endo, N. Multinucleation followed by an acytokinetic cell division in myxofibrosarcoma with giant cell proliferation. *J. Exp. Clin. Cancer Res.* **2009**, *28*, 44. [CrossRef] [PubMed]
6. Boşca, A.B.; Ilea, A.; Eovrea, A.S.; Constantin, A.M.; Ruxanda, F.; Rus, V.; Raţiu, C.; Miclăuş, V. Multinucleated Giant Cells Polymorphism in Epulis. *Bull. Univ. Agric. Sci. Vet. Med. Cluj.-Napoca. Agric.* **2015**, *72*, 47–52. [CrossRef]
7. Herring, M.; Gardner, A.; Glover, J. A single-staged technique for seeding vascular grafts with autogenous endothelium. *Surgery* **1978**, *84*, 498–504. [PubMed]
8. Zang, J.H.; Cavet, G.; Sabry, J.H.; Wagner, P.; Moores, S.L.; Spudich, J.A. On the role of myosin-II in cytokinesis: division of Dictyostelium cells under adhesive and nonadhesive conditions. *Mol. Biol. Cell* **1997**, *8*, 2617–2629. [CrossRef] [PubMed]
9. Webster, M.; Witkin, K.L.; Cohen-Fix, O. Sizing up the nucleus: nuclear shape, size and nuclear-envelope assembly. *J. Cell Sci.* **2009**, *122*, 1477–1486. [CrossRef] [PubMed]
10. Zink, D.; Fischer, A.H.; Nickerson, J.A. Nuclear structure in cancer cells. *Nat. Rev. Cancer* **2004**, *4*, 677. [CrossRef] [PubMed]
11. Kohli, R.; Mittal, K.L. *Developments in Surface Contamination and Cleaning—Vol 6: Methods of Cleaning and Cleanliness Verification*, 1st ed.; Elsevier Science: Waltham, MA, USA, 2013; p. 169.
12. Shi, Q.; King, R.W. Chromosome nondisjunction yields tetraploid rather than aneuploid cells in human cell lines. *Nature* **2005**, *437*, 1038. [CrossRef] [PubMed]
13. Draviam, V.M.; Xie, S.; Sorger, P.K. Chromosome segregation and genomic stability. *Curr. Opin. Genet. Dev.* **2004**, *14*, 120–125. [CrossRef] [PubMed]
14. Santaguida, S.; Amon, A. Short- and long-term effects of chromosome mis-segregation and aneuploidy. *Nat. Rev. Mol. Cell Biol.* **2015**, *16*, 473. [CrossRef] [PubMed]
15. Levy, D.L.; Heald, R. Nuclear Size Is Regulated by Importin α and Ntf2 in Xenopus. *Cell* **2010**, *143*, 288–298. [CrossRef] [PubMed]
16. Camps, J.; Erdos, M.R.; Ried, T. The role of lamin B1 for the maintenance of nuclear structure and function. *Nucleus* **2015**, *6*, 8–14. [CrossRef] [PubMed]
17. Martin, R.; Nieto, S.; Santamaria, L. Stereologic estimates of volume-weighted mean nuclear volume in colorectal adenocarcinoma: correlation with histologic grading, Dukes' staging, cell proliferation activity and p53 protein expression. *Gen. Diagn. Pathol.* **1997**, *143*, 29–38. [PubMed]
18. Jackson, B.; Peyrollier, K.; Pedersen, E.; Basse, A.; Karlsson, R.; Wang, Z.; Lefever, T.; Ochsenbein, A.M.; Schmidt, G.; Aktories, K.; et al. RhoA is dispensable for skin development, but crucial for contraction and directed migration of keratinocytes. *Mol. Biol. Cell* **2011**, *22*, 593–605. [CrossRef] [PubMed]

19. Wilson, E.B. *The Cell in Development and Inheritance*, 3rd ed.; Macmillan Company: New York, NY, USA, 1925; pp. 727–739.

20. Yamamoto, T.; Horiguchi, H.; Kamma, H.; Ogata, T.; Fukasawa, M.; Ikezawa, T.; Inage, Y.; Akaogi, E.; Mitsui, K.; Hori, M. The effect of nuclear DNA content on nuclear atypia and clinicopathological factors in non-small cell lung carcinoma. *J. Jpn. Soc. Clin. Cytol.* **1993**, *32*, 846–852. [CrossRef]

21. Omelchenko, T.; Vasiliev, J.M.; Gelfand, I.M.; Feder, H.H.; Bonder, E.M. Mechanisms of polarization of the shape of fibroblasts and epitheliocytes: Separation of the roles of microtubules and Rho-dependent actin-myosin contractility. *Proc. Natl. Acad. Sci. USA* **2002**, *99*, 10452–10457. [CrossRef] [PubMed]

22. Babich, A.; Li, S.; O'Connor, R.S.; Milone, M.C.; Freedman, B.D.; Burkhardt, J.K. F-actin polymerization and retrograde flow drive sustained PLCγ1 signaling during T cell activation. *J. Cell Biol.* **2012**, *197*, 775–787. [CrossRef] [PubMed]

23. Kharitonova, M.A.; Vasiliev, J.M. Length control is determined by the pattern of cytoskeleton. *J. Cell Sci.* **2004**, *117*, 1955–1960. [CrossRef] [PubMed]

24. Jones, B.C.; Kelley, L.C.; Loskutov, Y.V.; Marinak, K.M.; Kozyreva, V.K.; Smolkin, M.B.; Pugacheva, E.N. Dual Targeting of Mesenchymal and Amoeboid Motility Hinders Metastatic Behavior. *Mol. Cancer Res.* **2017**, *15*, 670–682. [CrossRef] [PubMed]

25. Kazmers, N.H.; Ma, S.A.; Yoshida, T.; Stern, P.H. Rho GTPase signaling and PTH 3–34, but not PTH 1–34, maintain the actin cytoskeleton and antagonize bisphosphonate effects in mouse osteoblastic MC3T3-E1 cells. *Bone* **2009**, *45*, 52–60. [CrossRef] [PubMed]

3

Measurement of Carcinoembryonic Antigen in Clinical Serum Samples Using a Centrifugal Microfluidic Device

Zhigang Gao [1,†], Zongzheng Chen [2,†], Jiu Deng [1], Xiaorui Li [1], Yueyang Qu [1], Lingling Xu [1], Yong Luo [1,*], Yao Lu [3], Tingjiao Liu [4], Weijie Zhao [1,*] and Bingcheng Lin [1,3]

[1]   School of Pharmaceutical Science and Technology, Dalian University of Technology, Dalian 116024, China; gzg1980@dlut.edu.cn (Z.G.); dengjiu@mail.dlut.edu.cn (J.D.); xrli@mail.dlut.edu.cn (X.L.); yyqu@mail.dlut.edu.cn (Y.Q.); nongxuexueshi@gmail.com (L.X.); bclin@dicp.ac.cn (B.L.)

[2]   Integrated Chinese and Western Medicine Postdoctoral research station, Jinan University, Guangzhou 510632, China; chenmond@foxmail.com

[3]   Dalian Institute of Chemical Physics, Chinese Academy of Sciences, Dalian 116023, China; luyao@dicp.ac.cn

[4]   College of Stomatology, Dalian Medical University, Dalian 116024, China; tingjiao@dlmedu.edu.cn

*   Correspondence: yluo@dlut.edu.cn (Y.L.); zyzhao@dlut.edu.cn (W.Z.)

†   These authors have equally contributed to this work.

Abstract: Carcinoembryonic antigen (CEA) is a broad-spectrum tumor marker used in clinical applications. The primarily clinical method for measuring CEA is based on chemiluminescence in serum during enzyme-linked immunosorbent assays (ELISA) in 96-well plates. However, this multi-step process requires large and expensive instruments, and takes a long time. In this study, a high-throughput centrifugal microfluidic device was developed for detecting CEA in serum without the need for cumbersome washing steps normally used in immunoreactions. This centrifugal microdevice contains 14 identical pencil-like units, and the CEA molecules are separated from the bulk serum for subsequent immunofluorescence detection using density gradient centrifugation in each unit simultaneously. To determine the optimal conditions for CEA detection in serum, the effects of the density of the medium, rotation speed, and spin duration were investigated. The measured values from 34 clinical serum samples using this high-throughput centrifugal microfluidic device showed good agreement with the known values (average relative error = 9.22%). These results indicate that the high-throughput centrifugal microfluidic device could provide an alternative approach for replacing the classical method for CEA detection in clinical serum samples.

Keywords: centrifugal microfluidic device; CEA detection; density medium; fluorescent chemiluminescence

1. Introduction

Carcinoembryonic antigen (CEA) is a polysaccharide-protein complex with a molecular weight that ranges from 180 to 220 kD, and has 28 potential N-linked glycosylation sites. CEA is primarily produced by the embryonic intestinal mucous membranes prior to birth. Thus, the concentration of CEA is usually very low in the serum of a healthy adult. However, the serum concentration of CEA can become elevated in the presence of several types of cancer, such as lung [1,2], breast [3,4], colorectal [5,6], or gastric [7] cancers, as well as colon adenocarcinoma [8]. This means that CEA can be considered a broad-spectrum biomarker for cancer diagnosis and prognosis.

A variety of immunoassay methods have been developed for detecting CEA in serum, such as enzyme-linked immunosorbent assays (ELISA) [9], radioimmunoassays [10], fluorescence immunoassays [11], chemiluminescence immunoassays [12] and amperometric immunoassays [13]. However, a common drawback of these testing methods is that multiple washing steps are required. These repeated washing steps can give rise to increasing measuring errors, which decreases the efficiency while requiring complex instrumentation. Recently, a wash-free one-step immunoassay [14] was developed using a centrifugal microfluidic device, which has great potential for use in clinical applications. This immunoassay method is based on the principle of centrifugal density gradient equilibrium, which takes place inside a microfluidic device. Analytes with fluorescent labels were separated from the bulk serum in one step, using the centrifugal force, through the dense medium located in the microchannels. Afterwards, the fluorescence microbeads, which aggregated at the end of microchannel, could be collected for quantitative analysis.

Following this strategy, Interleukin 6 was rapidly measured (within 15 min) in whole blood by Ulrich et al. [14]. Chung-Yan Koh et al. accomplished the ultrasensitive detection of botulinum toxin in a 2 µL unprocessed sample in 30 min from sample to answer [15]. These studies showed that it is possible to develop a rapid, accurate, high-throughput centrifugal microfluidic chip for the detection of CEA in serum.

In this study, chitosan, which is safe and has good biocompatibility, was used as the dense medium in the centrifugal microfluidic. When combined with ELISA testing, the CEA could be separated by the action of the centrifugal force produced by the rotation, and the concentration of CEA could be detected using a semi-quantitative fluorescence method. This enables the rapid and convenient detection of CEA in serum with high throughput.

2. Materials and Methods

2.1. Design and Manufacture of the Centrifugal Microfluidic Device

A polydimethylsiloxane (PDMS, Sylgard 184, DowDuPont Inc., Midland, MI, USA) glass microfluidic device was designed, as shown in Figure 1A. The height, width, and length of the individual microchannels were 150 µm, 4.2 mm and 1.5 cm, respectively. The diameter of the inlet hole was 5 mm. The distance between the center of the chip and the inlet hole was 6.5 cm. With this geometry, the micro-channels were patterned in PDMS using replica molding. The mold was prepared by spin-coating a thin layer of negative photoresist (SU-8, MicroChem, Corp., Westborough, MA, USA) onto a single side of a polished silicon wafer, which was patterned using UV exposure. Next, the micro-channel layer was obtained by pouring PDMS with a 10:1 (w/w) base-to-crosslinker ratio onto the mold to a thickness of approximately 3 mm. After curing the elastomer for 2 h at 80 °C, the PDMS slab was peeled from the mold, and was then punched and hermetically bonded to a coverslip by plasma oxidation.

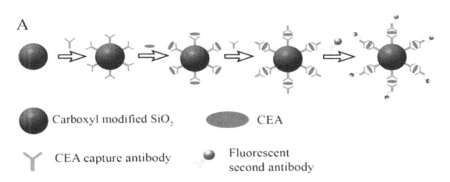

Figure 1. *Cont.*

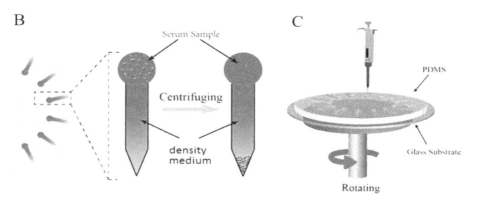

Figure 1. Design of the centrifugal microfluidic device. (**A**) schematic representation of the sandwiched immunocomplex formed by the binding of the target analyte; (**B**) schematic of the centrifugal microfluidic platform immunoassay, depicting the multiplexed analysis of the serum; (**C**) operating principle of the centrifugal microfluidic device.

2.2. Medium Density Screening

Based on the sedimentation process, a theoretical calculation pertaining to the relationship between the density of a material and the centrifugal sedimentation has been proposed [16]. In the case of particle transport in fluids, as in a sedimentation processes, the particles are subject to a viscous force, called drag (F_d). It is given by:

$$F_d = C_d \frac{\rho_{\text{fluid}}}{2} u^2 A_{\text{particle}},$$ (1)

where ρ_{fluid} and u are the density and velocity of the fluid relative to a particle, respectively, A_{particle} is the particle cross-sectional area, and C_d is the drag coefficient. In the laminar flow regime (Stoke's drag), the drag coefficient is proportional to the fluid viscosity μ and inversely proportional to its velocity u relative to the particle, so that for a spherical particle with radius r, the drag force is

$$F_S = 6\pi\mu r u.$$ (2)

Based on this, materials with intermediate densities, but various viscosities were tested. The isolating effects of Percoll (Aladdin Inc., Los Angeles, CA, USA) at a concentration at 1.13 g/mL, 7% or 14% dextran (Aladdin Inc.), as well as 1% or 2% chitosan (Aladdin Inc.) were compared in this study. To start, 1.4 g of dextran and 0.01 g Poloxamer (127 F) were dissolved in 9.8 mL hot water, and then mixed with 0.2 mL 5% bovine serum albumin (BSA) solution and stored at 4 °C. Then, 2 g chitosan powder was dissolved in a 0.1 M hydrochloric acid solution for 24 h using a centrifugal mixer. Finally, the solution was used as the dense medium to be added to the centrifugal microfluidic channel.

2.3. Optimization of the Rotation Speed and Spin Time

After the channels of the microfluidic device were cleaned with Phosphate Buffered Saline (PBS), 10 µL of 1% BSA (Aladdin Inc.) were added, and the devices were stored in a refrigerator at 4 °C to block the protein binding sites on the PDMS. Prior to adding 5 µL of 2% chitosan into the microfluidic device, the channels were washed five times with PBS, and stored in a 4 °C refrigerator until just before use. Then, 30 µL carboxyl-modified silica microspheres (Mozhidong Ldt., Beijing, China) were added to a 500 µL centrifuge tube, diluted to 200 µL, and then packaged with 10 µL of the primary antibodies (18.1 g/mL, Abcam, London, UK). After incubation on a table concentrator at room temperature for 2 h, and being stored at 4 °C in a refrigerator overnight, the beads with antibodies became stabilized. Then, the bead–antibody complexes were washed three times with PBS (pH 7.4), and diluted to 200 µL. Then, 5 µL BSA at a concentration at 5% was added to the solution, which was incubated at room temperature on a table concentrator for 2 h to block the remaining protein binding sites. Then,

30 ng/mL CEA samples (Abcam), with labeled primary antibodies and fluorescence labeled secondary antibodies, were successively added into microchannels with syringes or pipettes. The microfluidic device was centrifuged at various angular velocities (1000, 1500, 2000, 2500, 3000, 3500 or 4000 rpm) or at 2500 rpm for various spin durations (60, 90, 120, 150, 180 or 240 s). Afterwards, fluorescence images were obtained using a fluorescence microscope (IX71, Olympus, Tokyo, Japan) that used a high-power mercury lamp as the fluorescence light source and an exposure time of 3.5 s. After the fluorescence images were obtained, the fluorescence intensity values, with the background subtracted, were read by ImageJ software (version 2.1, National Institutes of Health, Bethesda, MD, USA). Then, statistical analyses were performed based on the particular requirements.

2.4. Establishing a CEA Standard Curve

CEA antigen samples at various concentrations, with labeled primary antibodies and fluorescence-labeled secondary antibodies, were successively added and incubated. Finally, the microfluidic device was centrifuged for 150 s at 2500 rpm in a horizontal centrifuge. At the same time, fluorescence images were obtained using a fluorescence microscope with exposure time of 3.5 s. The fluorescence images were analyzed with ImageJ software to establish a standard curve between the concentration of CEA and the corresponding fluorescence intensity.

2.5. Detection of CEA in Human Serum

BSA blocked bead–antibody complexes, and labeled primary antibodies and fluorescence-labeled secondary antibodies were added to the centrifuge microfluidic device and incubated at room temperature for 2 h. Then, clinical serum samples, which were collected and provided by the Affiliated Hospital of Dalian Medical University from both healthy and cancer person, were added to the centrifuge chip, and spun at 2500 rpm for 2.5 min. After obtaining the fluorescence images using the fluorescence microscope and processing with the ImageJ software, the standard concentration curve were used to obtain the experimental CEA concentrations.

2.6. Statistical Analysis

The SPSS 18.0. (IBM, New York, NY, USA) was used for mean value and standard deviation calculation as well as significance testing.

3. Results

3.1. Design, Fabrication, and Verification of the Centrifugal Microfluidic Device

Figure 1 shows the centrifugal microfluidic platform for detecting CEA using a sedimentation-based immunoassay. The sample was mixed with a detection cocktail consisting of silica microbeads (1 μm diameter), which were coated with specific antibodies for the target of interest, in this case, CEA. The detection antibodies were labeled with a fluorescent tag, which binds to the capture beads in the presence of the corresponding antigen (Figure 1A). After the serum samples were mixed with the antibody-conjugated capture beads and fluorescent detection antibodies in solution, they were added to a preloaded dense medium. The beads were pushed to the bottom of the channel to form pellets by the centrifugal force. Eventually, the target analytes separated from the rest of the sample (Figure 1B). The entire process of CEA detection could be completed in one step, as shown in Figure 1C. The samples were added at the entrance of the centrifugal microfluidic platform, which was split into 14 radially arranged pencil-like microchannels. Then, the target analyte could be detected using a sedimentation-based immunoassay. This simple, one-step centrifugal microfluidic platform provides high analytical accuracy and repeatability, which cannot be achieved by processes that require multiple steps.

To validate the effectiveness of the chemiluminescence immunoassay used in this device, CEA standard samples were measured using a double-antibody sandwich ELISA with the conventional method and the centrifugal microfluidic device. The proposed method was shown to be equivalent to the conventional method based on the linearity of the response (see supplementary material in the supporting information).

3.2. Medium Screening and Structure Optimization of the Microfluidic Device

Based on Equation (2), we screened various media to determine the optimal density and viscosity, as one of the critical aspects in this study. Percoll, dextran (7% or 14%), and chitosan (1% or 2%) were tested as dense media, as shown in Figure 2. It was suggested that the microbeads could not be separated in a Percoll solution at a concentration of 1.13 g/mL (Figure 2A). However, if the sample is whole blood with a density of 1.09 to 1.11 g/mL of red blood cells, Percoll can separate red blood cells from plasma. Although dextran can separate the microbeads from solution as a clinical plasma substitute, the separating effect is not as good as with the chitosan solution (Figure 2B,C). Because the concentration of the dense medium solution is 1%, the modified antigen antibody beads can become separated at the end of the microchannel. Furthermore, the rest of the solution will have been mixed with the medium because this is beyond the abilities of the separation process (Figure 2D,E). In addition, if the concentration of the dense medium is 2%, the modified antigen antibody beads can pass through the medium to reach the bottom of the channel. Therefore, a chitosan solution with a concentration of 2% was selected as the dense medium in the centrifugal microfluidic device to separate the microbeads modified by antigen antibodies in solution.

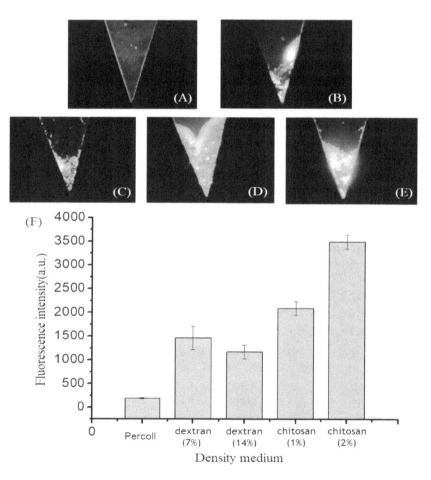

Figure 2. Effect of the dense medium on isolation efficiency in the centrifugal microfluidic platform. Separating effects of (**A**) Percoll, dextran ((**B**) 7% or (**C**) 14%), and chitosan ((**D**) 1% or (**E**) 2%) as dense media and (**F**) their histogram comparison.

3.3. Effects of Rotation Speed and Spin Duration on the Detection of CEA

The effects of rotation speed and spin duration were also considered in this study. In the centrifugal microfluidic device with chitosan as the dense medium, the effects of various angular velocities on the isolation power of CEA standard samples (25 ng/mL) were investigated.

In Figure 3A, the fluorescence intensity of aggregated microbeads increased as the rotation speed increased from 1000 to 2500 rpm. However, even if the rotation speed was set to greater than 2500 rpm, the fluorescence intensity of the aggregated microbeads did not increase, and instead plateaued at a constant value. This indicates that spinning at 2500 rpm caused all the microbeads in the bulk serum to migrate to the end of the microchannel. Thus, 2500 rpm was used as the rotation speed for CEA detection.

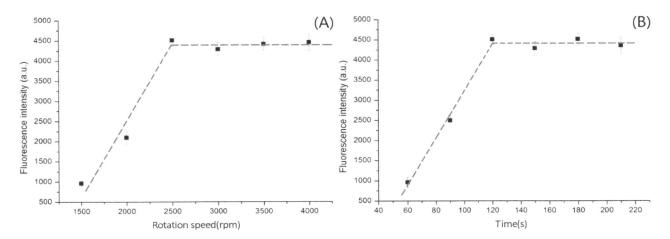

Figure 3. Effects of rotation speed and spin duration on carcinoembryonic antigen (CEA) isolation. (**A**) the effect of rotation speed on CEA isolation; (**B**) the effect of spin duration on CEA isolation.

Similarly, the effects of various spin durations of the centrifugal microfluidic device using chitosan as the dense medium on the isolation of CEA in a standard sample (25 ng/mL) were investigated at 2500 rpm. As shown in Figure 3B, in the first two minutes, the microbeads were gradually separated to the end of the microchannel, and the fluorescence intensity increased over time. After two minutes, the microbeads in the sample were almost completely in the detection area, and the fluorescence intensity was constant thereafter. To have a margin of safety, 2.5 min was selected as the centrifugal spin duration.

3.4. CEA Detection in Human Serum Samples

CEA standard samples with various concentrations were measured using this device, and the relationship between CEA concentration (x) and the fluorescence intensity (y) was established with a standard curve ($y = 1647.3x + 5432.9$). It is suggested that the analytical sensitivity of the standard curve is 1673.4. Based on Figure 4, the repeatability at each concentration was good ($n = 4$), and the curve was linear within the CEA concentration range of 0.7–22.5 ng/mL ($R^2 = 0.993$). Thus, these equations can be used as a standard curve for sample detection, including human serum samples.

CEA in clinical human serum samples with known concentrations were measured using the centrifugal microfluidic device, and comparisons between the known and measured concentrations are shown in Table 1 and Figure 4. It can be seen from the table that the sample testing errors from 90% of the samples are less than 20%, and the average relative error was only 9.22%. This indicates that the detection results obtained by this device were reliable. In addition, as shown in Figure 5A, in these tests, excluding the poor repeatability of certain outlier samples, the repeatability of the remaining samples was good for CEA concentrations in the range of 0.5 ng/mL to 27 ng/mL. In addition, it was determined from Figure 5B that, when the carcinoembryonic antigen concentration was less than

2.0 ng/mL, the detection concentration was consistent with the known concentration, and when the concentration of the serum sample was higher than 10 ng/mL, there were some slight differences between the actual and measured concentrations.

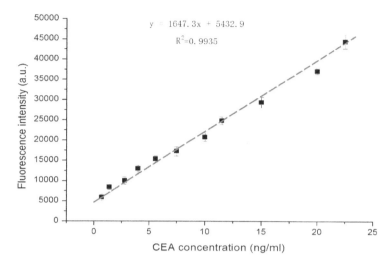

Figure 4. Relationship between fluorescence intensity of aggregated microbeads and CEA concentration in the serum.

Table 1. Results from 32 clinical serum samples.

No.	Known Value (ng/mL)	Measured Value (ng/mL), $n = 3$	Relative Error
1	12.94	12.82 ± 0.33	0.96%
2	3.69	3.82 ± 0.26	3.52%
3	0.71	0.58 ± 0.52	18.59%
4	2.4	2.43 ± 0.21	1.45%
5	5.76	6.10 ± 0.30	5.87%
6	2.75	2.94 ± 0.15	7%
7	0.91	1.03 ± 0.29	13.14%
8	2.55	3.31 ± 0.10	29.96%
9	2.01	2.04 ± 0.07	1.55%
10	2.02	2.23 ± 0.85	10.50%
11	2.52	2.47 ± 0.22	1.99%
12	8.01	7.46 ± 0.29	6.86%
13	14.07	13.59 ± 0.69	3.43%
14	24.16	24.54 ± 0.93	1.59%
15	9.12	9.48 ± 0.39	3.99%
16	26.54	25.69 ± 3.57	3.19%
17	3.35	3.29 ± 0.28	1.66%
18	2.98	3.27 ± 0.48	9.61%
19	1.34	1.57 ± 0.10	17.39%
20	9.63	9.48 ± 0.44	1.59%
21	2.04	2.08 ± 0.19	1.94%
22	4.58	4.60 ± 0.31	0.36%
23	0.91	0.93 ± 0.11	1.91%
24	0.53	0.55±0.15	4.67%
25	2.72	3.05 ± 0.37	12.31%
26	1.71	1.63 ± 0.46	4.48%
27	0.25	0.30 ± 0.08	21.68%
28	2.24	2.83 ± 0.57	26.23%
29	1.38	1.29 ± 0.18	6.55%
30	2.17	2.73 ± 0.51	25.8%
31	0.66	0.52 ± 0.36	21.22%
32	1.81	2.24 ± 0.97	24.02%

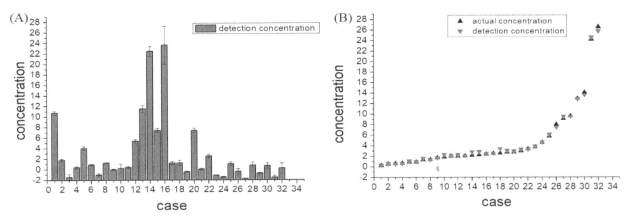

Figure 5. CEA detection in clinical human serum samples. (**A**) the repeatability of actual samples; (**B**) comparison of known and measured concentrations.

The CEA detection results using the centrifugal microfluidic device and the hospital instruments were compared. As shown in Table 2, when excluding samples 7, 18 and 26, the p-value of samples were above 0.05. This suggests that there were no significant differences between the detection method of the centrifugal microfluidic device and the hospital's method.

Table 2. p-values between paired samples.

Samples	p-Value	Samples	p-Value	Samples	p-Value
1	0.299	12	0.655	23	0.514
2	0.752	13	0.728	24	0.953
3	0.497	14	0.114	25	0.112
4	0.655	15	0.13	26	0.032
5	0.474	16	0.761	27	0.162
6	0.748	17	0.662	28	0.545
7	0.016	18	0.001	29	0.394
8	0.389	19	0.164	30	0.255
9	0.762	20	0.084	31	0.471
10	0.437	21	0.32	32	0.668
11	0.453	22	0.71	–	–

4. Discussion

A centrifugal microfluidic chip was constructed for detecting CEA in clinical serum samples. The device is based on a sandwiched immunoassay with biocompatible chitosan as the dense medium. It is driven by centrifugal force to implement rapid, high-throughput detection of serum CEA and other biomarkers. This centrifugal microfluidic chip does not require any washing steps, and can simplify the experimental procedure with increased accuracy and efficiency, compared with traditional immunoassays. Thus, this centrifugal microfluidic device can be expected to be used for CEA determination in hospitals.

The dense medium used in this microfluidic device was 2% chitosan to eliminate the need for the complicated washing steps of the traditional detection method. This device was able to separate the analyte from the solution in a one-step centrifugal process. Therefore, the samples could be detected directly and easily. In addition, the 14 individual pencil channels acted as parallel systems on the centrifugal microfluidic chip, with a relative standard deviation (RSD) value of just 4.95%.

The rotation speed and spin duration were optimized for the microfluidic device. It was determined that 2500 rpm for 150 s was able to completely move the analytes of the samples to the detection area. Thus, this microfluidic device can improve upon the current clinical detection methods.

Finally, the CEA detection results obtained from this centrifugal microfluidic device were compared and verified with clinical values. Thirty clinical serum samples were measured based on the standard curve established between the CEA concentration and fluorescence intensity. The detection error in 90% of the samples was less than 20% (Table 1), and the repeatability of the samples was good over the range of concentrations of 0.5 ng/mL to 27 ng/mL. Although a few samples showed low reproducibility, this might have been because the CEA was not uniformly distributed in the serum, and the volume of samples added to microfluidic device was microscale, thus making the contents to be measured in each sample unstable.

In conclusion, this study describes a centrifugal microfluidic device that was developed for detecting CEA. This method uses density gradient centrifugation and is free of washing steps, and is thus more accurate than traditional ELISA methods. It also can achieve high-throughput detection, with the potential to be used in central labs.

Figure S1: Chip channel parallelism measurement, Figure S2: Standard curve for determination of protein content, Figure S3: The comparison of fluorescence concentration curve between conventional ELISA method and centrifugal microfluidic device. (A) conventional ELISA method; (B) centrifugal microfluidic device.

Author Contributions: Z.G., Y.L. (Yong Luo), W.Z., B.L., Y.L. (Yao Lu) and T.L. conceived and designed the experiments; Z.G., X.L., and L.X. performed the experiments; Z.G., J.D., Y.L. (Yong Luo) and L.X. analyzed the data; Z.C., Y.Q., W.Z., B.L., Y.L. (Yao Lu) and T.L. contributed reagents/materials/analysis tools; Z.G., Z.C. and Y.L. (Yong Luo) wrote the paper.

Acknowledgments: The authors would like to appreciate Affiliated Hospital of Dalian Medical University to provide CEA Clinical samples.

References

1.   Braik, T.; Gupta, S.; Poola, H.; Jain, P.; Beiranvand, A.; Lad, T.E.; Hussein, L. Carcino embryonic antigen (CEA) elevation as a predictor of better response to first line pemetrexed in advanced lung adenocarcinoma. *J. Thorac. Oncol.* **2012**, *7*, S310.

2.   Yu, D.H.; Li, J.H.; Wang, Y.C.; Xu, J.G.; Pan, P.T.; Wang, L. Serum anti-p53 antibody detection in carcinomas and the predictive values of serum p53 antibodies, carcino-embryonic antigen and carbohydrate antigen 12–5 in the neoadjuvant chemotherapy treatment for III stage non-small cell lung cancer patients. *Clin. Chim. Acta* **2011**, *412*, 930–935. [CrossRef] [PubMed]

3.   Bao, H.; Yu, D.; Wang, J.; Qiu, T.; Yang, J.; Wang, L. Predictive value of serum anti-p53 antibodies, carcino-embryonic antigen, carbohydrate antigen 15-3, estrogen receptor, progesterone receptor and human epidermal growth factor receptor-2 in taxane-based and anthracycline-based neoadjuvant chemotherapy in locally advanced breast cancer patients. *Anti-Cancer Drug* **2008**, *19*, 317–323.

4.   Thriveni, K.; Krishnamoorthy, L.; Ramaswamy, G. Correlation study of carcino embryonic antigen & cancer antigen 15.3 in pretreated female breast cancer patients. *India J. Clin. Biochem.* **2007**, *22*, 57–60.

5.   Cierpinski, A.; Stein, A.; Ruessel, J.; Ettrich, T.; Schmoll, H.J.; Arnold, D. Prognostic impact of carcino embryonic antigen (CEA), carbohydrate antigen (CA 19–9), and lactate dehydrogenase (LDH) decrease in patients with metastatic colorectal cancer (mCRC) receiving a bevacizumab- or cetuximab-chemotherapy combination. *Onkologie* **2011**, *34*, 250.

6.   Wang, Y.R.; Yan, J.X.; Wang, L.N. The diagnostic value of serum carcino-embryonic antigen, alpha fetoprotein and carbohydrate antigen 19-9 for colorectal cancer. *J. Cancer Res. Ther.* **2014**, *10*, 307–309. [PubMed]

7.   Lai, H.; Jin, Q.; Lin, Y.; Mo, X.; Li, B.; He, K.; Chen, J. Combined use of lysyl oxidase, carcino-embryonic antigen, and carbohydrate antigens improves the sensitivity of biomarkers in predicting lymph node metastasis and peritoneal metastasis in gastric cancer. *Tumor Biol.* **2014**, *35*, 10547–10554. [CrossRef] [PubMed]

8.   Szajda, S.D.; Snarska, J.; Jankowska, A.; Roszkowska-Jakimiec, W.; Puchalski, Z.; Zwierz, K. Cathepsin D and carcino-embryonic antigen in serum, urine and tissues of colon adenocarcinoma patients. *Hepatogastroenterology* **2008**, *55*, 388–393. [PubMed]

9.   Zhao, L.; Xu, S.; Fjaertoft, G.; Pauksen, K.; Hakansson, L.; Venge, P. An enzyme-linked immunosorbent assay for human carcinoembryonic antigen-related cell adhesion molecule 8, a biological marker of granulocyte activities in vivo. *J. Immunol. Methods* **2004**, *293*, 207–214. [CrossRef] [PubMed]

10.   Chester, S.J.; Maimonis, P.; Vanzuiden, P.; Finklestein, M.; Bookout, J.; Vezeridis, M.P. A new radioimmunoassay

detecting early stages of colon cancer: a comparison with CEA, AFP, and Ca 19-9. *Dis. Markers* **1991**, *9*, 265–271. [PubMed]

11. Yan, F.; Zhou, J.; Lin, J.; Ju, H.; Hu, X. Flow injection immunoassay for carcinoembryonic antigen combined with time-resolved fluorometric detection. *J. Immunol. Methods* **2005**, *305*, 120–127. [CrossRef] [PubMed]
12. Lin, J.; Yan, F.; Hu, X.; Ju, H. Chemiluminescent immunosensor for CA19-9 based on antigen immobilization on a cross-linked chitosan membrane. *J. Immunol. Methods* **2004**, *291*, 165–174. [CrossRef] [PubMed]
13. Zhang, S.; Yang, J.; Lin, J. 3,3′-diaminobenzidine (DAB)-H_2O_2-HRP voltammetric enzyme-linked immunoassay for the detection of carcionembryonic antigen. *Bioelectrochemistry* **2008**, *72*, 47–52. [CrossRef] [PubMed]
14. Schaff, U.Y.; Sommer, G.J. Whole blood immunoassay based on centrifugal bead sedimentation. *Clin. Chem.* **2011**, *57*, 753–761. [CrossRef] [PubMed]
15. Koh, C.-Y.; Schaff, U.Y.; Piccini, M.E.; Stanker, L.H.; Cheng, L.W.; Ravichandran, E.; Singh, B.-R.; Sommer, G.J.; Singh, A.K. Centrifugal microfluidic platform for ultrasensitive detection of botulinum toxin. *Anal. Chem.* **2015**, *87*, 922–928. [CrossRef] [PubMed]
16. Strohmeier, O.; Keller, M.; Schwemmer, F.; Zehnle, S.; Mark, D.; Von Stetten, F.; Zengerle, R.; Paust, N. Centrifugal microfluidic platforms: advanced unit operations and applications. *Chem. Soc. Rev.* **2015**, *44*, 6187–6229. [CrossRef] [PubMed]

4

Mechanophenotyping of B16 Melanoma Cell Variants for the Assessment of the Efficacy of (-)-Epigallocatechin Gallate Treatment Using a Tapered Microfluidic Device

Masanori Nakamura *, Daichi Ono and Shukei Sugita

Department of Electrical and Mechanical Engineering, Nagoya Institute of Technology, Nagoya 466-8555, Japan; 30413043@stn.nitech.ac.jp (D.O.); sugita.shukei@nitech.ac.jp (S.S.)
* Correspondence: masanorin@nitech.ac.jp

Abstract: Metastatic cancer cells are known to have a smaller cell stiffness than healthy cells because the small stiffness is beneficial for passing through the extracellular matrix when the cancer cells instigate a metastatic process. Here we developed a simple and handy microfluidic system to assess metastatic capacity of the cancer cells from a mechanical point of view. A tapered microchannel was devised through which a cell was compressed while passing. Two metastasis B16 melanoma variants (B16-F1 and B16-F10) were examined. The shape recovery process of the cell from a compressed state was evaluated with the Kelvin–Voigt model. The results demonstrated that the B16-F10 cells showed a larger time constant of shape recovery than B16-F1 cells, although no significant difference in the initial strain was observed between B16-F1 cells and B16-F10 cells. We further investigated effects of catechin on the cell deformability and found that the deformability of B16-F10 cells was significantly decreased and became equivalent to that of untreated B16-F1 cells. These results addressed the utility of the present system to handily but roughly assess the metastatic capacity of cancer cells and to investigate drug efficacy on the metastatic capacity.

Keywords: microfluidics; mechanophenotyping; cancer; metastatic potential

1. Introduction

Metastasis is the spread of cancer cells from the primary site of origin to other sites of the body. When cancer cells metastasize, some cells known as circulating tumor cells (CTC), penetrate the endothelium and the basement membrane and pass through a tiny gap in the extracellular matrix [1–3]. It is therefore thought that having smaller stiffness is beneficial for cancer cells to instigate the metastatic process [4]. In support of this, only few studies show that cancer cells are stiffer, and a large majority of experiments indicate that cancerous cells are softer than their benign counterparts and that cellular rigidity decreases with the progression of the disease—as summarized in Aliber et al. [4]—although it remains unclear whether such cell softening is a universal feature [5].

Various tests were conducted to mechanically characterize living cells including cancer cells [6–15]. Mechanical studies on cancer cells and related cancer biology are thoroughly reviewed in Darling et al. [16], Aliber et al. [4], and Chaudhuri et al. [17]. Using atomic force microscopy, Cross et al. [8] demonstrated that metastatic cancer cells taken from the pleural fluids of patients with suspected lung, breast, and pancreas cancer have stiffness as much as 70% smaller than the benign cells. Remmerbach et al. [11] measured the compliance of cells from cell lines and primary samples of healthy donors and cancer patients using a microfluidic optical stretcher. They found that cancer cells were on average 3.5 times more compliant than those of healthy donors. Swaminathan et al. [12] showed that cancer cells with the highest migratory and invasive potential are five times less stiff than cells with the lowest potential. Furthermore, they reported that invasiveness decreased when cell stiffness, by restoring expression of the metastasis suppressor TβRIII/betaglycan, increased. It was also reported that the more motile and metastatic cancer cells were, the softer they were, indicating that nanomechanical stiffness was inversely correlated with the migration potential of the cancer cell [13,14]. These results suggest that the cell stiffness is a reliable quantitative indicator or a good biomarker of migration and the invasive potential of cancer cells. However, the conventional methods of mechanical tests such as atomic force microscopy, optical tweezers, and micropipette aspiration are time-consuming, labor-intensive, and often require difficult manipulation and mastery skills although they give relatively accurate data [18]. Additionally, each method has its own drawback. For instance, atomic force microscopy requires a cell adhering to a basement. Micropipette aspiration involves difficult manipulation and fine adjustment of pressure. In order to use the cell stiffness as a biomarker of the metastatic potential of cancer cells in clinical practice, more viable methods are demanded.

Microfluidic devices have high throughputs in selecting cancer cells and assessing their metastatic functions [19–24]. For example, Hou et al. [22] and Khoo et al. [23] established a spiral microfluidic channel to separate CTCs from blood cells. Tse et al. [24] evaluated the mechanical properties of cells sampled from malignant pleural effusions using a crossed microfluidic channel, proposed by Gossett et al. [25]. These studies addressed a great potential of microfluidic techniques to handily characterize the mechanical properties of cancer cells in clinical practice.

Epigallocatechin gallate (EGCG) is a major component of green tea. Taniguchi et al. [26] reported that EGCG inhibited the spontaneous metastasis of B16-F10 cells and B16-BL6 cells to the lungs of mice. EGCG binds to various proteins and both DNA and RNA molecules [27], it also inhibits binding of ligands and tumor promoters to their receptors in the cell membrane, and the receptor signaling pathway of epidermal growth factor (EGF) [28]. EGCG also works as an immune check point inhibitor [29]. EGCG acts on the cell membrane of cancer cells, hardens the cell membrane [30], and suppresses cancer cell migration and invasion [31]. EGCG blocks induction of carcinogenic factors by hardening the cell membrane and inhibits metastasis of cancer cells [32]. Taking these facts together, it is considered that hardening of cancer cells with EGCG could be another way of inhibiting metastasis of cancer cells.

Better and more appropriate cancer therapies, including a choice of drugs (weak or strong) with minimal side effects, could be applied if the metastatic potentials of the circulating tumor cells were easier to evaluate in clinical practice. The aim of the present study is therefore to investigate the mechanical properties of cancer cells, in particular highlighting internal cytoskeletal structures and changes brought by EGCG treatment. A microflow channel of a simple design was used to evaluate cell stiffness. Here we used two cell types that are known to have different metastatic potential and investigated whether these cells can be differentiated from their viscoelastic properties. The same assessment process was also applied to untreated and EGCG-treated cells to see whether effectiveness of EGCG treatment can be detected using the same procedure as used in differentiating the metastatic potential.

2. Materials and Methods

2.1. Cell Sample

Mouse melanoma cell lines B16-F1 and B16-F10 were used. B16-F1 was obtained by a one-time selective procedure and B16-F10 by a ten-time selective procedure using Fidler's method [33], meaning that B16-F10 was a select group of cancer cells having greater invasive and metastatic capacity than B16-F1. The characteristics of the cells were reported in Fidler [33], Poste et al. [34], and Nakamura et al. [35]. The cells were cultured in DMEM (05919, Nissui, Tokyo, Japan) containing 10% fetal bovine serum (172012, Sigma-Aldrich, St. Louis, MO, USA) in a humidified atmosphere of 5% of CO_2 at 37 °C.

Trypsin (25200-056, Gibco, Gaithersburg, MD, USA) was added to the cells that were semi-confluent to detach them from dishes. After the cells were washed with phosphate buffered saline (PBS(-)), cell samples with a concentration of 3–4 $\times$ 10^5 cells/ml were prepared.

2.2. Microflow Channel

Lee et al. [36] and Lima's group [37,38] used hyperbolic-shaped contraction for the ability to impose a constant strain rate along the centerline of the contraction, as well as to achieve high extensional and shear flows. Although the hyperbolic-shaped contraction was efficient for causing cell deformation, here we used a linearly tapered microflow channel, as shown in Figure 1a. The geometry of the channel is similar to that in TruongVo et al. [39], who also used it to characterize breast cancer cells. The channel has four ports: (a) Inlet for cell flow, (b) and (c) inlets for sheath flow, and (d) outlet. In design, the main flow channel has a taper with an inlet width of 40 μm, an outlet width of 15 μm, and a length of 200 μm. The height of the main channel is 20 μm, providing a rectangular cross-section.

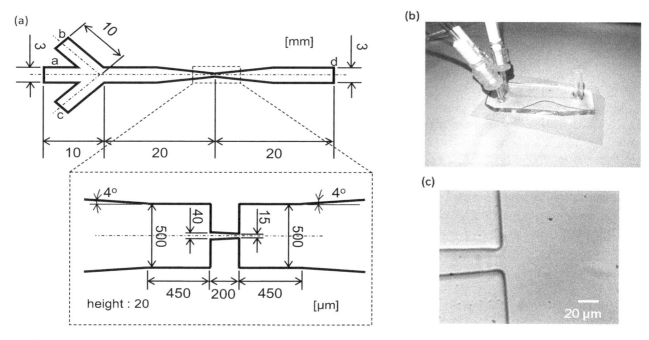

Figure 1. (**a**) Schematic drawing of the microflow channel—a, inlet port for cell flow; b and c, inlet ports for sheath flow; and d, outlet. (**b**) A fabricated microfluidic device and (**c**) a magnified view of the tip of the microflow channel.

The flow channel was fabricated according to standard photolithography and soft lithography techniques. The negative photoresist pattern was fabricated on a silicon wafer (Matsuzaki, Tokyo, Japan) with SU8- 3050 (Nippon Kayaku, Tokyo, Japan). PDMS prepolymer (Sylgard 184 silicone elastomer kit, Toray Dow Corning, Tokyo, Japan) was poured onto the silicon wafer and baked at 80 °C for 1 h. Plasma treatment was used to chemically bond the PDMS mold to a glass slide with a thickness of 0.12–0.17 mm (C050701, Matsunami, Bellingham, WA, USA). The fabricated microfluidic device and the microscopic image of the tapered part are shown in Figure 1b,c, respectively. In the final product, the width of the tip was 20 μm and the channel height was 32 μm.

2.3. Experimental Setup

Figure 2 provides a schematic illustration of the experimental setup. The experimental setup mainly consists of an inverted microscope (IX-71, Olympus, Tokyo, Japan), a high-speed camera (FASTCAM Mini AX200, Photron, Tokyo, Japan), syringe pumps (KDS-210, KD Scientific, Holliston, MA, USA), and a flow channel. Cells were introduced to the flow channel by one of the syringe pumps. Along with cell flow, sheath flow was also introduced to direct cells to the center of the channel. The total flow rate of the cell flow and sheath flows was set to 66 μL/min that gave approximately 1.5 m/s at the tip of the tapered channel. The ratio of the flowrate between cell flow and sheath flow was 1:6. A cell shape at the tip of the taper and its downstream was recorded with a high-speed camera at a frame rate of 100,000 fps via an objective lens of 60x (N.A. 0.7, LUCPlanFLN 60x, Olympus). The cell height $h(t)$—defined as cell length in a direction perpendicular to the flow, exemplified in Figure 3—was measured using image analysis software (ImageJ 1.48v, National Institutes of Health, Bethesda, MD, USA).

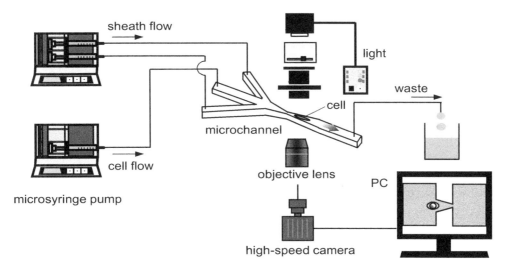

Figure 2. Schematic illustration of the experimental setup. The microflow channel was placed under the microscope and cell deformation was recorded with a high-speed camera.

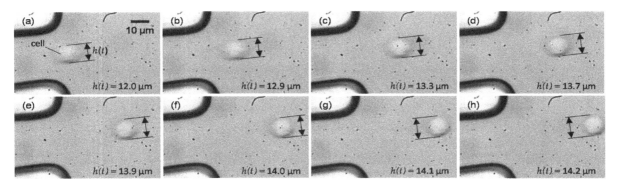

Figure 3. A time series of snapshots of a cell showing how the cell was recovering its shape after it had left the tip of the tapered channel (**a**). The time interval between consecutive snapshots (**b**–**h**) is 20 μs. The scale bar in Figure 3a applies to all images.

2.4. Mechanical Characterization of a Cell

Cells leaving the tapered channel are released from compressive forces and gradually recover to their original shape. Here, the compression strain $\varepsilon(t)$ of a cell at time t after leaving the tapered channel—was defined by the following formula:

$$\varepsilon(t) = \frac{h_\infty - h(t)}{h_\infty} \tag{1}$$

where $h(t)$ is the cell height at time t, and h_∞ is the cell height in the last frame where the cell is sufficiently far from the tip of the tapered channel.

The recovery process of the cell diameter was expressed with a Kelvin–Voigt model that has a purely viscous damper with a viscosity of μ and a purely elastic spring with a spring constant k

connected in parallel. When a cell leaves the tapered channel, it is released from the compressive force. Under this condition, the compressive strain of the cell, $\varepsilon(t)$, is expressed with the following formula:

$$\varepsilon(t) = \varepsilon_0 \exp\left(-\frac{t}{\tau}\right) \tag{2}$$

where τ is a time constant of shape recovery and equal to μ/k.

2.5. EGCG Treatment

EGCG is the main polyphenolic constituent of green tea [26]. Reportedly, EGCG inhibits tumor promotion induced by teleocidin in a two-stage carcinogenesis experiment on mouse skin [40] and duodenal carcinogenesis with N-ethyl-N'-nitro-IV-nitrosoguanidine [41]. It is also reported that EGCG inhibits lung colonization of B16-F10 cells and spontaneous metastasis of B16-BL6 cells from the foot to the lung [26]. Clinical trials have demonstrated that green tea catechins including EGCG are effective for cancer prevention [42–45]. Here, EGCG was used to stiffen cells by following a protocol described in Fujiki and Okuda [46]. An EGCG culture medium of 200 μM/L was prepared by diluting an EGCG/PBS(-) solution of 25 mM/L in DMEM. Cells were cultured with the EGCG culture medium for 4 h. After the culture, the cells were removed from dishes by treatment with trypsin, which was followed by centrifuge and removal of the medium. Finally, EGCG-treated cells were suspended in PBS(-) such that the cell concentration became 3–4 × 10^5 cells/mL.

2.6. Staining

The cell nucleus and actin filaments of B16-F1 and B16-F10 cells were stained. Staining was conducted for both cells that were attached to dishes and cells that were floating. The latter group was prepared by detaching the cells from the dishes with trypsin and leaving them for 30 min at room temperature until the cells become stably spherical. In the following staining processes, the floating cells were always centrifuged at a relative centrifugal force of 17.9 g for 5 min at washing and liquid exchange. First, cells were fixed with 10% neutral buffered formalin for 10 min at room temperature then washed with PBS(-). The cells were then permeated with 0.2% Triton X-100 in PBS(-) for 10 min then washed. This was followed by blocking with 4% albumin from bovine serum (Wako)/PBS(-) solution for 15 min then washing. For staining actin filaments, cells were treated with Alexa Fluor 488 phalloidin, diluted to 1:200 times with PBS(-) in a dark room for 30 min at room temperature. For staining the cell nucleus, cells were treated with Hoechst 33342 diluted to 1:10,000 with 0.2% BSA/PBS(-) solution in a dark room for 30 min at room temperature. Images were obtained using a confocal laser scanning microscope (FV3000, Olympus) with a 60x oil immersion objective lens (N.A. 1.35, UPLSAPO60XO, Olympus). A laser (OBIS, Coherent, Santa Clara, CA, USA) with an excitation wavelength of 488 nm and 405 nm was used to observe actin filaments and cell nuclei, respectively.

2.7. Statistical Method

Student's unpaired t-test was used in all statistical analyses. A significance level of 0.05 was used.

3. Results

Figure 3 shows a series of snapshots of a B16-F10 cell flowing downstream from the tip of the tapered channel. Note that the snapshots in Figure 3 were the ones obtained every two snapshots that were recorded. The cell size at rest was 15.4 ± 1.6 μm for B16-F1 cells and 15.4 ± 1.4 μm for B16-F10 cells, and no statistical difference was found in cell size between them. As seen, the cell that was compressed at the tip gradually recovered its shape to being spherical as it flowed further downstream. A temporal variation of the compressive strain of the cell, $\varepsilon(t)$, is shown in Figure 4 where Figure 4a–d is for untreated B16-F1 cells, untreated B16-F10 cells, EGCG-treated B16-F1 cells, and EGCG-treated B16-F10 cells, respectively. Note that the graphs in Figure 4 are a representative case of each cell and treatment condition. All the figures demonstrate an exponential decrease in $\varepsilon(t)$ as a function of time.

Fitting Equation (2) to the data in Figure 4 clearly indicates that a change in the compressive strain could be represented by the Kelvin–Voigt model.

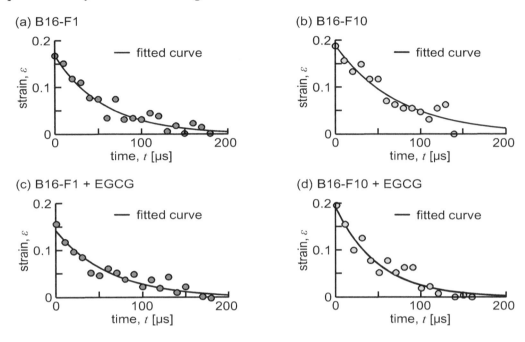

Figure 4. Time variations of the compressive strain of the cell. (**a**) Untreated B16-F1, (**b**) untreated B16-F10, (**c**) epigallocatechin gallate (EGCG)-treated B16-F1, and (**d**) EGCG-treated B16-F10.

Figure 5 compares the initial compression strain, ε_0, when a cell was at the tip of the taper. The mean $\pm$ SD of ε_0 was 0.15 ± 0.06 for untreated B16-F1 cells, 0.17 ± 0.09 for untreated B16-F10 cells, 0.15 ± 0.03 for EGCG-treated B16-F1 cells, and 0.18 ± 0.05 for EGCG-treated B16-F10 cells. No statistical difference was found in ε_0 between any combinations.

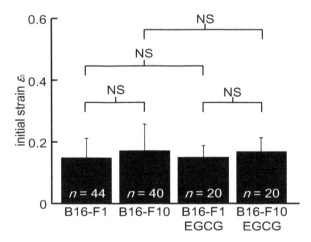

Figure 5. A comparison of the initial compressive strain, ε_0. n: Number of cells.

A comparison of a time constant of the shape recovery τ is presented in Figure 6. The mean $\pm$ SD of τ was 50 ± 15 µs for untreated B16-F1 cells, 70 ± 23 for untreated B16-F10 cells, 59 ± 22 µs for EGCG-treated B16-F1 cells, and 60 ± 12 µs for EGCG-treated B16-F10 cells. A statistical difference in τ was found in a pair of untreated B16-F1 cells vs. untreated B16-F10 cells ($p < 0.05$) and untreated B16-F1 vs EGCG-treated B16-F1 cells ($p < 0.05$), while no statistical difference was noted in a pair of untreated B16-F10 cells vs. EGCG-treated B16-F10 cells and EGCG-treated B16-F1 cells vs EGCG-treated B16-F10 cells.

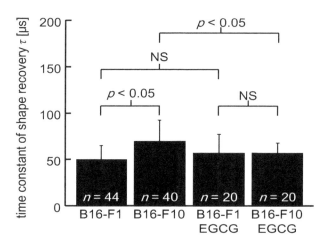

Figure 6. A comparison of the time constant of shape recovery τ. n: Number of cells.

Figure 7 provides fluorescent images of cellular nuclei and the actin filaments of cells. Figure 7a,b show the cells that remained adhered to dishes, and Figure 7c,d show the cells that were detached from the dishes. Cell lines were B16-F1 for a and c, and B16-F10 for b and d. The detached cells appeared to be spherical, while those adhering to dishes spread with extending processes. In looking at Figure 7a,b, we found that when the cells adhere to dishes, B16-F1 cells had thicker actin filaments than B16-F10 cells, although both cell lines showed fibrous structure of actin filaments. To confirm this perceptual finding, thickness of actin filaments was evaluated with the standard deviation of a Gaussian function fitted to the intensity profile across stress fibers. This is because the spatial resolution of 0.083 μm/pixel in the present images is not fine enough to measure the thickness of actin filaments with a certain accuracy. The evaluation was conducted for three locations for each of the actin filaments arrowed in Figure 7. The results demonstrated 2.15 ± 0.71 pixels for B16-F1 cells and 0.99 ± 0.14 pixels for B16-F10 cells ($p < 0.05$), supporting the perceptual finding of a difference in the thickness. For the cells that were detached from the dishes, the fibrous structure disappeared and no remarkable difference in the structure and amount of actin filaments was noticed between B16-F1 cells and B16-F10 cells.

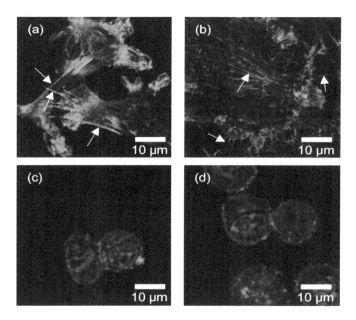

Figure 7. Fluorescent images of actin filaments (green) and nuclei (blue). (**a**) Adhered B16-F1 cells, (**b**) adhered B16-F10 cells, (**c**) floating B16-F1 cells, and (**d**) floating B16-F10 cells. Arrows in (**a,b**) indicate actin filaments whose thickness was evaluated.

4. Discussion

Microfluidic devices have been used in prior studies to find circulating tumor cells in blood. Recently, Tse et al. [24] invented a microfluidic device of a crossed flow channel at the junction where a cell was deformed by counter striking flows. They successfully classified cells based on cell deformability and took the initiative in diagnosing malignant pleural effusions by microfluidics. Raj et al. [47] fabricated a microfluidic device comprised of multiple parallel microconstrictions. They introduced a theoretical model of cell flow and deformation in the channels and succeeded in quantifying cell elasticity. The present study is situated in part as an extension of these studies. As demonstrated in Figure 6, we found that a time constant of shape recovery could be a useful index to rate the metastatic potentials of cancer cells. Moreover, the time constant could be useful to assess drug-screening applications where biophysical changes occur in cells. The present microfluidic system is totally label-free, which would relieve clinicians from the tangled procedure of labeling and reduce their workload. The microfluidic system proposed here is simple, but its use is not limited to screening of metastatic cells, it has the potential to be used in many areas of medicine other than cancer diagnostics. Although some improvements such as quantification of cell viscoelasticity is necessary, extensive applications of the present system will enable rapid mechanophenotyping of various cells.

Since a tapered portion of the channel was sufficiently long compared to cell size, viscous deformation was assumed to have completed before a cell left the taper. In other words, in the current system, it was considered that the effect of cell viscosity on cell deformation or shape at the tip of the taper was considered to be small and the initial strain ε_0 was determined mostly by cell elasticity. As shown in Figure 5, the initial strain ε_0 of B16-F1 cells was almost the same as that of B16-F10 cells, leading to an assumption that there was no difference in cell elasticity between B16-F1 cells and B16-F10 cells. Moreover, as shown in Figure 6, B16-F10 cells had a significantly larger time constant τ than B16-F1. As time constant τ is a ratio of the viscosity to the elasticity of a cell, μ/k, the assumption that there was no difference in cell elasticity between B16-F1 cells and B16-F10 cells indicated that B10-F10 cells had larger cell viscosity than B10-F1 cells. In light of a biological viewpoint that more metastatic and invasive cells should be softer to pass through a narrow gap in extracellular matrix, larger cell viscosity could be unbeneficial for metastatic cells. The biological relevance of larger viscosity for more metastatic cells remains inconclusive and should be clarified in future research.

The width of the flow channel at the exit of the tapered channel was 20 μm. This width might not be small enough to cause large deformation to cells if we consider that the cell size was 15.4 μm in diameter on average. In fact, as shown in Figure 5, we did not find a statistically significant difference in cell stiffness between B16-F1 and B16-F10 cells in the present experimental condition. Two possible reasons were considered. First, loaded cell deformation was not large enough to reflect a difference in cell stiffness. Second, B16-F1 and B16-F10 cells have a comparable level of stiffness in the floating state. Experiments with larger loading by using a device with smaller width will answer this question. At the same time however, narrowing the channel increases the risk of clogging with cells or other debris. Taking into account the practical applications of the proposed channel, clogging has to be avoided. As shown in the present study, a statistically significant difference in the time constant was noticed even with the current width. In this sense, though it was limited to the cell types examined here, the width of 20 μm was considered to be sufficient.

The sheath flow was established in the present flow channel. The sheath flow is necessary as the cell is much smaller than the taper tip and it is important to control cells at a particular position. In this sense, the sheath flow was redundant in the current experiment because the channel width of the taper tip was comparable with cell size.

Although cells flowed along the centerline of the flow channel at the tip, they may have had some rotational motions when they were released into a large pool beyond the taper tip. Due to deformation, cells would have not stayed in the centerline, although they moved downstream by inertia. As a consequence, fluid shear was exerted on cells such that they exhibited rotational motions. Once cells are out of the centerline, they experience a shear-induced lift force that drives them toward channel walls [48]. As deformed cells recover their shape, a time period of the rotation decreases [49], meaning that cells rotate more quickly. However, we did not observe significant cell rotation when looking at cell behaviors in the present experiment. This could be because the experiment's duration was not long enough to observe cell rotation. As shown in Figures 3 and 4, cell deformations were tracked for only 200 μs in the present experiment. During that period of time, the cell traveled approximately 30 μm, which is 1.5 times as large as a cell size. The cell rotation would have introduced fluctuating errors in cell height, thereby giving errors in the measurement of the time constant of shape recovery. In fact, the time variation of cell height shown in Figure 4a showed fluctuating behaviors. Further experiments are needed to assess the effect of cell rotations on the time constant of shape recovery.

Actin filaments are concerned with the structural strength, shape stability, and deformation behaviors of cells [50–53]. As seen in Figure 7a,b, in adherent cells, B16-F1 cells appeared to have thicker actin fibers than B16-F10 cells. This observation was consistent with Sadano et al. [54], who found that actin fibers provide cells with mechanical integrity and structurally support the plasma membrane. In this sense, B16-F1 cells that were rich in actin fibers should be stiffer than B16-F10 cells. This speculation was congruent with Watanabe et al. [14], who demonstrated larger elasticity in B16-F1 than B16-F10 using atomic force microscopy. In contrast, the present results demonstrated no difference in cell elasticity between B16-F1 cells and B16-F10 cells. In fact, cell deformation might not be large enough to reflect a difference in elasticity in the present experimental condition. But, assuming that cells were sufficiently deformed, we attribute a discrepancy between Watanabe et al. [14] and the present result to a difference in cell state—cells analyzed in this study were detached from dishes and were suspended in PBS(-). In suspended cells, actins did not have firm fiber structures. The cell detachment from a dish caused depolymerization of filamentous actins (F-actin) into the monomeric globular form of actin (G-actin) as a part of cytoskeletal remodeling. In fact, filamentous structures were not found in floating B16-F1 cells (Figure 7c) anymore, and no remarkable difference was noticed in the structure and amount of actin filaments between B16-F1 cells and B16-F10 cells. These observations indicated that the leveling in cell elasticity of B16-F1 cells and B16-F10 cells was due to the loss of F-actin by cell detachment. Depolymerization of F-actin would have resulted in an increase in the amount of G-actin. Dispersion of G-actin, or a solid particulate phase in a liquid phase of cytoplasm might have resulted in changing the rheological properties of cytoplasm. As shown in Figure 6, the viscosity of B16-F10 cells was larger than that of B16-F1 cells. This would imply that an increase in G-actin provides cytoplasm with its pseudoplastic nature, by which apparent viscosity decreased with increased stress. Future studies should warrant these speculations.

As shown in Figures 5 and 6, for B16-F1 cells, no changes in ε_0 and shape recovery time constant τ were observed, regardless of the catechin treatment. In contrast, the shape recovery time constant τ of B16-F10 cells was significantly decreased by catechin treatment and was almost the same value as that of B16-F1 cells, indicating that the catechin treatment promoted fast shape recovery of the B16-F10 cells. On the other hand, Figure 5 showed no change in ε_0 of B16-F10 cells between catechin-treated and untreated groups. Since a fluid force is continuously applied to the cells while passing through the tapered part of the flow channel, ε_0 is hardly influenced by the cell viscosity and is thought to be solely determined by cell stiffness. If so, the decrease in the shape recovery time constant τ is thought to be due to the decrease in cell viscosity μ by catechin treatment. Although the mechanism of how catechin brings a change in the viscosity of cancer cells is unclear, these results suggest that it would be possible to evaluate drug efficacy, at least in highly metastatic cancer cells, using the shape recovery time constant τ.

Cells were potentially dead after they passed through microflow channels. A significant loss of cancer cell viability can occur at shear stress levels above 10 Pa [55]. In the present experimental condition, the maximum shear stress of a channel flow was roughly estimated to be 638 Pa under the assumption of the Poiseuille flow. In the study by Zhou et al. [55], cell viability was 83% for the maximum shear stress calculated to be 199 Pa. Their flow channels with smaller maximum shear stress levels reduced cell viability, although a direct application of their results to our study is difficult as their channel is different from the present flow channel in design. However just for cancer cell screening, cells were not necessarily viable after they passed through the flow channel. Cell viability must be cared if filtration, concentration or sorting of cells are included in the scope of application.

Microfluidic techniques and devices offer rapid high throughput in cell mechanophenotyping compared to conventional analytical techniques such as atomic force microscopy (AFM), microaspiration, and optical tweezers [23,24,56–59]. In AFM, cell samples need to be indented one by one with care, although it allows researchers to map the mechanical properties of a single cell and provide information on cellular structures including cytoskeletal structure. One of the drawbacks of AFM is that it is applicable only to cells that adhere to the base or dish, and thus the use of AFM for floating cancer cells in circulation is not appropriate. Microaspiration and optical tweezers are more conventional approaches for the mechanical characterization of cells. These techniques provide both local and global mechanical properties of cells but are laborious and require partial technical skill. In our experience, it takes more than an hour to measure a few cells. Microfluidic techniques, including that used in the present study, reduce such laboratory workload. A comparison of microfluidic techniques with AFM, microaspiration, and optical tweezers for measuring red blood cell deformability is summarized in Bento et al. [18]. In microfluidic techniques, cells can be continuously scanned once cell flow is supplied. Combined with imaging analysis, cell mechanophenotyping can be automated. As the present system is not equipped with the automatic imaging analysis, cell deformability was assessed manually after the experiment. Yet, indices of the cell deformability such as the time constant were immediately obtained once a cell was identified in a series of recorded images—after some assessments of image quality. Future improvement of imaging analysis will achieve rapid mechanophenotyping of cancer cells.

Spring constant and viscosity coefficient cannot be determined independently with only the present experiment data. Tajikawa et al. [60] and Kohri et al. [61] studied red blood cells using a similar experimental setup, measured the Young's modulus of red blood cells by a uniaxial tensile test in a separate experiment and estimated the spring constant. This approach however, requires the cell type to be known in advance, and it cannot be applied to this study where it is desired to identify an unknown cell type and evaluate its metastatic potential. Recently, Raj et al. [62] developed a method to estimate the Young's modulus of the cell. A different approach to estimate the Young's modulus of floating cells is also given in TruongVo et al. [39], who used a flow channel similar to the present design. If the spring constant k can be determined from the Young's modulus of the cell using the method of Raj et al. [62] and TruongVo et al. [39], the viscosity coefficient μ can then be estimated from the shape recovery time constant τ and a more detailed analysis of the cell's mechanical properties can be made.

In the present experiment, the exposure time was 10 μs and the spatial resolution was 0.083 μm/pixel. Because of these conditions, some images were blurred and the boundary of cells was not clear. In the present analysis, cell shape was manually determined. This may have resulted in errors in measuring the cell height and in turn estimating the time constant of shape recovery. If a cell whose diameter at rest is 15.4 μm is imaged and its diameter is measured as 14.8 μm, the compressive strain for this case is approximately 0.039. If a cell diameter is measured two pixels larger, the diameter is quantified as 14.966 μm and the compressive strain is calculated as 0.028. This yields approximately 10% error in the compressive strain. Careful tuning of the exposure time and the use of better spatial resolution will improve the accuracy of the measurement such that an even tiny difference in the mechanical properties between cells is appreciated.

5. Conclusions

The present study proposes a method to evaluate metastatic potential by evaluating the viscoelastic properties of cancer cells on a tapered microchannel. The shape recovery time constant τ became larger as cancer cells had higher metastatic potential. The results suggested that it would be possible to evaluate the metastatic potential of cancer cells using the shape recovery time constant τ.

The method is simple, but its use is not limited to screening of metastatic cells. It can be extensively applied to various medical and biological areas other than cancer diagnostics, such as the assessment of drug efficacy. Although further improvements are necessary, the present method will help with rapid mechanophenotyping and screening of metastatic cancer cells in clinical practice.

Author Contributions: Conceptualization, M.N.; methodology, M.N. and D.O.; formal analysis, D.O.; resources, M.N.; writing—original draft preparation, D.O. and M.N.; writing—review and editing, S.S. and M.N.; supervision, M.N.; project administration, M.N.; funding acquisition, M.N.

References

1.   Orr, F.W.; Wang, H.H.; Lafrenie, R.M.; Scherbarth, S.; Nance, D.M. Interactions between cancer cells and the endothelium in metastasis. *J. Pathol.* **2000**, *190*, 310–329. [CrossRef]

2.   Eger, A.; Mikulits, W. Models of epithelial–mesenchymal transition. *Drug Dis. Today Dis. Models* **2005**, 57–63. [CrossRef]

3.   Chambers, A.F.; Groom, A.C.; MacDonald, I.C. Dissemination and growth of cancer cells in metastatic sites. *Nat. Rev. Cancer* **2002**, *2*, 563–572. [CrossRef]   *2,*

4.   Alibert, C.; Goud, B.; Manneville, J.B. Are cancer cells really softer than normal cells? *Biol. Cell* **2017**, *109* 167–189. [CrossRef]

5.   Jonietz, E. Mechanics: The forces of cancer. *Nature* **2012**, *491*, S56–S57. [CrossRef]

6.   Binnig, G.; Quate, C.F.; Gerber, C. Atomic force microscope. *Phys. Rev. Lett.* **1986**, *56*, 930–933. [CrossRef]   ,

7.   Hochmuth, R.M. Micropipette aspiration of living cells. *J. Biomech.* **2000**, *33*, 15–22. [CrossRef]

8.   Cross, S.E.; Jin, Y.S.; Rao, J.Y.; Gimzewski, J.K. Nanomechanical analysis of cells from cancer patients. *Nat. Nanotechnol.* **2007**, *2*, 780–783. [CrossRef] [PubMed]

9.   Suresh, S. Nanomedicine: Elastic clues in cancer detection. *Nat. Nanotechnol.* **2007**, *2*, 748–749. [CrossRef]

10.   Zhang, H.; Liu, K.; Soc, J.R. Optical tweezers for single cells. *J. R. Soc. Interface* **2008**, *5*, 671–690. [CrossRef] [PubMed]

11.   Remmerbach, T.W.; Wottawah, F.; Dietrich, J.; Lincoln, B.; Wittekind, C.; Guck, J. Oral cancer diagnosis by mechanical phenotyping. *Cancer Res.* **2009**, *69*, 1728–1732. [CrossRef]   ]

12.   Swaminathan, V.; Mythereye, K.; O'Brien, E.T.; Berchuck, A.; Blobe, G.C.; Superfine, R. Mechanical stiffness grades metastatic potential in patient tumor cells and in cancer cell line. *Cancer Res.* **2011**, *71*, 5075–5080. [CrossRef] [PubMed]

13.   Plodinec, M.; Loparic, M.; Monnier, C.A.; Obermann, E.C.; Zanetti-Dallenbach, R.; Oertle, P.; Hyotyla, J.T.; Aebi, U.; Bentires-Alj, M.; Lim, R.Y.H.; et al. The nanomechanical signature of breast cancer. *Nat. Nanotechnol.* **2012**, *7*, 757–765. [CrossRef]

14.   Watanabe, T.; Kuramochi, H.; Takahashi, A.; Imai, K.; Katsuta, N.; Nakayama, T.; Fujiki, H.; Suganuma, M. Higher cell stiffness indicating lower metastatic potential in B16 melanoma cell variants and in (-)-epigallocatechin gallate-treated cells. *J. Cancer Res. Clin. Oncol.* **2012**, *138*, 859–866. [CrossRef]

15.   Hayashi, K.; Iwata, M. Stiffness of cancer cells measured with an AFM indentation method. *J. Mech. Behav. Biomed. Mater.* **2015**, *49*, 105–111. [CrossRef]

16.   Darling, E.M.; Di Carlo, D. High-throughput assessment of cellular mechanical properties. *Annu. Rev. Biomed. Eng.* **2015**, *17*, 35–62. [CrossRef]

17.   Chaudhuri, P.K.; Low, B.C.; Lim, C.T. Mechanobiology of tumor growth. *Chem. Rev.* **2018**, *118*, 6499–6515. [CrossRef] [PubMed]

18.   Bento, D.; Rodrigues, R.O.; Faustino, V.; Pinho, D.; Fernandes, C.S.; Pereira, A.I.; Garcia, V.; Miranda, J.M.; Lima, R. Deformation of red blood cells, air bubbles, and droplets in microfluidic devices: Flow visualizations and measurements. *Micromachines* **2018**, *9*, 151. [CrossRef] [PubMed]

19.   Tan, S.J.; Yobas, L.; Lee, G.Y.H.; Ong, C.N.; Lim, C.T. Microdevice for the isolation and enumeration of cancer cells from blood. *Biomed. Microdevices* **2009**, *11*, 883–892. [CrossRef]

20.   Chen, J.; Li, J.; Sun, Y. Microfluidic approaches for cancer cell detection, characterization, and separation. *Lab Chip* **2012**, *12*, 1753–1767. [CrossRef]

21.   Ma, Y.H.V.; Middleton, K.; You, L.; Sun, Y. A review of microfluidic approaches for investigating cancer extravasation during metastasis. *Microsys. Nanoeng.* **2018**, *4*, 17104. [CrossRef]

22. Hou, H.W.; Warkiani, M.E.; Khoo, B.L.; Li, Z.R.; Soo, R.A.; Tan, D.S.W.; Lim, W.T.; Han, J.; Bhagat, A.A.S.; Lim, C.T. Isolation and retrieval of circulating tumor cells using centrifugal forces. *Sci. Rep.* **2013**, *3*, 1259. [CrossRef]

23. Khoo, B.L.; Warkiani, M.E.; Tan, D.S.W.; Bhagat, A.A.S.; Irwin, D.; Lau, D.P.; Lim, A.S.T.; Lim, K.H.; Krisna, S.S.; Lim, W.T.; et al. Clinical validation of an ultra high-throughput spiral microfluidics for the detection and enrichment of viable circulating tumor cells. *PLoS ONE* **2014**, *9*, e99409. [CrossRef]

24. Tse, H.T.; Gossett, D.R.; Moon, Y.S.; Masaeli, M.; Sohsman, M.; Ying, Y.; Mislick, K.; Adams, R.P.; Rao, J.; Di Carlo, D. Quantitative diagnosis of malignant pleural effusions by single-cell mechanophenotyping. *Sci. Transl. Med.* **2013**, *5*, 212ra163. [CrossRef]

25. Gossett, D.R.; Henry, T.K.; Lee, S.A.; Ying, Y.; Lindgrenc, A.G.; Yang, O.O.; Rao, J.; Clark, A.T.; Carlo, D.D. Hydrodynamic stretching of single cells for large population mechanical phenotyping. *Proc. Natl. Acad. Sci. USA* **2012**, *109*, 7630–7635. [CrossRef]

26. Taniguchi, S.; Fujiki, H.; Kobayashi, H.; Go, H.; Miyado, K.; Sadano, H.; Shimokawa, R. Effect of (-)-epigallocatechin gallate; the main constituent of green tea; on lung metastasis with mouse B16 melanoma cell lines. *Cancer Lett.* **1992**, *65*, 51–54. [CrossRef]

27. Kuzuhara, T.; Sei, Y.; Yamaguchi, K.; Suganuma, M.; Fujiki, H. DNA and RNA as new binding targets of green tea catechins. *J. Biol. Chem.* **2006**, *281*, 17446–17456. [CrossRef]

28. Sah, J.F.; Balasubramanian, S.; Eckert, R.L.; Rorke, E.A. Epigallocatechin-3-gallate inhibits epidermal growth factor receptor signaling pathway. Evidence for direct inhibition of ERK1/2 and AKT kinases. *J. Biol. Chem.* **2004**, *279*, 12755–12762. [CrossRef] [PubMed]

29. Rawangkan, A.; Wongsirisin, P.; Namiki, K.; Iida, K.; Kobayashi, Y.; Shimizu, Y.; Fujiki, H.; Suganuma, M. Green tea catechin is an alternative immune checkpoint inhibitor that inhibits PD-L1 expression and lung tumor growth. *Molecules* **2018**, *23*, 2071. [CrossRef] [PubMed]

30. Tsuchiya, H.; Nagayama, M.; Tanaka, T.; Furusawa, M.; Kashimata, M.; Takeuchi, H. Membrane-rigidifying effects of anti-cancer dietary factors. *Biofactors* **2002**, *16*, 45–56. [CrossRef] [PubMed]

31. Fang, C.Y.; Wu, C.C.; Hsu, H.Y.; Chuang, H.Y.; Huang, S.Y.; Tsai, C.H.; Chang, Y.; Tsao, G.S.W.; Chen, C.L.; Chen, J.Y. EGCG inhibits proliferation, invasiveness and tumor growth by up-regulation of adhesion molecules, suppression of gelatinases activity, and induction of apoptosis in nasopharyngeal carcinoma cells. *Int. J. Mol. Sci.* **2015**, *16*, 2530–2558. [CrossRef] [PubMed]

32. Takahashi, A.; Watanabe, T.; Mondal, A.; Suzuki, K.; Kururu-Kanno, M.; Li, Z.; Yamazaki, T.; Fujiki, H.; Suganuma, M. Mechanism-based inhabitation of cancer metastasis with (-)-epigallocatechin gallate. *Biochem. Biophys. Res. Commun.* **2014**, *443*, 1–6. [CrossRef] [PubMed]

33. Fidler, I.J. Selection of successive tumour lines for metastasis. *Nat. New Biol.* **1973**, *242*, 148–149. [CrossRef] [PubMed]

34. Poste, G.; Doll, J.; Hart, I.R.; Fidler, I.J. In vitro selection of murine B16 melanoma variants with enhanced tissue-invasive properties. *Cancer Res.* **1980**, *40*, 1636–1644. [PubMed]

35. Nakamura, K.; Yoshikawa, N.; Yamaguchi, Y.; Kagota, S.; Shinozuka, K.; Kunitomo, M. Characterization of mouse melanoma cell lines by their mortal malignancy using an experimental metastatic model. *Life Sci.* **2002**, *70*, 791–798. [CrossRef]

36. Lee, S.S.; Yim, Y.; Ahn, K.H.; Lee, S.J. Extensional flow-based assessment of red blood cell deformability using hyperbolic converging microchannel. *Biomed. Microdevices* **2009**, *11*, 1021–1027. [CrossRef]

37. Yaginuma, T.; Oliveira, M.S.N.; Lima, R.; Ishikawa, T.; Yamaguchi, T. Human red blood cell behavior under homogeneous extensional flow in a hyperbolic-shaped microchannel. *Biomicrofluidics* **2013**, *7*, 054110. [CrossRef] [PubMed]

38. Rodrigues, R.O.; Lopes, R.; Pinho, D.; Pereira, A.I.; Garcia, V.; Gassmann, S.; Sousa, P.C.; Lima, R. In vitro blood flow and cell-free layer in hyperbolic microchannels: Visualizations and measurements. *BioChip J.* **2016**, *10*, 9–15. [CrossRef]

39. TruongVo, T.N.; Kennedy, R.M.; Chen, H.; Chen, A.; Berndt, A.; Agarwal, M.; Zhu, L.; Nakshatri, H.; Wallace, J.; Na, S. Microfluidic channel for characterizing normal and breast cancer cells. *J. Micromech. Microeng.* **2017**, *27*, 035017. [CrossRef]

40. Yoshizawa, S.; Horiuchi, T.; Fujiki, H.; Yoshida, T.; Okuda, T.; Sugimura, T. Antitumor promoter activity of (-)-epigallocatechin gallate, the main constituent of "tannin" in green tea. *Phytother. Res.* **1987**, *1*, 44–47. [CrossRef]

41.   Fujita, Y.; Yamane, T.; Tanaka, M.; Kuwata, K.; Okuzumi, J.; Takahashi, T.; Fujiki, H.; Okuda, T. Inhibitory
      effect of (-)-epigallocatechin gallate on carcinogenesis with IV-ethyl-IV'-nitro-N-nitrosoguanidine in mouse
      duodenum. *Jpn. J. Cancer Res.* **1989**, *80*, 503–505. [CrossRef]
42.   Bettuzzi, S.; Brausi, M.; Rizzi, F.; Castagnetti, G.; Peracchia, G.; Corti, A. Chemoprevention of human prostate
      cancer by oral administration of green tea catechins in volunteers with highgrade prostate intraepithelial
      neoplasia: A preliminary report from a one-year proof-of-principle study. *Cancer Res.* **2006**, *66*, 1234–1240.
      [CrossRef]
43.   Tsao, A.S.; Liu, D.; Martin, J.; Tang, X.M.; Lee, J.J.; El-Naggar, A.K.; Wistuba, I.; Culotta, K.S.; Mao, L.;
      Gillenwater, A.; et al. Phase II randomized, placebocontrolled trial of green tea extract in patients with
      high-risk oral premalignant lesions. *Cancer Prev. Res.* **2009**, *2*, 931–941. [CrossRef] [PubMed]
44.   Singh, B.N.; Shankar, S.; Srivastava, R.K. Green tea catechin, epigallocatechin-3-gallate (EGCG): Mechanisms,
      perspectives and clinical applications. *Biochem. Pharmacol.* **2011**, *82*, 1807–1821. [CrossRef] [PubMed]
45.   Yang, C.S.; Wang, X. Green tea and cancer prevention. *Nutr. Cancer* **2010**, *62*, 931–937. [CrossRef]
46.   Fujiki, H.; Okuda, T. (−)-Epigallocatechin gallate. *Drugs Future* **1992**, *17*, 462–464. [CrossRef]
47.   Raj, A.; Dixit, M.; Doble, M.; Sen, A.K. A combined experimental and theoretical approach towards
      mechanophenotyping of biological cells using a constricted microchannel. *Lab Chip* **2017**, *17*, 3704–3716.
      [CrossRef]
48.   Zhou, J.; Papautsky, I. Fundamentals of inertial focusing in microchannels. *Lab Chip* **2013**, *13*, 1121–1132.
      [CrossRef]
49.   Masaeli, M.; Sollier, E.; Amini, H.; Mao, W.; Camacho, K.; Doshi, N.; Mitragotri, S.; Alexeev, A.; Di Carlo, D.
      Continuous inertial focusing and separation of particles by shape. *Phys. Rev. X* **2012**, *2*, 031017. [CrossRef]
50.   Peeters, E.A.G.; Bouten, C.V.C.; Oomens, C.W.J.; Bader, D.L.; Snoeckx, L.H.E.H.; Baajiens, F.P.T. Anisotropic,
      three-dimensional deformation of single attached cells under compression. *Ann. Biomed. Eng.* **2004**, *32*,
      1443–1452. [CrossRef]
51.   Hu, S.; Eberhard, L.; Chen, J.; Love, J.L.; Butler, J.P.; Fredberg, J.J.; Whitesides, G.M.; Wang, N. Mechanical
      anisotropy of adherent cells probed by a three-dimensional magnetic twisting device. *Am. J. Physiol. Cell
      Physiol.* **2004**, *287*, C1184–C1191. [CrossRef]
52.   Kumar, S.; Mexwell, I.Z.; Heisterkamp, A.; Polte, T.R.; Lele, T.P.; Salanga, M.; Mazur, E.; Ingber, D.E.
      Viscoelastic retraction of single living stress fibers and its imoact on cell shape, cytoskeletal organization,
      and extracellular matrix mechanics. *Biophys. J.* **2006**, *90*, 3762–3773. [CrossRef] [PubMed]
53.   Titushkin, I.; Cho, M. Modulation of cellular mechanics during osteongenic differentiation of human
      mesenchymal stem cells. *Biophys. J.* **2007**, *93*, 3693–3702. [CrossRef] [PubMed]
54.   Sadano, H.; Shimokawa-Kuroki, R.; Taniguchi, S. Intracellular localization and biochemical function of
      variant β-Actin, which inhibits metastasis of B16 melanoma. *Cancer Res.* **1994**, *85*, 735–743. [CrossRef]
55.   Zhou, J.; Giridhar, P.V.; Kasper, S.; Papautsky, I. Modulation of rotation-induced lift force for cell filtration in
      a low aspect ratio microchannel. *Biomicrofluidics* **2014**, *8*, 044112. [CrossRef]
56.   Liu, Z.; Huang, F.; Du, J.; Shu, W.; Feng, H.; Xu, X.; Cheng, Y. Rapid isolation of cancer cells using microfluidic
      deterministic lateral displacement structure. *Biomicrofluidics* **2013**, *7*, 0011801. [CrossRef]
57.   Du, G.; Fang, Q.; den Toonder, J.M.J. Microfluidics for cell-based high throughput screening platformsd—A
      review. *Anal. Chim. Acta* **2016**, *903*, 36–50. [CrossRef]
58.   Jiang, J.; Zhao, H.; Shu, W.; Tian, J.; Huang, Y.; Song, Y.; Wang, R.; Li, E.; Slamon, D.; Hou, D.; et al. An
      integrated microfluidic device for rapid and high-sensitivity analysis of circulating tumor cells. *Sci. Rep.*
      2017, *7*, 42612. [CrossRef] [PubMed]
59.   Nivedita, N.; Garg, N.; Lee, A.P.; Papautsky, I. A high throughput microfluidic platform for size-selective
      enrichment of cell populations in tissue and blood samples. *Analyst* **2017**, *142*, 2558–2569. [CrossRef]
60.   Tajikawa, T. Quantitative evaluation of erythrocyte deformability by using micro-visualization
      technique—Measurement of time constant of shape recovery process as a visco-elastic specification of
      each blood cells. *J. Vis. Soc. Jpn.* **2014**, *34*, 16–21. (In Japanese)
61.   Kohri, S.; Kato, Y.; Tajikawa, T.; Yamamoto, Y.; Bando, K. Measurement of erythrocyte deformability by
      uniaxial stretching—Measurement of apparent Young's modulus and time constant of shape recovering.
      Trans. Jpn. Soc. Med. Biol. Eng. **2015**, *53*, 1–7. (In Japanese)
62.   Raj, A.; Sen, A.K. Entry and passage behavior of biological cells in a constricted compliant microchannel.
      R. Soc. Chem. **2018**, *8*, 20884–20893. [CrossRef]

5

High-Precision Lens-Less Flow Cytometer on a Chip

Yuan Fang [1,2], Ningmei Yu [1,*], Yuquan Jiang [1] and Chaoliang Dang [1]

[1] School of Automation and Information Engineering, Xi'an University of Technology, Xi'an 710048, China; fangyuanmy@163.com (Y.F.); yqjiang@xaut.edu.cn (Y.J.); dangclkk@163.com (C.D.)
[2] School of Electrical and Electronic Engineering, Baoji University of Arts and Sciences, Baoji 721016, China
* Correspondence: yunm@xaut.edu.cn

Abstract: We present a flow cytometer on a microfluidic chip that integrates an inline lens-free holographic microscope. High-speed cell analysis necessitates that cells flow through the microfluidic channel at a high velocity, but the image sensor of the in-line holographic microscope needs a long exposure time. Therefore, to solve this problem, this paper proposes an S-type micro-channel and a pulse injection method. To increase the speed and accuracy of the hologram reconstruction, we improve the iterative initial constraint method and propose a background removal method. The focus images and cell concentrations can be accurately calculated by the developed method. Using whole blood cells to test the cell counting precision, we find that the cell counting error of the proposed method is less than 2%. This result shows that the on-chip flow cytometer has high precision. Due to its low price and small size, this flow cytometer is suitable for environments far away from laboratories, such as underdeveloped areas and outdoors, and it is especially suitable for point-of-care testing (POCT).

Keywords: cell analysis; lens-less; microfluidic chip; twin-image removal; POCT

1. Introduction

Cell analysis using an optical microscope or a flow cytometer is an important technique in biology and medicine [1]. Optical microscopes can obtain focus images of cells for biomedical applications, and flow cytometers can collect the signature of a large number of cells in liquid specimens with high analysis speed. However, these instruments are unsuitable for outdoor and undeveloped areas because of their high price and large size. Currently, there is a need for a small and inexpensive cell analysis device that combines the properties of the above two devices.

Over the past decade, lens-less imaging has been considered a good way to reduce the volume and cost of cell analysis tools. Seung Ah Lee and Guoan Zheng designed opto-fluidic microscopes using a complementary metal oxide semiconductor (CMOS) image sensor (CIS) and a microfluidic channel [2–7]. To weaken the shadow-imaging diffraction, the distance between the cells and the surface of the image sensor must be shorter than 2 μm. These researchers mounted a micro-channel on a CIS by removing the protective glass and Bayer filter. To improve the spatial resolution of cell images obtained with a 4× object lens, they used a multi-frame, super-resolution algorithm based the sub-pixel movement of cells flowing through the micro-channel. At the same time, Aydogan Ozcan and Serhan O. Isikman designed numerous lens-free on-chip microscopes based on incoherent digital holography [8–25]. The lens-free on-chip microscopes capture digital diffractive images of cells by using an in-line holographic structure. The diffractive images were used to reconstruct clear images of the cells using angular spectrum theory [26], and the resultant clear cell images are comparable to those obtained by a 10× object lens with a numerical aperture of ~0.1–0.2. Later, Se-Hwan Paek and Sungkyu Seo proposed a new method to classify different types of cells using digital diffractive images [27–30]. Mei Yan and Hao Yu conducted a blood cell analysis with a single-frame super resolution [31]. The concept of a lens-less microscopy technique is a novel idea for the miniaturization of flow cytometry, but the accuracy and speed of cell counting in such a method are challenges. At present, most devices based on a lens-less platform use only one frame to count cells, and this leads to inaccurate cell counting [27]. It is not easy to distinguish between cells and dust using a static image, which has a great influence on the ability to count with high precision.

In this manuscript, we propose an on-chip flow cytometer system based on lens-less imaging and a microfluidic control technique to improve the speed of cell analysis. The system causes cells to flow through a micro-channel in a polydimethylsiloxane (PDMS) microfluidic chip above a CIS. A near-coherent light source is mounted above the microfluidic chip (~5 cm), and diffraction shadow images of cells generated by the near-coherent light source are then captured by the CIS. To obtain clear images of cells, a phase iterative reconstruction algorithm is used for image diffraction [32]. In addition, the system can obtain a very accurate image without cells absented for background removal. After the background is removed, images of each segmented cell can be acquired from the whole image more precisely. Therefore, we can more accurately extract features from each cell image and quickly classify and count cells.

Because of the low intensity of near-coherent light caused by a pinhole, the exposure time of the image sensor in the system is longer than 400 ms. Therefore, there is stronger motion blur while the cells are quickly flowing in the micro-channel. To solve this problem, this manuscript proposes a method in which the cells in the micro-channel are imaged simultaneously in a large field of view (FOV) instead of with a flow cytometer method in which the cells pass through the testing area at high speed. In other words, the method takes advantage of the larger FOV of the CIS to reduce the cell flow velocity. To utilize the large FOV of the CIS, we design an "S" channel shape. As a result, we can ensure that the CIS captures the maximum possible number of cells in a frame. In addition, the cells in current frame flow out of the micro-channel completely before the next exposure of the CIS. Thus, all the cells in each frame are new cells, and the cells in each individual frame can be evaluated to increase the number of tested cells. Regarding cost, the CIS is commonly used in industrial cameras and mobile phones, so the price is very low (below $10). The microfluidic chip comprises a PDMS channel and a piece of thin glass (0.18 mm), making it very cheap and easy to replace. Overall, this manuscript proposes an on-chip cytometer that can test blood cells, bacteria, and other micro-particles in liquids. Because of the low price and small volume, the system is especially suitable for places far away from the laboratory and undeveloped areas and for family health tests.

2. Materials and Methods

2.1. System Setup

The flow cytometer utilized a lens-less imaging technique based on an in-line holography structure, and the overall structure is shown in Figure 1.

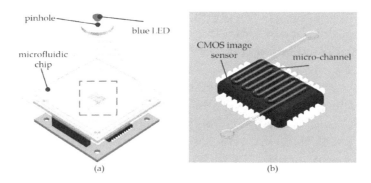

Figure 1. The structure of an on-chip flow cell counting system: (**a**) The general structure of the system; (**b**) the micro-channel on the image sensor (CIS) surface in the red box in (**a**).

As shown in Figure 1, the flow cytometer comprised a greyscale CIS (Aptina MT9P031, Micron Technology, Pennsylvania, ID, USA), a PDMS microfluidic chip and a blue light-emitting diode (LED) light source (central wavelength of ~465 nm). The pixel size of the CIS was 2.2 μm, the effective pixel size was 2592 H × 1944 V (5.7 mm × 4.2 mm), and the imaging area reached ~24.4 mm². To obtain holographic diffraction patterns on the surface of the CIS, the blue light LED was located 5 cm above the surface of the image sensor. In addition, there was a plate with a pinhole (diameter of 0.1 mm) at the front of the LED to obtain a coherent light source. To utilize the large FOV of the CIS, an S-type micro-channel was designed that could easily determine the volume of liquid samples and count the maximum possible number of cells in a frame. Moreover, the concentration of cells in a specimen could be calculated accurately, similar to a classic cell counting chamber. We used a PDMS channel and a piece of thin glass bonded together to obtain a microfluidic chip to capture the holograms of cells (the diffractive shadow images of cell) and fix the microfluidic chip on the surface of the CIS. We briefly introduce the fabricated process of the microfluidic below.

The photoresist (SU-8 2015, Microchem, Westborough, MA, USA) and a silicon wafer (4 inches in diameter) were used to fabricate positive model. The 3 mL of photoresist was dropped in the centrality of a wafer, and the photoresist film was 30 μm in thickness after using the spin coater at 1500 r/min for 15 s. Then, the silicon wafer was pre-baked for 15 min at 95 °C. The pre-designed channel photolithography plate was used for exposure on the lithography machine for 125 s. Next, the exposed wafer was after-baked for 3 min at 95 °C, and developed for 3 min. Then, we poured 30 g of liquid PDMS on the positive film, and put it in baking box for 40 min at 95 °C to solidify. The solidified PDMS layer and a piece of thin glass were bonded by vacuum plasma technique. Finally, the PDMS layer was drilled the holes of the inlet and outlet to finish the microfluidic chip.

However, since a microfluidic chip was used, a cell sample could be continuously detected, similar to a flow cytometer, as shown in Figure 2.

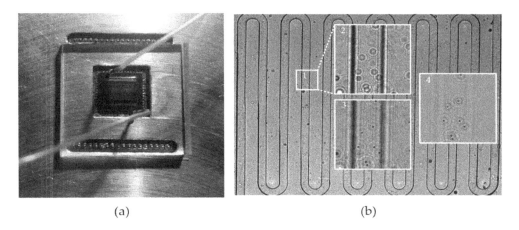

(a)   (b)

Figure 2. The proposed flow cytometer: (**a**) The flow cytometer system; (**b**) the holograms of the microfluidic chip captured by the system. Box 2 is an amplificatory image of box 1, and box 3 is a diffractive reconstruction image of box 2. Box 4 is the image of box 3 with the background removed, where the red circles mark the cells.

Next, we prepared an experimental platform to obtain the features and parameters of the proposed system. In addition, we found that the exposure time of the image sensor in this system was greater than 400 ms. Unfortunately, motion blur is caused by the movement of cells in the sample when the image sensor is operating during the exposure time. Therefore, we considered that instead of the cells flowing through the detection area at high speed, a large number of cells passed through the exposure region at one time. In other words, the system utilized the large FOV of the CIS to obtain a large number of images of cells from each frame. To avoid the motion blur caused by cell flowing, we used a method of periodically controlling the flow velocity of the specimen. There was only one inlet and one outlet in the micro-channel, ensuring that the flow of all the tested cells out of the micro-channel and that of the new cells flow into the micro-channel took a short time. To obtain a sufficient processing time for the image processing algorithm, the new cells were injected into the micro-channel during the image processing period. Subsequently, all the tested cells flowed out the micro-channel, and then the flow of the cells stopped and the cell images were captured by the image sensor. With several repetitions, the device was able to collect the maximum possible number of cell signatures to improve the accuracy of the analysis.

2.2. Sample Preparation

The flow cytometer is suitable for samples with a large number of cells, such as blood. Therefore, we performed an experiment with whole blood. The concentration range of red blood cells (RBCs) in whole blood is from ~4×10^{12}/L to 5.5×10^{12}/L. To ensure the reconstruction of the wavefront in the in-line holography system, we had to reduce the concentration of cells in the whole blood. According to the experiments, we found that 1:400 was a suitable volume dilution to count blood cells. When RBCs were tested, the dilution ratio was 1:400, corresponding to 10 µL of whole blood diluted with 4 mL of phosphate buffer saline (PBS, 0.0067 M PO_4), and the resulting solution was pumped into the microfluidic chip for testing.

The concentration of white blood cells (WBCs) in whole blood is 4×10^9/L–10×10^9/L, and the ratio of WBCs to RBCs is close to 1:1000. When WBCs were tested, 200 µL of a whole blood sample was diluted with 400 µL of RBC lysis buffer and this was then injected into the micro-channel after one minute of delay. The study was approved by the School of Automation and Information Ethics Committee, Xi'an University of Technology.

2.3. Reconstruction of Lens-Less Holographic Images

The lens-less imaging technique utilizes an in-line holographic structure proposed by Gabor [33] to reconstruct the image of the cell plane. The lens-less holographic imaging system is mainly composed of a blue LED light source, a pinhole plate, a microfluidic chip and a CIS, as shown in Figure 3.

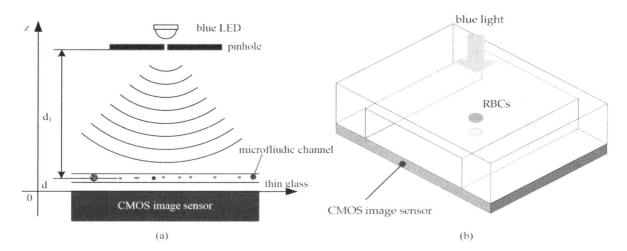

Figure 3. Graphic sketch of an in-line holographic microscope: (**a**) the structure of the lens-less holographic imaging system; (**b**) the procedure for capturing the lens-less hologram by the CIS.

Because of the infinitesimal size of blood cells (~2–15 µm), the shadows of the blood cells on the surface of the CIS are diffraction images. Due to the influence of diffraction phenomenon, the shorter the wavelength of light source is, the higher the spatial resolution of the microscopic image becomes. In the most commonly used LED of single frequency light sources, a blue light source has the shortest wavelength. So we chose a blue LED as the light source. For convenience, we assumed that the cell plane was the object plane and that the surface of CIS was the image plane. The distance from the pinhole to the object plane was d_1, and the distance from the object plane to the image plane was d ($d_1 \gg d$). According to the angular spectrum theory of diffraction, we can reconstruct an image of the object plane by recording the image plane. We assumed that the transmittance of the sample was $O(x, y)$ and that the complex amplitude of the wavefront through the object plane was as below:

$$U_d(x, y) = 1 - O(x, y) \tag{1}$$

Here, the image plane is assumed as the plane of $z = 0$, and the object plane is assumed as the plane of $z = d$. According to the Rayleigh–Sommerfeld diffraction theory, the transfer function of light waves in two planes separated by a distance d is defined as:

$$H_d(\varepsilon, \eta) = \begin{cases} \exp\left[jd\frac{2\pi}{\lambda}\sqrt{1 - (\lambda\varepsilon)^2 - (\lambda\eta)^2} \right], & \varepsilon^2 + \eta^2 < \frac{1}{\lambda^2} \\ 0, & otherwise \end{cases} \tag{2}$$

Here, ε and η denote the coordinates of a frequency domain and have been transformed by x and y into a spatial domain. λ is the wavelength of the light source. According to the transfer function, we can obtain the complex amplitude of the image plane:

$$U_0(x, y) = H_d^+[1 - O(x, y)] \tag{3}$$

where H_d^+ and H_d^- represent the optical forward and backward propagation operators, which carry out a fast Fourier transform and an inverse fast Fourier transform, respectively, belonging to a convolution operator. d denotes the distance of the light propagation; in other words, it is the distance between the object plane and the image plane. $+$ and $-$ denote forward propagation and backward propagation along the z-axis, respectively. The light intensity in the holographic plane recorded by the image sensor is the square of the amplitude of the light wave, and the light intensity is as below:

$$I_0(x, y) = |U_0(x, y)|^2 \tag{4}$$

In Equation (4), $U_0(x,y)$ is the complex amplitude of the actual light wave in the image plane, but the image sensor can receive only the light intensity, I_0, and the phase is discarded. Normally, image sensor acquisition of the holographic plane light intensity is a linear process, so the light intensity information collected by image sensor can be expressed as:

$$I_s(x, y) = \alpha + \beta I_0(x, y) \tag{5}$$

The amplitude of the light wave in the object plane can be obtained by the reconstruction of the distance image at the back of the image plane:

$$U_r(x, y) = H_d^+[I_s(x, y)] \tag{6}$$

With Equations (1)–(6), we obtain Equation (7):

$$U_r(x, y) = D - O^*(x, y) - H_{2d}^+[O(x, y)] + H_d^+\left\{ |H_d^+[O(x, y)]|^2 \right\} \tag{7}$$

In Equation (7), the first term is the direct current (DC) component; the second term is the focus image; the third term is the holographic image, which is the focus image backward propagated a distance of $2d$; and the fourth term is the intermodulation. The second and third terms constitute the twin image, which still appears after the forward transfer reconstruction of the diffraction plane and is difficult to separate. In fact, the twin-image phenomenon, which is caused by the absence of a light phase, is a major problem in the in-line holographic system. In addition, we used micro-bead images obtained with a $10\times$ objective lens to simulate the twin-image problem (Figure 4).

(a) (b) (c)

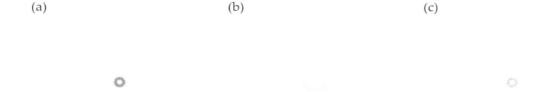

Figure 4. The twin-image problem: (**a**) a 7 μm micro-bead image was used to simulate the reconstruction of lens-less holographic images. (**b**) By simulating the holographic imaging with Equations (1)–(4), we retained the amplitude of the complex number and discarded the phase to simulate the recording procedure of a CIS. (**c**) We used Equation (6) to reconstruct the focus image of object plane, but it was polluted by the twin-image phenomenon.

According to Gabriel Koren's research [32], we can use only one diffractive to reconstruct a focus image of the object plane and suppress the twin-image phenomenon. In our proposed algorithm, only a holographic diffraction image and a cell-absent background image were needed to reconstruct the phase and obtain a focus image of the object plane. The general steps were as follows:

Step 1: Using the square root of the light intensity and the initial value of the phase (generally 0), reversely transfer the diffractive pattern of the image plane back to the object plane by the transfer function to obtain the focus image. However, the initial estimation of the object plane seriously suffers from the twin-image phenomenon. Thus, it is necessary to use the following steps to suppress the twin images. The main operation of the reconstruction process is similar to the frequency domain filter in digital image processing. The transfer function of the filter is shown by Equation (2), and the reconstruction algorithm of the object plane is shown below:

$$U_r^1(x,y) = H_d^- \left[\sqrt{I_s(x,y)} \right]$$ (8)

Step 2: The region information of the object is extracted from the preliminary estimated object image, which is used for the object plane constraint. Classic image segmentation algorithms, such as the gradient boundary extraction algorithm and the threshold segmentation algorithm can be used to find the object plane constraint. Because of the low signal-to-noise ratio (SNR) of the image extracted by the CIS, the threshold segmentation algorithm is more reliable. The threshold is 0.34 in this manuscript; in other words, the grey value of cell regions on the object plane is usually less than 0.34.

Step 3: The cell region is the C region, and the background is the non-C region. Through an iterative algorithm, the cell regions are close to the real image, and the twin-image phenomenon will be weakened on the object plane. The algorithm is

$$U_r^{(i+1)}(x,y) = \begin{cases} m \times D(x,y), x,y \notin C \\ U_r^i(x,y), x,y \in C \end{cases}$$ (9)

where $D(x,y)$ is the background image, which is obtained by the image sensor without cells, and m is shown with

$$m = mean\left(U_r^i(x,y)\right)/mean(D(x,y))$$ (10)

Step 4: The new complex amplitude of the image is obtained by the forward transfer operation. The phase of the newly calculated complex amplitude is retained, and the amplitude is replaced by the original known image plane amplitude. This process is called the image plane constraint:

$$U_0^i(x,y) = \left|U_0^1(x,y)\right| \times \exp\left(j \times \varphi_0^i(x,y)\right) \tag{11}$$

The iteration can be completed by repeating the third and fourth steps and can converge after 5–6 iterations. To obtain the missing phase, the algorithm iterates between two planes (object plane and image plane) through the amplitude and makes the iteration convergent using the object plane constraint (Equation (9)) and the image plane constraint (Equation (11)). However, the algorithm converges rapidly in the initial several iterations, and then the convergence is almost stagnant. Furthermore, there is a large error in the estimation of the initial phase when the distance between the object plane and the image plane has a deviation in an actual system. Therefore, the classic phase recovery algorithm is necessary to improve an actual system. The manuscript proposes an initial phase constraint algorithm based on the classic algorithm, in which Equation (8) is replaced by Equation (12):

$$U_r^1 = H_d^- \left[\sqrt{I_s(x,y)} \times \exp\left(j \times \left(1 - \sqrt{I_s(x,y)}\right)\right)\right]. \tag{12}$$

In general, there is no linear relationship between the amplitude and phase in a complex number. However, the phase changes of near-coherent light passing through a cell are related to the cell transmittance, and the cell transmittance is also expressed in amplitude. Therefore, there is a weak correlation between amplitude and phase. Using this property, we can estimate the initial phase of the iteration by transmittance. Through the initial phase constraint, the iterative convergent speed is faster, the reconstruction precision is higher, and the anti-jamming ability is stronger.

To test the performance of the algorithm, we used a dyed leucocyte captured by a 20× object lens microscope to perform a simulation. Using Equations (1)–(5) to establish a diffractive degradation model, we obtained the diffractive pattern of the leucocytes. To replicate our flow cytometer, we chose the same parameters as the actual system for simulation. The central wavelength of the light source was 465 nm, the distance between the object plane and the image plane was 0.875 mm, and the pixel size was 2.2 μm. The iterative algorithm without the initial phase constraint was compared to the iterative algorithm with the initial phase constraint, and the result is shown in Figure 5.

To test the performance of the two methods, we calculated the root-mean-square error (RMSE) for the reconstructed image of the object plane and original image. Finally, the proposed algorithm was used to reconstruct the cell image on the object plane and compared with the original image to calculate the RMSE:

$$RMSE = \sqrt{\frac{1}{MN}\sum_{m=1}^{M}\sum_{n=1}^{N}\left(\left|U_r^i(x,y)\right| - \left|U_d(x,y)\right|\right)^2} \tag{13}$$

According to the distance between the object plane and image plane, we conducted two groups of comparative experiments. The first was without deviation, and the second was with 20% deviation. The RMSEs of the two method were calculated by Matlab (Version: 2016b, MathWorks, Endogenous, MA, USA) and are shown in Figure 6.

In Figure 6, the 'phase constraint' is our proposed method, and the 'non-phase constraint' is the classic method. The proposed method has a faster convergence rate and a lower error rate, making it more conducive to counting and analyzing cells. As shown in Figures 5 and 6, by comparing the two groups with the two methods, we found that the iteration method with initial phase constraints had a faster iteration speed. In the case of a 20% distance deviation, the proposed method was able to restore the cell image, whereas the original method could not restore the image effectively, which has a great influence on the actual system. Moreover, when all the parameters were accurate, the proposed method converged faster, and the RMSE of image reconstruction was smaller. The results in Figure 6 show that our proposed method can greatly reduce the time consumption of the image processing algorithm and provide a guarantee for the real-time implementation of the system.

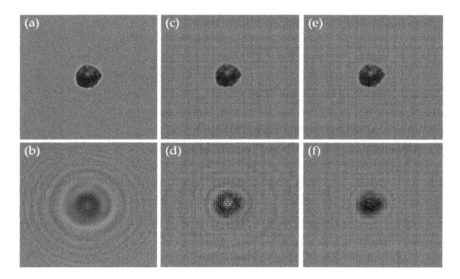

Figure 5. The result of our proposed method and classic method without a phase constraint. (**a**) The image captured by a 20× object lens microscope; (**b**) the diffractive image on the image plane; (**c**) the image reconstructed by Gabriel Koren's method with 0% deviation in distance; (**d**) the image reconstructed by Gabriel Koren's method with 20% deviation in distance; (**e**) the image reconstructed by our modified method with 0% deviation in distance; (**f**) the image reconstructed by our modified method with 20% deviation in distance.

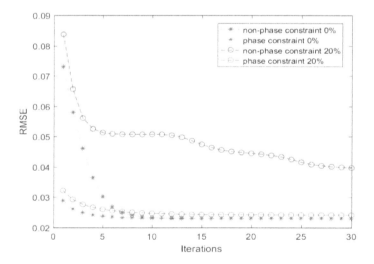

Figure 6. The root-mean-square error (RMSE) of our proposed method and the classic method without a phase constraint.

Finally, we used a frame image of whole blood cells captured by the lens-less flow cytometer to test the computation time. We used Matlab to reconstruct the holographic image, and the hardware was graphics workstation (Xeon E5-2600, 16 GB DIMM DDR4, Intel, Santa Clara, CA, USA). The time consumed for one iteration was about 2 s with the classic method of phase iterative reconstruction, and the proposed method took ~0.1 s longer than the classic method. However, the method we proposed only needed 5 iterations, and the classic method needed 10 times to achieve the same reconstruction effect. Therefore, the time consumed by the propose method was ~12.82 s, and that of the classic one was ~24.42 s. In other words, it means that the proposed method reduced the computational time by

~48%. In general, the two algorithms have almost the same computational complexity. Our algorithm only adds one phase constraint to the first image reconstruction, but its time computation is ~0.19 s.

2.4. Blood Cell Analysis Method

In the on-chip flow cytometer, the blood cells flow in the micro-channel above the image sensor, and their holographic diffraction image is transmitted onto the sensor surface by the near-coherent light source. To reduce the cost and volume of the device, an ordinary blue LED with a limited light intensity was used. The light on the plane of the cells is further weakened because the light is illuminated through a pinhole. Therefore, the exposure time of the image sensor needs to be longer than 400 ms to capture a bright enough hologram. If the blood cells move during the exposure time of the CIS, there is a motion blur, as shown in Figure 7a. To solve this problem, we used a pulse injection method, which is shown in Figure 7b.

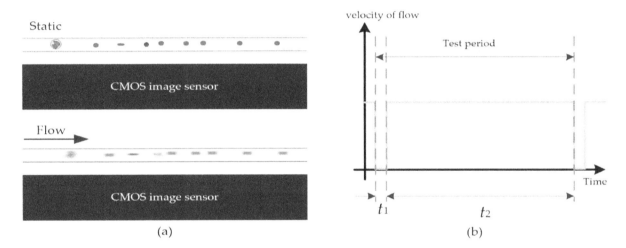

Figure 7. The pulse flow control mode: (**a**) The flow of cells stops in the micro-channel during the CIS exposure time to capture a holographic image of the cells. (**b**) When the system is processing images of cells captured in the last exposure, the tested cells flow out of the micro-channel, and the new cells flow into the micro-channel.

In Figure 7, t_1 is the exposure time, and t_2 is the injection time. This process can be controlled by a micro-pump. Due to the high precision of micro-pump control, the injection time and stationary time of the blood cells can be fixed. Therefore, the algorithm can be processed according to fixed parameters. After an experiment, accurate cell image collection and injection of new samples in micro-pump mode can be ensured.

In addition, instead of the micro-pump method, a hand-push model can be used to reduce the cost and volume of the device. In the hand-push model, the motion state of the cells in the microfluidic chip can be detected by the image processing algorithm. The system acquisition accuracy can generally be guaranteed with $t_1 > 5$ s and $t_2 > 20$ s. The state of cell motion in the microfluidic chip is detected by the RMSE between two frames.

In addition, there are two important problems, which relate to cell overlap. The first is the cell overlap in the holographic image. As mentioned earlier, the raw image captured by the lens-less platform is a holographic image, so the size of a diffractive image of the cell is ~4 times bigger than that of a focus image. The inevitable cell image overlap was solved by the phase iterative reconstruction algorithm. The other problem relates to the position of cell overlap and the 3D structure of the micro-channel leads to the shadow image overlap. The problem is difficult to solve by digital image processing algorithms. Therefore, we used a diluted cell sample to solve the problem. According to the experiment, the 1:400 dilution ratio is an acceptable ratio for the blood cells, and cell overlap is almost impossible at 1:1000 dilution. Considering the speed of counting, we chose a 1:400 dilution.

The microfluidic chip was mounted above the CIS so that we could easily obtain the background image without cells. In addition, we then injected a fluid sample of cells into the micro-channel to record the holograms and reconstruct the focus images of the cells. The location and size of the cells were determined by threshold segmentation with images with background interference removed. According to our experiment, the flow velocity was 100 μL/min. Because of the infinitesimal volume of the micro-channel (0.246 μL), the digital injection pump was able to replace all cells in the channel less than 1s. However, it took ~15 s to 20 s for the cells in the fluid to become static. Fortunately, were able to use this time to process the cell image. Since the pixel number of the CIS was about 5.04 million, the computer took ~16 s to process the full resolution image.

The on-chip flow cytometry capability of this method, together with its ease of use, may offer a highly precise and lower cost alternative to existing whole blood analysis tools, urine analysis tools and plankton analysis tools, especially for point-of-care biological and medical tests.

3. Results and Discussion

To test the performance of our proposed system, we performed an experiment with whole blood cells. In the results section, we show the results of focus image reconstruction for cell counting in our proposed system.

Figure 8 shows that the images of the cells were captured by removing the background in the reconstructed image and that the quantity and size of the sample were determined by the image threshold segmentation algorithm. The system obtained an accurate background image, effectively removed the background effect, accurately acquired the location of the sample, and greatly improved the counting accuracy. Finally, the cell concentration was calculated based on the number of cells and the volume of the micro-channel. The micro-channel was 30 μm in height, 150 μm in width, and ~54.6 mm in length; thus, it was easy to calculate its volume as ~0.246 μL and projective area as 8.19 mm^2.

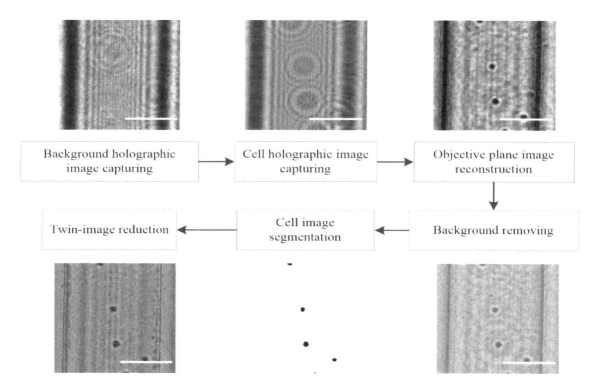

Figure 8. The reconstruction of the focus cell images flow path. To better observe the effect of holographic image reconstruction, which is a small segment of the whole image, all scale bars indicate 100 μm.

Then, we used different concentrations of the whole blood samples to test the linearity and the accuracy of the proposed method. We diluted seven groups of different concentrations of blood cells with a dilution ratio to perform an experiment. The results of this experiment are indicated in Figure 9.

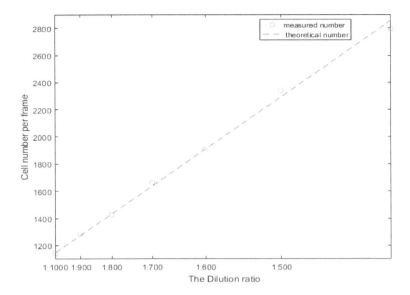

Figure 9. The result of linearity of different concentrations.

Ultimately, we used whole blood cells to count RBCs and WBCs in order to verify the effectiveness of the cell counting procedure. According to the above preparation method, diluted whole blood cells and lysed whole blood cells were divided twice. In addition, we needed to substract the concentration of WBCs from the concentration of whole blood cells to get the concentration of RBCs. Then, the test results of the proposed system were compared with those of an automatic blood cell analyser (BC-5180, Mindray, Shenzhen, China), and the results are shown in Table 1.

Table 1. The result of different sample concentrations.

Sample No.	Tools	White Blood Cells (WBCs) Concentration	Error	Red Blood Cells (RBCs) Concentration	Error
1	Our system BC-5180	6.83×10^9/L 6.93×10^9/L	1.4%	5.22×10^{12}/L 5.35×10^{12}/L	2.4%
2	Our system BC-5180	4.80×10^9/L 4.86×10^9/L	1.2%	5.28×10^{12}/L 5.36×10^{12}/L	1.5%
3	Our system BC-5180	6.33×10^9/L 6.29×10^9/L	0.6%	4.64×10^{12}/L 4.73×10^{12}/L	1.9%
4	Our system BC-5180	5.10×10^9/L 5.22×10^9/L	2.3%	4.61×10^{12}/L 4.68×10^{12}/L	1.5%
5	Our system BC-5180	6.78×10^9/L 6.96×10^9/L	2.6%	4.87×10^{12}/L 4.74×10^{12}/L	2.7%

Table 1 shows that the average fractional errors of RBC and WBC counting were 2% and 1.6%, respectively. In other words, the relative error between the proposed system and the whole blood cell counter was less than 2%. This accuracy indicates the potential for applying the proposed system to the early detection of some liquid samples, such as blood tests, urine tests, semen tests, and microbiological tests. In areas where the use of large-scale, high-precision instruments is inconvenient, such as the outdoors, the battlefield, and underdeveloped areas, the tool proposed here can enable early and real-time detection.

4. Conclusions

The current paper improved the twin-image recovery algorithm in a coaxial holography system and increased the convergence speed of the iterative algorithm. In addition, this paper proposed a flow cytometer based on lens-less holographic microscopy that improved the counting accuracy to 2.3%. The on-chip flow cytometer based on a pulse injection method can continuously count cells and continuously collect a large number of cell images for subsequent cell analysis. Ultimately, this on-chip flow cytometer is very suitable for use in underdeveloped areas and areas far away from the laboratory because of its low price and tiny size and is in full compliance with the current development trend of point-of-care testing (POCT).

Author Contributions: Yuan Fang conceived and designed the experiments; Yuan Fang and Yuquan Jiang performed the experiments; Yuan Fang and Chaoliang Dang analysed the data; Ningmei Yu contributed reagents/materials/analysis tools; Yuan Fang wrote the paper.

Acknowledgments: This work was supported by the National Natural Science Foundation of China (No. 61471296), the National Natural Science Foundation of China (No. 61771388) and the key research project of Baoji University of Arts and Sciences (No. 209010439).

References

1. Tang, W.; Tang, D.; Ni, Z.; Xiang, N.; Yi, H. Microfluidic impedance cytometer with inertial focusing and liquid electrodes for high-throughput cell counting and discrimination. *Anal. Chem.* **2017**, *89*, 3154–3161. [CrossRef] [PubMed]

2. Zheng, G. Innovations in Imaging System Design: Gigapixel, Chip-Scale and Multi-Functional Microscopy. Ph.D. Thesis, California Institute of Technology, Pasadena, CA, USA, 2013.

3. Lee, A.S. Bright-Field and Fluorescence Chip-Scale Microscopy for Biological Imaging. Ph.D. Thesis, California Institute of Technology, Pasadena, CA, USA, 2014.

4. Lee, S.A.; Yang, C. A smartphone-based chip-scale microscope using ambient illumination. *Lab Chip* **2014**, *14*, 3056–3063. [CrossRef] [PubMed]

5. Lee, S.A.; Leitao, R.; Zheng, G.; Yang, S.; Rodriguez, A.; Yang, C. Color capable sub-pixel resolving optofluidic microscope and its application to blood cell imaging for malaria diagnosis. *PLoS ONE* **2011**, *6*, e26127. [CrossRef] [PubMed]

6. Zheng, G.; Lee, S.A.; Yang, S.; Yang, C. Sub-pixel resolving optofluidic microscope for on-chip cell imaging. *Lab Chip* **2010**, *10*, 3125–3129. [CrossRef] [PubMed]

7. Zheng, G.; Lee, S.A.; Antebi, Y.; Elowitz, M.B.; Yang, C. The ePetri dish, an on-chip cell imaging platform based on subpixel perspective sweeping microscopy (SPSM). *Proc. Natl. Acad. Sci. USA* **2011**, *108*, 16889–16894. [CrossRef] [PubMed]

8. Greenbaum, A.; Luo, W.; Khademhosseinieh, B.; Su, T.-W.; Coskun, A.F.; Ozcan, A. Increased space-bandwidth product in pixel super-resolved lensfree on-chip microscopy. *Sci. Rep.* **2013**, *3*, 1717. [CrossRef]

9. Isikman, S.O.; Bishara, W.; Mudanyali, O.; Sencan, I.; Su, T.-W.; Tseng, D.K.; Yaglidere, O.; Sikora, U.; Ozcan, A. Lensfree on-chip microscopy and tomography for bio-medical applications. *IEEE J. Sel. Top. Quantum Electron.* **2011**, *18*, 1059–1072. [CrossRef] [PubMed]

10. Weidling, J.; Isikman, S.O.; Greenbaum, A.; Ozcan, A.; Botvinick, E. Lens-free computational imaging of capillary morphogenesis within three-dimensional substrates. *J. Biomed. Opt.* **2012**, *17*, 126018. [CrossRef] [PubMed]

11. Oh, C.; Isikman, S.O.; Khademhosseinieh, B.; Ozcan, A. On-chip differential interference contrast microscopy using lensless digital holography. *Opt. Express* **2010**, *18*, 4717–4726. [CrossRef] [PubMed]

12. Mudanyali, O.; Tseng, D.; Oh, C.; Isikman, S.O.; Sencan, I.; Bishara, W.; Oztoprak, C.; Seo, S.; Khademhosseini, B.; Ozcan, A. Compact, light-weight and cost-effective microscope based on lensless incoherent holography for telemedicine applications. *Lab Chip* **2010**, *10*, 1417–1428. [CrossRef] [PubMed]

13. Tseng, D.; Mudanyali, O.; Oztoprak, C.; Isikman, S.O.; Sencan, I.; Yaglidere, O.; Ozcan, A. Lensfree microscopy on a cellphone. *Lab Chip* **2010**, *10*, 1787–1792. [CrossRef] [PubMed]

14. Seo, S.; Isikman, S.O.; Sencan, I.; Sencan, I.; Mudanyali, O.; Su, T.-W.; Bishara, W.; Erlinger, A.; Ozcan, A. High-throughput lens-free blood analysis on a chip. *Anal. Chem.* **2010**, *82*, 4621–4627. [CrossRef] [PubMed]

15. Bishara, W.; Su, T.W.; Coskun, A.F.; Ozcan, A. Lensfree on-chip microscopy over a wide field-of-view using pixel super-resolution. *Opt. Express* **2010**, *18*, 11181–11191. [CrossRef] [PubMed]
16. Mudanyali, O.; Oztoprak, C.; Tseng, D.; Erlinger, A.; Ozcan, A. Detection of waterborne parasites using field-portable and cost-effective lensfree microscopy. *Lab Chip* **2010**, *10*, 2419–2423. [CrossRef] [PubMed]
17. Su, T.W.; Erlinger, A.; Tseng, D.; Ozcan, A. Compact and light-weight automated semen analysis platform using lensfree on-chip microscopy. *Anal. Chem.* **2010**, *82*, 8307–8312. [CrossRef] [PubMed]
18. Khademhosseinieh, B.; Biener, G.; Sencan, I.; Ozcan, A. Lensless on-chip color imaging using nano-structured surfaces and compressive decoding. In Proceedings of the 2011 Conference on Lasers and Electro-Optics, Baltimore, MD, USA, 1–6 May 2011.
19. Zhu, H.; Yaglidere, O.; Su, Ti.; Tseng, D.; Ozcan, A. Cost-effective and compact wide-field fluorescent imaging on a cell-phone. *Lab Chip* **2011**, *11*, 315–322. [CrossRef] [PubMed]
20. Coskun, A.F.; Sencan, I.; Su, T.W.; Ozcan, A. Wide-field lensless fluorescent microscopy using a tapered fiber-optic faceplate on a chip. *Analyst* **2011**, *136*, 3512–3518. [CrossRef] [PubMed]
21. Coskun, A.F.; Sencan, I.; Su, T.W.; Ozcan, A. Lensfree fluorescent on-chip imaging of transgenic Caenorhabditis elegans over an ultra-wide field-of-view. *PLoS ONE* **2011**, *6*, e15955. [CrossRef] [PubMed]
22. Bishara, W. Holographic pixel super-resolution in portable lensless on-chip microscopy using a fiber-optic array. *Lab Chip* **2011**, *11*, 1276–1279. [CrossRef] [PubMed]
23. Isikman, S.O.; Bishara, W.; Sikora, U.; Yaglidere, O.; Yeah, J.; Ozcan, A. Field-portable lensfree tomographic microscope. *Lab Chip* **2011**, *11*, 2222–2230. [CrossRef] [PubMed]
24. Isikman, S.O.; Bishara, W.; Zhu, H.; Ozcan, A. Optofluidic tomography on a chip. *Appl. Phys. Lett.* **2011**, *98*, 161109. [CrossRef] [PubMed]
25. Isikman, S.O.; Bishara, W.; Mavandadi, S.; Yu, F.W.; Feng, S.; Lau, R.; Ozcan, A. Lens-free optical tomographic microscope with a large imaging volume on a chip. *Proc. Natl. Acad. Sci. USA* **2011**, *108*, 7296–7301. [CrossRef] [PubMed]
26. Nordin, G.P.; Mellin, S.D. Limits of scalar diffraction theory and an iterative angular spectrum algorithm for finite aperture diffractive optical element design. *Opt. Express* **2001**, *8*, 705–722.
27. Roy, M.; Jin, G.; Seo, D.; Nam, M.-H.; Seo, S. A simple and low-cost device performing blood cell counting based on lens-free shadow imaging technique. *Sens. Actuators B Chem.* **2014**, *201*, 321–328. [CrossRef]
28. Lee, J.; Kwak, Y.H.; Paek, S.-H.; Han, S.; Seo, S. CMOS image sensor-based ELISA detector using lens-free shadow imaging platform. *Sens. Actuators B Chem.* **2014**, *196*, 511–517. [CrossRef]
29. Jin, G.; Yoo, I.H.; Pack, S.P.; Yang, J.W.; Ha, U.H.; Paek, S.H.; Seo, S. Lens-free shadow image based high-throughput continuous cell monitoring technique. *Biosens. Bioelectron.* **2012**, *38*, 126–131. [CrossRef] [PubMed]
30. Seo, D.; Oh, S.; Lee, M.; Hwang, Y.; Seo, S. A field-portable cell analyzer without a microscope and reagents. *Sensors* **2017**, *18*, 85. [CrossRef] [PubMed]
31. Huang, X.; Jiang, Y.; Liu, X.; Xu, H.; Han, Z.; Rong, H.; Yang, H.; Yan, M.; Yu, H. Machine learning based single-frame super-resolution processing for lensless blood cell counting. *Sensors* **2016**, *16*, 1836. [CrossRef] [PubMed]
32. Koren, G.; Polack, F.; Joyeux, D. Iterative algorithms for twin-image elimination in in-line holography using finite-support constraints. *J. Opt. Soc. Am. A* **1993**, *10*, 423–433. [CrossRef]
33. Gabor, D. A new microscopic principle. *Nature* **1948**, *161*, 777–778. [CrossRef] [PubMed]

6

A Microfluidic Deformability Assessment of Pathological Red Blood Cells Flowing in a Hyperbolic Converging Microchannel

Vera Faustino [1,2], Raquel O. Rodrigues [1], Diana Pinho [1,2,3,*,†], Elísio Costa [4], Alice Santos-Silva [4], Vasco Miranda [5], Joana S. Amaral [6,7] and Rui Lima [2,8]

[1] Center for MicroElectromechanical Systems (CMEMS-UMinho), University of Minho, Campus de Azurém, 4800-058 Guimarães, Portugal; id5778@alunos.uminho.pt (V.F.); d8605@dei.uminho.pt (R.O.R.)

[2] MEtRICs, Mechanical Engineering Department, University of Minho, Campus de Azurém, 4800-058 Guimarães, Portugal; rl@dem.uminho.pt

[3] Research Centre in Digitalization and Intelligent Robotics (CeDRI), Instituto Politécnico de Bragança, Campus de Santa Apolónia, 5300-253, Portugal

[4] UCIBIO-REQUINTE, Faculty of Pharmacy of University of Porto, Rua de Jorge Viterbo Ferreira, 4150-755 Porto, Portugal; emcosta@ff.up.pt (E.C.); assilva@ff.up.pt (A.S.-S.)

[5] Dialysis Clinic of Gondomar, Rua 5 de Outubro, 4420-086 Gondomar, Portugal; mail@vascomiranda.com

[6] CIMO, Centro de Investigação de Montanha, Instituto Politécnico de Bragança, Campus de Sta. Apolónia, 5300-253 Bragança, Portugal; jamaral@ipb.pt

[7] REQUIMTE-LAQV, Pharmacy Faculty, University of Porto, 4099-002 Porto, Portugal

[8] CEFT, Faculdade de Engenharia da Universidade do Porto (FEUP), R. Dr. Roberto Frias, 4200-465 Porto, Portugal

* Correspondence: diana@ipb.pt

† Current affiliation: INL—International Iberian Nanotechnology Laboratory, Av. Mestre José Veiga, 4715-330 Braga, Portugal.

Abstract: The loss of the red blood cells (RBCs) deformability is related with many human diseases, such as malaria, hereditary spherocytosis, sickle cell disease, or renal diseases. Hence, during the last years, a variety of technologies have been proposed to gain insights into the factors affecting the RBCs deformability and their possible direct association with several blood pathologies. In this work, we present a simple microfluidic tool that provides the assessment of motions and deformations of RBCs of end-stage kidney disease (ESKD) patients, under a well-controlled microenvironment. All of the flow studies were performed within a hyperbolic converging microchannels where single-cell deformability was assessed under a controlled homogeneous extensional flow field. By using a passive microfluidic device, RBCs passing through a hyperbolic-shaped contraction were measured by a high-speed video microscopy system, and the velocities and deformability ratios (DR) calculated. Blood samples from 27 individuals, including seven healthy controls and 20 having ESKD with or without diabetes, were analysed. The obtained data indicates that the proposed device is able to detect changes in DR of the RBCs, allowing for distinguishing the samples from the healthy controls and the patients. Overall, the deformability of ESKD patients with and without diabetes type II is lower in comparison with the RBCs from the healthy controls, with this difference being more evident for the group of ESKD patients with diabetes. RBCs from ESKD patients without diabetes elongate on average 8% less, within the hyperbolic contraction, as compared to healthy controls; whereas, RBCs from ESKD patients with diabetes elongate on average 14% less than the healthy controls. The proposed strategy can be easily transformed into a simple and inexpensive diagnostic microfluidic system to assess blood cells deformability due to the huge progress in image processing and high-speed microvisualization technology.

Keywords: microfluidic devices; cell deformability; chronic renal disease; diabetes; red blood cells (RBCs); hyperbolic microchannel; blood on chips

1. Introduction

Blood is a complex and an extremely information-rich fluid that can be used to diagnose different kinds of blood diseases with multiple biophysical techniques and tools [1,2]. Under normal healthy conditions, the red blood cells (RBCs) comprise about 42% in adult females and 47% in adult males of the total blood volume [3]. As RBCs are the most abundant cells in blood, their deformable properties strongly influence the blood rheological properties, particularly in microvessels with complex geometries and diameters of less than 300 μm [4]. Several research works have found that complex microgeometries, such as contractions [5,6] and bifurcations [2,7–9], promote the presence of strong shear and extensional flows that elongate the RBCs without reaching the rupture.

Ever since the RBCs deformability became a potential biomarker for blood diseases, such as malaria [10,11], sickle cell disease [1,12], and diabetes [13–15], several techniques have been developed to measure the biomechanical properties of the RBCs. Additionally, there have been several reviews that discuss different kind of experimental methods to measure the RBC deformability [1,2,16–18]. The available methods can be divided in two main kinds, i.e., the high-throughput methods that measure high concentrations or diluted suspensions of RBCs, and the single-cell techniques. The most popular high-throughput methods, which include the conventional rotational viscometer [19–21], ektacytometer [9,14] and micro-pore filtration assay [9], have been used to measure the blood viscosity and other rheological properties, but they are generally expensive, labor intensive, and do not provide a direct and detailed source of information on the mechanical properties of the RBCs. A recent study that was performed by Sosa et al. [9] has shown that the results from the micro-pore filtration and ektacytometry were often in disagreement, and that neither of them represent the actual blood flow conditions occurring in microvascular networks. Other methods, known as single-cell techniques, which include the micropipette aspiration and optical tweezers, are also extremely popular for measuring the mechanical properties of the RBC membrane [1,13]. However, these techniques also have several drawbacks, such as a low-throughput, labor intensive, and static process. Additionally, it is argued that these methods do not represent the actual RBC deformability that happens during microcirculation [2].

The progress in microfabrication made fabricating microfluidic devices with the ability to directly visualize, measure, and control the motion and deformation of RBCs flowing through constricted [19,22–24] and bifurcated microchannels [7,9,24] possible. The distinctive advantage of the microfluidic devices, such as the need of small sample's volumes and their ability to reproduce more realistic conditions of the microcirculation, have promoted a vast amount of studies on the cell motion and deformability, mainly under the shear flow effect [3,6,16,20,25–27]. Some examples are the deformability measurements that were performed under transient high shear stress in sudden constriction channels, [16,28] and in microchannels with dimensions that were comparable to cell size [2,16]. Besides the shear flow effect, the extensional flow and the combination of both can be often found in the microcirculation system, such as in microstenosis and microvascular networks. Hence, during the last decade, several extensional blood flow studies have been performed in cross slot devices [29,30] and in microfluidic devices with hyperbolic channels [31–36]. Recent studies that were performed in cross slot devices [37] and sudden constriction channels [26] have shown that cells entrance location and angular orientation strongly affect the cells deformability. On the other hand, extensional flows, where cells are deformed at almost constant strain rates, has been demonstrated to be a microfluidic methodology that is capable of efficiently and accurately probing singe-cell deformability with high throughputs [16,29].

Additionally, the ability of hyperbolic-shaped contraction channels to generate constant strain-rates makes them a promising strategy for measuring RBCs deformability under a well-controlled microenvironment. Taking these advantage into account, the present study investigates the ability of hyperbolic microfluidic channels to measure the deformation and cell motion of RBCs that were obtained from healthy and diseased individuals (having end-stage kidney disease (ESKD), with or without diabetes type II) and exploits the relevance of this flow technique to be used as a viable tool suitable for detecting and diagnosing RBC related diseases.

Chronic kidney disease (CKD) is a pathological condition that results from a gradual, permanent loss of kidney function over time, usually, months to years, which can lead to an end-stage kidney disease (ESKD) [38]. This condition is associated with a decreased quality of life [39], increased hospitalization [39,40], cardiovascular complications, such asangina, left ventricular hypertrophy (LVH), and chronic heart failure, and increased mortality [41,42].

The remainder of this paper is organized, as follows: Section 2 comprises several subsections to explain the experimental framework around blood samples, setups used to acquire the data, and methods used to analyze it. Sections 3 and 4 presents and results and discussion, respectively.

2. Materials and Methods

2.1. Patients

In this study, a total of 20 ESKD patients under online hemodiafiltration (OL-HDF) that voluntary accepted to participate in the study, have been tested. From those, eight additionally showed diabetic nephropathy. Patients were excluded if they: (1) did not accept to participate in the study; (2) were under 18 years old; (3) were cognitively impaired; (4) had a severe speech or hearing impairment; (5) were in the dialysis program for less than three months; and, (6) presented malignancy, autoimmune, inflammatory, or infectious diseases.

The control group included seven healthy volunteers presenting normal haematological and biochemical values, with no history of renal or inflammatory diseases, and, as far as possible, age- and gender-matched with ESKD patients. The controls did not receive any medication known to interfere with the studied variables. Blood samples (using EDTA as anticoagulant) were drawn from the fasting controls or before the second dialysis session of the week in ESKD patients.

All of the blood samples were obtained from dialysis patients at the hemodialysis clinic of Gondomar, in Porto, Portugal. Informed consent was obtained from all the participants and this study was approved by the clinic's ethics review board.

2.2. Microfluidic Device, Experimental Setup and Parameters

The polydimethylsiloxane (PDMS) microfluidic devices that were evaluated in this work were fabricated by using a conventional soft-lithographic technique [22]. To perform the deformability assessment, hyperbolic converging microchannels were fabricated with 382 μm of length (L_c), as well as maximum width of 400 μm (W_1) and minimum width of 20 μm (W_2) at the wide and narrow sizes, respectively (cf. Figure 1). This particular geometry corresponds to a hyperbolic contraction with a Hencky strain (ε_H) of ~3. Note that the ε_H can be defined as ln (W_1/W_2) [32]. The advantages of the use of this hyperbolic geometry for RBCs screening have already been ascribed in previous studies [43,44]. The hyperbolic contraction geometry was chosen, mainly due to the strong extensional flow that was generated in the middle of the microchannel, which is dominant over the shear flow. The cells by passing through the hyperbolic contraction are submitted to a strong extensional flow, where the velocity almost linearly increases, but the strain rate stays approximately constant. Note that the depth was about 50 μm along the full length of the device.

Figure 1b also shows the main advantage of using hyperbolic converging microchannels. At the entrance of these kinds of geometries, the RBCs tend to exhibit a linear increase of their velocities and consequently the strain rates within the hyperbolic contractions are close to a constant. This flow phenomenon imposes a homogenous mechanical fluid behaviour to the RBCs and avoids some possible motions (tumbling, twisting, and rolling rotations), often observed in abrupt contractions [26]. Hence, by using hyperbolic converging microchannels, most of the RBCs tend to elongate when they flow through the contraction. It is worth mentioning that RBCs motions, such as tumbling, twisting, and rolling rotations, were never observed during our experiments.

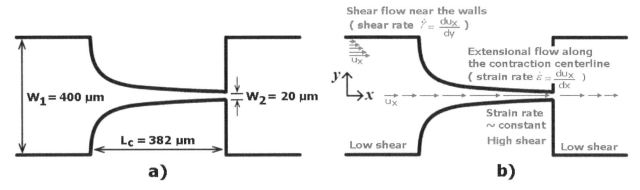

Figure 1. Microfluidic device fabricated in polydimethylsiloxane (PDMS) with a hyperbolic-shaped contraction to assess the of the red blood cells (RBCs) deformability: (**a**) main dimensions; (**b**) flow phenomena happening in this kind of geometry. Adapted with permission from [45].

The visualization and measurements of the motion of the RBCs were performed by means of a high-speed video microscopy system that includes an inverted microscope (IX71, Olympus, Tokyo, Japan) combined with a high-speed camera (Fastcam SA3, Photron, San Diego, CA, USA). The microfluidic device was placed on the microscope stage and the flow rate of the working fluids was kept constant at 3 µL/min. by using a syringe pump (PHD Ultra, Harvard Apparatus, Holliston, MA, USA) with a 1 mL disposable syringe (Terumo) (Figure 2). For all of the flow measurements, the average shear rate at the hyperbolic contraction region was about 1750 s^{-1}. The average or pseudo shear rate was calculated by $\overline{\gamma} = \frac{U}{D_h}$, where U is the mean velocity of the blood cells that were obtained at the contraction region, and D_h is the hydraulic diameter at the end of the contraction region.

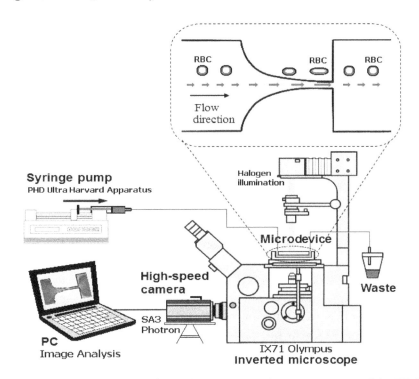

Figure 2. Experimental set-up used to perform the motion and measurements of the RBCs deformability.

The images of the RBCs flowing through the hyperbolic contraction were captured by the high-speed camera with a frame rate of 3000 frames/s and a shutter speed ratio of 1/75,000 s. These parameters were selected in order to obtain well defined RBCs and avoid possible image distortions that are caused by the high flow velocities at the contraction region. Table 1 shows the most of the relevant experimental parameters that were used to perform the RBCs deformability measurements.

Table 1. Main experimental parameters used to perform the RBCs deformability measurements.

Main Experimental Parameters	
Maximum width of the microchannel	400 μm
Minimum width of the microchannel	20 μm
Total length of the contraction region	382 μm
Depth of the microchannel	50 μm
Flow rate (syringe of 1 mL)	3 μL/min
Average shear rate	$1750\ s^{-1}$
Shear viscosity of the Dextran 40	4.5×10^{-3} Pa·s
Density of the Dextran 40	$1046\ kg/m^3$
Haematocrit of the working fluid	1%
Temperature of the working fluid	22 °C
Magnification (M)	40×
Numerical Aperture (NA)	0.75
Frame rate	3000 frames/s
Exposure time	1/75,000 s

2.3. Working Fluids

To perform the RBCs deformability studies, Dextran 40 (Sigma-Aldrich, Saint Louis, MO, USA) at 10% (*w/v*) solution containing 1% of haematocrit (Hct 1%, *v/v*) of RBCs was used as the working fluid. Briefly, venous blood samples from both patients and healthy donors were collected into 10 mL BD-Vacutainers (BD, Franklin Lakes, NJ, USA) tubes containing ethylenediaminetetraacetic acid (EDTA) to prevent coagulation. The RBCs and buffy coat were separated from the plasma after centrifugation (2500 rpm for 10 min., at 4 °C). The RBCs were then washed with physiological salt solution (PSS) and then centrifuged, with this procedure repeated twice. The RBCs were suspended in Dextran 40 to make several samples with low hematocrit levels of ~1% by volume (cf. Figure 3) to obtain the measurements of individual RBC flowing through hyperbolic contraction. Dextran 40 was used as substitute of the blood plasma, since it prevents not only the sedimentation of the RBCs during the experimental assays, but also the cell clogging phenomenon. All of the analyses were performed within a maximum period of 12 h, with blood samples being hermetically stored at 4 °C until being used in the flow experiments.

Image analysis was essential to obtain sharper, brighter, and clearer images of the RBCs flowing through the contraction, and to consequently obtain reliable velocity and deformability measurements, at the regions of interest (ROI) in both contraction and expansion regions, where the RBCs deform and recover to their normal circular shape, respectively (see Figure 3a and supplementary video). The first step of this process involves the capture of videos with a resolution of 1024 × 576 pixels at frame intervals of 330 μs at the end of the contraction region. Figure 4a shows a typical obtained image. In order to reduce static artifacts in the images, a background image (Figure 4b) was created from the original stack images, by averaging each pixel over the sequence of static images while using an ImageJ function, called *Z project*, and then subtracted from the stack images. This process eliminates all the static objects including the microchannel walls and some possible attached cells, which resulted in having at the end, only the RBCs of interest (Figure 4c). *Brightness/Contrast* adjustment was also applied to enhance the image quality. Finally, the greyscale images were converted to binary images adjusting the threshold level (Figure 4d). At this stage, an *Otsu* threshold method was applied and when required, the level was manually refined. This segmentation process generates objects of interest (RBCs) as black ellipsoidal objects against a white background. At the end, the flowing RBCs in the binary images were measured frame by frame manually, by using *Wand tool* function in ImageJ. The main output results of these measurements were the major and minor axis lengths of the RBCs and the x-y coordinates of their centroid.

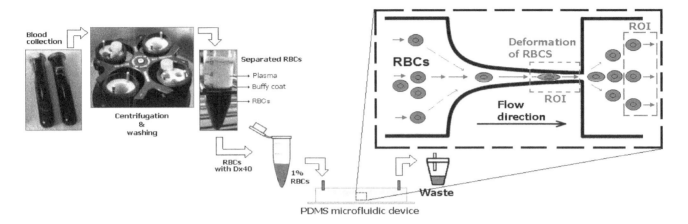

Figure 3. Schematic diagram from blood collection up to the flow microfluidic tests with RBCs. Samples with low hematocrit levels of ~1% were crucial in order to visualize individual RBC flowing through hyperbolic contraction. The ROI regions represent the regions of interest used to analyze the RBCs deformation index.

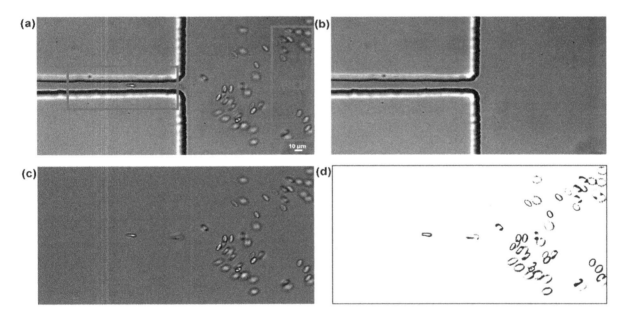

Figure 4. Images analysis sequence: (**a**) original image at the regions of interest (ROI) regions in which moving RBCs as well as microchannel boundaries are visible, (**b**) background image containing only static objects, (**c**) original image after background subtraction showing only moving RBCs, and (**d**) final binary image to perform measurements of the RBCs major and minor axis lengths.

The deformation ratio (DR) of all the measured RBCs was calculated and saved with the cell's positions, given by their x-y coordinates, using the set of data obtained for the cells at the regions of interest (ROI) at both constriction and expansion locations of the microchannel. In this study, DR was defined by the equation that is shown in Figure 5, where L_{major} and L_{minor} refer to the major and minor axis lengths of the RBC, respectively.

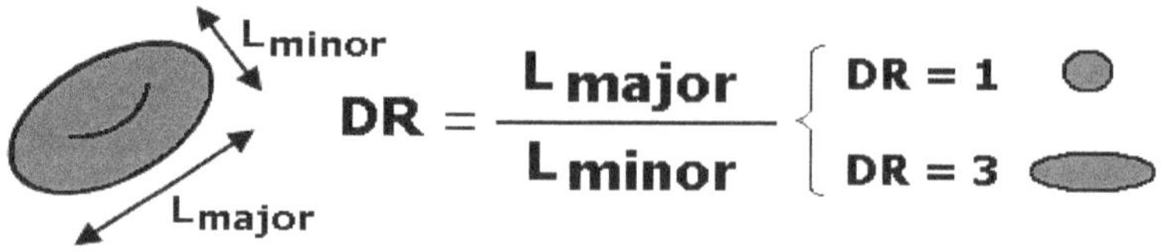

Figure 5. Definition of the deformation ratio, DR = L_{major}/L_{minor}, where L_{major} and L_{minor} are the major and minor axis lengths of the ellipse best fitted to the cell.

Although different automatic methods to track RBCs in microfluidic devices have been reported in the literature [45–49], further improvements still need to be achieved to perform reliable deformability measurements. Hence, in the present study, hundreds of RBCs were manually tracked by using the ImageJ plug-in, MTrackJ. By selecting this method, it is possible to easily track the cells by a centroid based strategy and obtain their centroid position (*x*-*y* coordinates), by carefully tracking individual RBCs and consequently determine their orientations and velocities within the hyperbolic contraction and downstream of the contraction region. In this study, measurements were only performed for the in focus cells flowing from the side, as it is possible to observe in the examples at the supplementary video. In this video, it is also possible to observe a RBC that flows from the top (the biconcave disc shape cell). However, the cells flowing with this orientation were not considered in our deformability measurements.

2.4. Statistical Analysis

The statistical analysis was performed by using one-way ANOVA (Microsoft Office Excel, version Office 365 ProPlus). Before performing the ANOVA analysis, the requirements regarding normal distribution were tested by means of the Shapiro–Wilk's test. In this test, the null hypothesis that the population is normally distributed was accepted since $p > 0.05$. Overall, for the constriction region, we have measured the deformability of 1769 RBCs corresponding to 12 ESKD patients and a total of 736 measured RBCs, eight ESKDD patients and a total of 444 measured RBCs, and seven healthy controls and a total of 589 measured RBCs. All of the statistical tests were performed at a 95% confidence level; differences with $p < 0.05$ were considered to be statistically significant, and were represented as asterisks (*).

3. Results and Discussion

The determination of the RBC velocities plays an essential role in confirming whether the cells are deformed under similar flow conditions. Hence, before the deformability assessment of each sample, velocity measurements were performed and compared. After analyzing the average velocities of each sample at the contraction region, it was decided to compare the RBC deformability for all of the samples having similar flow conditions, i.e., both shear and extensional flows. Figure 6 shows representative RBC trajectories that were manually tracked within the hyperbolic contraction and downstream of the contraction region.

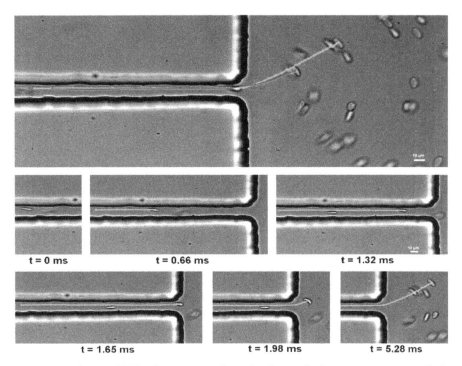

Figure 6. Trajectories of two RBCs flowing within the hyperbolic contraction and downstream of the contraction region (Upper part); detail of a representative trajectory of a RBC flowing near the microchannel wall at different times intervals (Bottom part).

Figure 7 shows the measurements of the velocity and DR of representative RBCs flowing through the hyperbolic-shaped contraction (ROI region) for both healthy donors and ESKD patients (see also supplementary video). The majority of the RBC velocities tend to slightly increase as they move through the exit of the contraction, and then they suffer a dramatic reduction of their velocities when flowing from the narrow to the wide region of the microchannel (cf. Figure 7a). Overall, the velocities of the RBCs of both control and ESKD patients present a similar qualitative flow behavior at the tested region of the device, which results in a good agreement in the deformability results obtained in all the samples (cf. Figure 7b). However, it should be noted that, quantitatively, the DR results indicate that the deformability of the ESKD RBCs under extensional flow tend to be smaller when compared to the control RBCs (cf. Figure 7b). These latter results are further confirmed with the measurements that were performed with several ESKD patients and healthy individual, as shown in Figure 8. Additionally, during all the flow visualization measurements at constriction region, the RBCs did not show any tumbling and rolling motion, which was mainly due to the uniform and strong extensional flow generated along the hyperbolic-shaped contraction. Note that, under shear flow, it is extremely common to observe RBCs flowing with complex dynamics, such as tumbling and rolling [26,46]. In the present study, the RBCs only exhibited such kind of complex flow motions at the expansion region, due to the dominant shear flow with respect to the extensional flow (cf. supplementary video). Hence, by using the proposed method, when the RBCs enter into the contraction region, they change from a circular to an elliptical shape, with a tendency to become increasingly elongated as they moved through the hyperbolic contraction. This latter flow behavior is possible to observe in Figure 7b. Additionally, in this figure, it can be observed that, at the downstream of the contraction region, the cells start to recover their nearly circular shape, exhibiting a DR that is close to one.

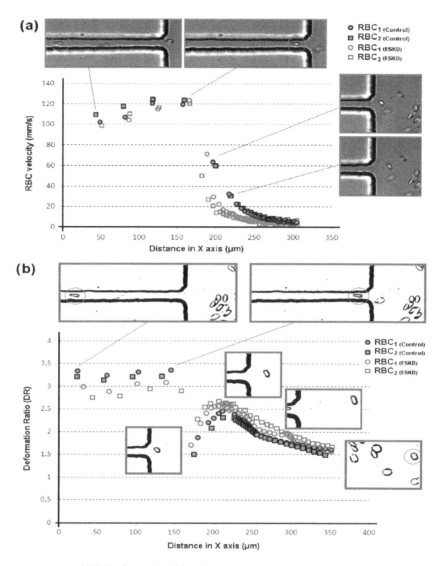

Figure 7. Measurements of RBCs from healthy donors and end-stage kidney disease (ESKD) patients, flowing within the hyperbolic contraction and downstream of the contraction region: (**a**) velocity measurements; (**b**) deformability measurements. The X axis represents the position of the cells centroid flowing through the microchannel.

Figure 8 shows the box plot of the deformation ratio (DR) for three different groups, i.e., samples of ESKD patients without diabetes type II (n = 12), samples of ESKD patients with diabetes (n = 8) type II, and samples from healthy donors (n = 7). For each patient sample, more than 60 RBCs with similar flow behavior were individually measured and analyzed at the hyperbolic constriction and recovering channel of the proposed microfluidic device (Figure 8). Additionally, Table 2 shows the data of the average DR and standard deviation (SD) of the RBCs deformation at both the contraction and expansion region for all of the tested samples. Overall, the deformability of ESKD patients (with and without diabetes) measured at the hyperbolic constriction is lower in comparison with the RBCs from the normal healthy controls ($p < 0.05$), as shown in Figure 8b. This difference is more evident when only the group of ESKD patients with diabetes is taken into consideration. For instance, RBCs from ESKD patients without diabetes elongates, on average, 8% less within the hyperbolic contraction when compared to healthy controls, whereas RBCs from ESKD patients with diabetes elongates on average 14% less than the healthy controls (cf. Figure 8b). On the other hand, all of the cells analyzed, both healthy and diseased, have been shown to have a similar DR (nearly to 1, i.e., close to a spherical-shape) at the expansion region of the microchannel (Figure 8c,d), where cells tend to recover to their normal circular shape due to the low shear rate and a negligible strain rate. Therefore, the results from the present study demonstrate that the RBCs DR measured by using the proposed microfluidic device can be considered as a sensitive mechanical biomarker, as it was able to detect changes in DR of the RBCs from patients with different diseases in comparison with healthy ones. Moreover, this study also corroborates other previous research works [13,14], where, by using different deformability measurement techniques, it was shown that elongation of RBCs from patients with diabetes is lower in comparison with the non-diabetic healthy controls.

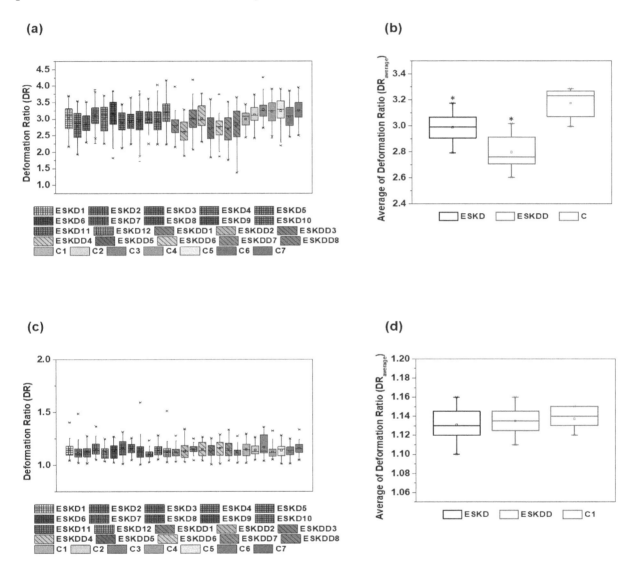

Figure 8. Box plot representation of RBC's deformation ratio (DR) measured by the proposed microfluidic device: (**a**) DR of individual donors, including ESKD patients, ESKD patients with diabetes and healthy donors (control) in the hyperbolic constriction, (**b**) Average DR of the groups of donors, including ESKD patients, ESKD patients with diabetes and healthy donors (control) in the hyperbolic constriction, (**c**) DR of individual donors, including ESKD patients, ESKD patients with diabetes and healthy donors (control) at the expansion region, (**d**) Average DR of the groups of donors, including ESKD patients, ESKD patients with diabetes and healthy donors (control at the expansion region. The asterisks (*) indicates statistically significant differences ($p < 0.05$) determined by Student's t test.

Table 2. Average DR and standard deviation (SD) of the flowing RBCs at both contraction and expansion region for each sample.

Blood Samples	Contraction Region DR		Expansion Region DR	
	Average	SD	Average	SD
ESKD1	3.03	0.34	1.12	0.08
ESKD2	2.79	0.36	1.10	0.09
ESKD3	2.86	0.26	1.13	0.06
ESKD4	3.11	0.25	1.14	0.08
ESKD5	3.03	0.39	1.12	0.06
ESKD6	3.15	0.37	1.15	0.07
ESKD7	2.89	0.31	1.15	0.08
ESKD8	2.93	0.26	1.16	0.05
ESKD9	2.94	0.35	1.13	0.10
ESKD10	3.02	0.24	1.10	0.05
ESKD11	2.96	0.32	1.14	0.06
ESKD12	3.17	0.35	1.13	0.08
ESKDD1	2.78	0.25	1.12	0.05
ESKDD2	2.60	0.27	1.13	0.07
ESKDD3	3.01	0.32	1.15	0.05
ESKDD4	3.02	0.32	1.13	0.08
ESKDD5	2.72	0.37	1.14	0.07
ESKDD6	2.74	0.28	1.16	0.08
ESKDD7	2.69	0.34	1.14	0.08
ESKDD8	2.81	0.43	1.11	0.06
C1	2.99	0.21	1.14	0.07
C2	3.12	0.23	1.13	0.06
C3	3.28	0.22	1.13	0.10
C4	3.23	0.27	1.12	0.06
C5	3.24	0.31	1.15	0.07
C6	3.07	0.30	1.14	0.07
C7	3.27	0.27	1.15	0.06

As previously mentioned, RBCs occupy almost half of the total blood volume and, under healthy conditions, they are highly deformable in order to pass through capillaries with dimensions several times lower than the RBCs size [16]. Hence, it is well known that the RBC deformability plays a crucial role in the rheological properties of blood in microvessels, i.e., the decrease of the RBC deformability might result in an increase of the blood viscosity and, consequently, in an increased tendency for microvascular complications and associated diseases. The results that are presented in this study indicate that the ESKD patients with and without diabetes have a tendency to decrease the RBCs deformability and, as a result, night have a substantial impact in the whole blood viscosity of these patient's health. This can result in an elicit hemolysis in the capillaries and premature sequestration of RBCs by the reticulo-endothelial system, and altering tissue oxygenation. However, a larger scale study is required to confirm whether the decrease of the RBC deformability contributes to the increase of the blood viscosity, or not.

4. Limitations and Future Directions

The primary goal of the present work was to investigate the ability of hyperbolic converging microchannels to be used as an alternative clinical tool that is suitable to detect and diagnose RBC related diseases. To accomplish it, high speed microfluidic studies were performed in a hyperbolic contraction microchannel with a uniform depth of about 50 μm. The selection of this depth was a compromise solution mainly due to the limitation of our high-speed video camera: although, by decreasing the microchannel depth, the orientation of the cells tend to be more stable, the difficulty to measure the RBCs deformability increases due to the extremely high velocities that were generated at this region. The major advantage of this geometrical modification is the ability to use simple automatic methods, which results in a significant increase of the number of cell measurements performed under similar flow conditions. Nevertheless, in this study, we opted for manual measurements to guarantee that only adequate cells were included.

Additionally, we would like to refer that recently, Schonbrun et al. [50] have shown that by using blue light the hemoglobin absorption makes cells extremely visible and easier to track in microchannels for low shear rates. Although this optical option looks promising, further research needs to be performed regarding the ability to measure blood cells at high shear rates. We consider that a combination of both strategies could result in a promising methodology to preform DR measurement of RBCs with high accuracy. The high-speed camera used due to its cost can be a limitation to consider the technique as a common tool; however, during the last two decades, the cost of this technology has been decreasing in an exponential way, thus we believe that it will be possible to have in a more affordable way a high-speed system in the future. Another way can be the use of compact CCD cameras due its capacity to achieve similar sensitivity and exposure, but in an affordable way.

5. Conclusions

RBCs deformability plays a crucial role in microcirculation and the loss of their deformability can be related to many pathologies. The present study investigated the ability of hyperbolic microfluidic channels to measure the deformation and RBC motion from the blood samples of patients with ESKD (with and without diabetes type II) compared to healthy individuals (used as control) and exploit the relevance of this method to be used as viable clinical tool suitable to detect and diagnose RBC related disease. This study has shown the potential of the proposed device to detect changes in DR of the RBCs from patients with different complications. Overall, the elongation of RBCs from the ESKD patients, with and without diabetes, was lower in comparison with the RBCs from the healthy controls, being the difference more evident for the group of ESKD patients with diabetes. Another important finding was related to the comparison of the cells at the expansion region, where the RBCs have recovered their normal circular shape. At this region, the cells were deformed under low shear rate and negligible strain rate. Under those conditions, we have not found any difference between the ESKD patients and the healthy controls. This latter result indicates that the RBCs need to be submitted to high mechanical stresses to deform the cells and, consequently, to detect different state of blood diseases.

Additionally, the results that are presented in this study indicate that the ESKD patients with and without diabetes have a tendency to decrease the RBCs deformability, which might have a substantial impact in the whole blood viscosity of these patients. However, a larger scale study would be necessary to confirm whether the decrease of the RBC deformability contributes to the increase of the blood viscosity, or not. Although the proposed microfluidic tool requires further improvements, the results that were obtained from the present study suggest that this technique is able to assure a simple and efficient cell deformability assessment at both physiological and pathological situations.

Figure S1: Images from a video where it is possible to observe that the RBCs rotation only happens at the expansion region of the microchannel, and Video S1: Visualization of RBCs flowing within the hyperbolic contraction and downstream of the contraction region.

Author Contributions: Conceptualization, R.L., J.S.A. and E.C. Methodology, R.L., J.S.A. and E.C.; Software, V.F. and R.L. Formal Analysis, R.L., V.F., D.P., R.O.R.; Investigation, R.L., J.S.A., V.F., D.P., R.O.R., E.C. and A.S.-S.; Resources, R.L., J.S.A., E.C., A.S.-S., and V.M.; Data Curation, R.L., V.F., D.P., R.O.R., J.S.A.; Writing—Original Draft Preparation, R.L., J.S.A., E.C., and R.O.R.; Writing—Review & Editing, R.L., D.P., R.O.R., J.S.A. Supervision, R.L., J.S.A., E.C. and A.S.-S.; Project Administration, R.L. and J.S.A.; Funding Acquisition, R.L. and J.S.

Acknowledgments: V.F. acknowledges the PhD scholarship SFRH/BD/99696/2014 attributed by FCT.

References

1. Lee, G.Y.; Lim, C.T. Biomechanics approaches to studying human diseases. *Trends Biotechnol.* **2007**, *25*, 111–118. [PubMed]
2. Tomaiuolo, G. Biomechanical properties of red blood cells in health and disease towards microfluidics. *Biomicrofluidics* **2014**, *8*, 051501. [PubMed]

3.   Siddhartha, T.; Kumar, Y.V.B.V.; Amit, P.; Suhas, S.J.; Amit, A. Passive blood plasma separation at the microscale: A review of design principles and microdevices. *J. Micromech. Microeng.* **2015**, *25*, 083001.

4.   Lima, R.; Ishikawa, T.; Imai, Y.; Yamaguchi, T. Blood Flow Behavior in Microchannels: Past, Current and Future Trends. In *Single and Two-Phase Flows on Chemical and Biomedical Engineering*; Dias, R., Martins, A.A., Lima, R., Mata, T.M., Eds.; Bentham Science: Sharjah, UAE, 2012; pp. 513–547.

5.   Abkarian, M.; Faivre, M.; Horton, R.; Smistrup, K.; Best-Popescu, C.A.; Stone, H.A. Cellular-scale hydrodynamics. *Biomed. Mater.* **2008**, *3*, 034011. [PubMed]

6.   Pinho, D.; Yaginuma, T.; Lima, R. A microfluidic device for partial cell separation and deformability assessment. *BioChip J.* **2013**, *7*, 367–374.

7.   Bento, D.; Fernandes, C.; Miranda, J.; Lima, R. In vitro blood flow visualizations and cell-free layer (CFL) measurements in a microchannel network. *Exp. Therm. Fluid Sci.* **2019**, *109*, 109847.

8.   Shevkoplyas, S.S.; Yoshida, T.; Gifford, S.C.; Bitensky, M.W. Direct measurement of the impact of impaired erythrocyte deformability on microvascular network perfusion in a microfluidic device. *Lab Chip* **2006**, *6*, 914.

9.   Sosa, J.M.; Nielsen, N.D.; Vignes, S.M.; Chen, T.G.; Shevkoplyas, S.S. The relationship between red blood cell deformability metrics and perfusion of an artificial microvascular network. *Clin. Hemorheol. Microcirc.* **2014**, *57*, 275–289.

10. Boas, L.V.; Faustino, V.; Lima, R.; Miranda, J.M.; Minas, G.; Fernandes, C.S.V.; Catarino, S.O. Assessment of the Deformability and Velocity of Healthy and Artificially Impaired Red Blood Cells in Narrow Polydimethylsiloxane (PDMS) Microchannels. *Micromachines* **2018**, *9*, 384.

11. Shelby, J.P.; White, J.; Ganesan, K.; Rathod, P.K.; Chiu, D.T. A microfluidic model for single-cell capillary obstruction by Plasmodium falciparum-infected erythrocytes. *Proc. Natl. Acad. Sci. USA* **2003**, *100*, 14618–14622.

12. Dao, M.; Lim, C.T.; Suresh, S. Mechanics of the human red blood cell deformed by optical tweezers. *J. Mech. Phys. Solids* **2003**, *51*, 2259–2280.

13. Agrawal, R.; Smart, T.; Nobre-Cardoso, J.; Richards, C.; Bhatnagar, R.; Tufail, A.; Shima, D.; Jones, P.H.; Pavesio, C. Assessment of red blood cell deformability in type 2 diabetes mellitus and diabetic retinopathy by dual optical tweezers stretching technique. *Sci. Rep.* **2016**, *6*, 15873. [PubMed]

14. Shin, S.; Ku, Y.-H.; Ho, J.-X.; Kim, Y.-K.; Suh, J.-S.; Singh, M. Progressive impairment of erythrocyte deformability as indicator of microangiopathy in type 2 diabetes mellitus. *Clin. Hemorheol. Microcirc.* **2007**, *36*, 253–261. [PubMed]

15. Tsukada, K.; Sekizuka, E.; Oshio, C.; Minamitani, H. Direct Measurement of Erythrocyte Deformability in Diabetes Mellitus with a Transparent Microchannel Capillary Model and High-Speed Video Camera System. *Microvasc. Res.* **2001**, *61*, 231–239.

16. Bento, D.; Rodrigues, R.O.; Faustino, V.; Pinho, D.; Fernandes, C.S.; Pereira, A.I.; Garcia, V.; Miranda, J.M.; Lima, R. Deformation of Red Blood Cells, Air Bubbles, and Droplets in Microfluidic Devices: Flow Visualizations and Measurements. *Micromachines* **2018**, *9*, 151.

17. Musielak, M. Red blood cell-deformability measurement: Review of techniques. *Clin. Hemorheol. Microcirc.* **2009**, *42*, 47–64.

18. Xue, C.; Wang, J.; Zhao, Y.; Chen, D.; Yue, W.; Chen, J. Constriction Channel Based Single-Cell Mechanical Property Characterization. *Micromachines* **2015**, *6*, 1794–1804.

19. Pinho, D.; Campo-Deaño, L.; Lima, R.; Pinho, F.T. In vitro particulate analogue fluids for experimental studies of rheological and hemorheological behavior of glucose-rich RBC suspensions. *Biomicrofluidics* **2017**, *11*, 054105.

20. Pinho, D.; Rodrigues, R.O.; Faustino, V.; Yaginuma, T.; Exposto, J.; Lima, R. Red blood cells radial dispersion in blood flowing through microchannels: The role of temperature. *J. Biomech.* **2016**, *49*, 2293–2298.

21. Sousa, P.C.; Carneiro, J.; Vaz, R.; Cerejo, A.; Pinho, F.T.; Alves, M.A.; Oliveira, M.S. Shear viscosity and nonlinear behavior of whole blood under large amplitude oscillatory shear. *Biorheology* **2013**, *50*, 269–282.

22. Faustino, V.; Catarino, S.O.; Lima, R.; Minas, G. Biomedical microfluidic devices by using low-cost fabrication techniques: A review. *J. Biomech.* **2016**, *49*, 2280–2292. [PubMed]

23. Wei, Y.; Zheng, Y.; Nguyen, J.; Sun, Y. Recent advances in microfluidic techniques for single-cell biophysical characterization. *Lab Chip* **2013**, *13*, 2464.

24. Catarino, S.O.; Rodrigues, R.O.; Pinho, D.; Miranda, J.M.; Minas, G.; Lima, R. Blood Cells Separation and

Sorting Techniques of Passive Microfluidic Devices: From Fabrication to Applications. *Micromachines* **2019**, *10*, 593.

25. Quinn, D.J.; Pivkin, I.; Wong, S.Y.; Chiam, K.H.; Dao, M.; Karniadakis, G.E.; Suresh, S. Combined simulation and experimental study of large deformation of red blood cells in microfluidic systems. *Ann. Biomed. Eng.* **2011**, *39*, 1041–1050. [PubMed]

26. Zeng, N.F.; Ristenpart, W.D. Mechanical response of red blood cells entering a constriction. *Biomicrofluidics* **2014**, *8*, 064123. [PubMed]

27. Zhao, R.; Marhefka, J.N.; Shu, F.; Hund, S.J.; Kameneva, M.V.; Antaki, J.F. Micro-Flow Visualization of Red Blood Cell-Enhanced Platelet Concentration at Sudden Expansion. *Ann. Biomed. Eng.* **2008**, *36*, 1130–1141. [PubMed]

28. Fujiwara, H.; Ishikawa, T.; Lima, R.; Matsuki, N.; Imai, Y.; Kaji, H.; Nishizawa, M.; Yamaguchi, T. Red blood cell motions in high-hematocrit blood flowing through a stenosed microchannel. *J. Biomech.* **2009**, *42*, 838–843.

29. Gossett, D.R.; Tse, H.T.K.; Lee, S.A.; Ying, Y.; Lindgren, A.G.; Yang, O.O.; Rao, J.; Clark, A.T.; Di Carlo, D. Hydrodynamic stretching of single cells for large population mechanical phenotyping. *Proc. Natl. Acad. Sci. USA* **2012**, *109*, 7630–7635.

30. Guillou, L.; Dahl, J.B.; Lin, J.-M.G.; Barakat, A.I.; Husson, J.; Muller, S.J.; Kumar, S. Measuring Cell Viscoelastic Properties Using a Microfluidic Extensional Flow Device. *Biophys. J.* **2016**, *111*, 2039–2050.

31. Lee, S.S.; Yim, Y.; Ahn, K.H.; Lee, S.J. Extensional flow-based assessment of red blood cell deformability using hyperbolic converging microchannel. *Biomed. Microdevices* **2009**, *11*, 1021–1027.

32. Rodrigues, R.O.; Bañobre-López, M.; Gallo, J.; Tavares, P.B.; Silva, A.M.T.; Lima, R.; Gomes, H.T. Haemocompatibility of iron oxide nanoparticles synthesized for theranostic applications: A high-sensitivity microfluidic tool. *J. Nanopart. Res.* **2016**, *18*, 1–17.

33. Rodrigues, R.O.; Lopes, R.; Pinho, D.; Pereira, A.I.; Garcia, V.; Gassmann, S.; Sousa, P.C.; Lima, R. In vitro blood flow and cell-free layer in hyperbolic microchannels: Visualizations and measurements. *BioChip J.* **2016**, *10*, 9–15.

34. Rodrigues, R.O.; Pinho, D.; Faustino, V.; Lima, R. A simple microfluidic device for the deformability assessment of blood cells in a continuous flow. *Biomed. Microdevices* **2015**, *17*, 108. [PubMed]

35. Yaginuma, T.; Oliveira, M.S.N.; Lima, R.; Ishikawa, T.; Yamaguchi, T. Human red blood cell behavior under homogeneous extensional flow in a hyperbolic-shaped microchannel. *Biomicrofluidics* **2013**, *7*, 54110. [PubMed]

36. Zografos, K.; Pimenta, F.; Alves, M.A.; Oliveira, M.S.N. Microfluidic converging/diverging channels optimised for homogeneous extensional deformation. *Biomicrofluidics* **2016**, *10*, 043508.

37. Henon, Y.; Sheard, G.J.; Fouras, A. Erythrocyte deformation in a microfluidic cross-slot channel. *RSC Adv.* **2014**, *4*, 36079.

38. Astor, B.C.; Muntner, P.; Levin, A.; Eustace, J.A.; Coresh, J. Association of kidney function with anemia: The Third National Health and Nutrition Examination Survey (1988–1994). *Arch. Intern. Med.* **2002**, *162*, 1401–1408.

39. Staples, A.O.; Wong, C.S.; Smith, J.M.; Gipson, D.S.; Filler, G.; Warady, B.A.; Martz, K.; Greenbaum, L.A. Anemia and risk of hospitalization in pediatric chronic kidney disease. *Clin. J. Am. Soc. Nephrol. CJASN* **2009**, *4*, 48–56.

40. Brines, M.; Grasso, G.; Fiordaliso, F.; Sfacteria, A.; Ghezzi, P.; Fratelli, M.; Latini, R.; Xie, Q.W.; Smart, J.; Su-Rick, C.J.; et al. Erythropoietin mediates tissue protection through an erythropoietin and common beta-subunit heteroreceptor. *Proc. Natl. Acad. Sci. USA* **2004**, *101*, 14907–14912.

41. Robinson, B.M.; Joffe, M.M.; Berns, J.S.; Pisoni, R.L.; Port, F.K.; Feldman, H.I. Anemia and mortality in hemodialysis patients: Accounting for morbidity and treatment variables updated over time. *Kidney Int.* **2005**, *68*, 2323–2330.

42. Yang, W.; Israni, R.K.; Brunelli, S.M.; Joffe, M.M.; Fishbane, S.; Feldman, H.I. Hemoglobin Variability and Mortality in ESRD. *J. Am. Soc. Nephrol. JASN* **2007**, *18*, 3164–3170. [PubMed]

43. Faustino, V.; Pinho, D.; Yaginuma, T.; Calhelha, R.C.; Ferreira, I.C.; Lima, R. Extensional flow-based microfluidic device: Deformability assessment of red blood cells in contact with tumor cells. *BioChip J.* **2014**, *8*, 42–47.

44.   Faustino, V.; Pinho, D.; Yaginuma, T.; Calhelha, R.C.; Kim, G.M.; Arana, S.; Ferreira, I.C.F.R.; Oliveira, M.S.N.; Lima, R. Flow of Red Blood Cells Suspensions through Hyperbolic Microcontractions. In *Visualization and Simulation of Complex Flows in Biomedical Engineering*; Lima, R., Imai, Y., Ishikawa, T., Oliveira, M.S., Eds.; Springer: Dordrecht, The Netherlands, 2014; pp. 151–163.

45.   Lima, R.A.; Saadatmand, M.; Ishikawa, T. Microfluidic Devices Based on Biomechanics. In *Integrated Nano-Biomechanics*; Yamaguchi, T., Ishikawa, T., Imai, Y., Eds.; Elsevier: Boston, MA, USA, 2018; pp. 217–263. [CrossRef]

46.   Forsyth, A.M.; Wan, J.; Ristenpart, W.D.; Stone, H.A. The dynamic behavior of chemically "stiffened" red blood cells in microchannel flows. *Microvasc. Res.* **2010**, *80*, 37–43. [PubMed]

47.   Pinho, D.; Lima, R.; Pereira, A.I.; Gayubo, F. Automatic tracking of labeled red blood cells in microchannels. *Int. J. Numer. Method Biomed. Eng.* **2013**, *29*, 977–987. [CrossRef] [PubMed]

48.   Rodrigues, V.; Rodrigues, P.J.; Pereira, A.I.; Lima, R. Automatic tracking of red blood cells in micro channels using OpenCV. In *AIP Conference Proceedings*; AIP Publishing: Melville, NY, USA, 2013; Volume 1558, p. 594. [CrossRef]

49.   Taboada, B.; Monteiro, F.; Lima, R. Automatic tracking and deformation measurements of red blood cells flowing through a microchannel with a microstenosis: The keyhole model. *Comput. Methods Biomech. Biomed. Eng. Imaging Vis.* **2016**, *4*, 229–237. [CrossRef]

50.   Schonbrun, E.; Malka, R.; Di Caprio, G.; Schaak, D.; Higgins, J.M. Quantitative Absorption Cytometry for Measuring Red Blood Cell Hemoglobin Mass and Volume. *Cytometry A* **2014**, *85*, 332–338. [CrossRef] [PubMed]

7

Blood Viscoelasticity Measurement Using Interface Variations in Coflowing Streams under Pulsatile Blood Flows

Yang Jun Kang ⓘ

Department of Mechanical Engineering, Chosun University, 309 Pilmun-daero, Dong-gu, Gwangju 61452, Korea; jkang2011@chosun.ac.kr

Abstract: Blood flows in microcirculation are determined by the mechanical properties of blood samples, which have been used to screen the status or progress of diseases. To achieve this, it is necessary to measure the viscoelasticity of blood samples under a pulsatile blood condition. In this study, viscoelasticity measurement is demonstrated by quantifying interface variations in coflowing streams. To demonstrate the present method, a T-shaped microfluidic device is designed to have two inlets (a, b), one outlet (a), two guiding channels (blood sample channel, reference fluid channel), and one coflowing channel. Two syringe pumps are employed to infuse a blood sample at a sinusoidal flow rate. The reference fluid is supplied at a constant flow rate. Using a discrete fluidic circuit model, a first-order linear differential equation for the interface is derived by including two approximate factors ($F_1 = 1.094$, $F_2 = 1.1087$). The viscosity and compliance are derived analytically as viscoelasticity. The experimental results showed that compliance is influenced substantially by the period. The hematocrit and diluent contributed to the varying viscosity and compliance. The viscoelasticity varied substantially for red blood cells fixed with higher concentrations of glutaraldehyde solution. The experimental results showed that the present method has the ability to monitor the viscoelasticity of blood samples under a sinusoidal flow-rate pattern.

Keywords: viscoelasticity; microfluidic device; coflowing streams; interface; linear differential equation; two approximate factors

1. Introduction

Cardiovascular diseases (CVDs) occur without any symptoms and can lead to unexpected death [1]. In other words, blood clotting or abnormal blood flow contributes to vasculature blockages. Currently, biochemical properties (i.e., biomarkers [2,3] or DNA [4]) are used to diagnose CVDs. However, the biochemical approach has not been considered an effective tool for early detection of CVDs, because it does not provide information on blood flows or blood clotting. Instead of the biochemical approach, a biophysical approach is required to quantify abnormal blood flows in narrow-sized vessels. Blood samples collected from patients with CVDs or disorders exhibit changes in cells (i.e., red blood cells (RBCs) [5] or platelets [6]) or plasma proteins [3,7]. To detect CVDs effectively, it is necessary to quantify the contributions of cells or plasma proteins. Blood flows in microcirculation are determined by the mechanical properties of blood samples. In addition, blood vessel walls (i.e., shape and size) contribute to varying blood flows substantially. These properties include viscosity, elasticity, RBC aggregation, and RBC deformability. According to recent reports, a blood sample collected from a patient with CVD showed significantly different biophysical properties when compared with a normal blood sample [2,8,9]. For this reason, the mechanical properties of blood samples have been used to monitor the status or progress of CVDs. Additionally, the mechanical properties have been quantified under dynamic blood flows [10]. Under ex vivo closed-circuit conditions, blood flows vary periodically over time. When a flow regulator is integrated into the fluidic circuit, a periodic flow pattern is regulated to a constant flow pattern [11]. The viscosity of the blood sample is then quantified by using reverse flow-switching phenomena under a constant blood flow. Additionally, blood viscosity is obtained by monitoring the interface in coflowing streams, while the flow rates of the blood sample and reference fluid remain constant at the same flow rate with two syringe pumps [12,13]. However, because the blood sample includes viscoelasticity (viscosity and elasticity) under a periodic flow condition, it is necessary to quantify the viscoelasticity of the blood sample without a flow regulator (i.e., periodic flow rate).

Recently, a microfluidic platform has been suggested for effectively manipulating a small volume of blood sample in microfluidic channels. A microfluidic channel has been used to investigate hemorheological properties of blood samples. Under a microfluidic platform, several techniques have been suggested to quantify the viscoelasticity of blood samples. Guido et al. have measured membrane viscoelasticity by measuring the velocity and shape of a single RBC in converging or diverging flow [14]. Kim et al. measured RBC stretching with viscoelastic cell focusing [15]. The method was then used to characterize differences in RBC deformability. Lee et al. measured the viscosity and elasticity of blood samples by infusing steady and transient blood flows sequentially [16]. The viscosity and time constant were obtained sequentially by controlling the flow rate of the reference fluid and blood sample, respectively. Here, the time constant was quantified by monitoring temporal variation of a bridge channel filled with a human blood sample at a transient blood flow. The elasticity of the blood sample was quantified by using the linear Maxwell model (elasticity = viscosity/time constant). Kang reported that viscosity and elasticity of blood samples can be obtained sequentially under a periodic on–off blood flow condition [17]. Monitoring the interface in a coflowing stream enabled blood viscoelasticity to be obtained at an interval of a specific period.

More recently, the author suggested a viscoelasticity measurement method under a sinusoidal blood flow rate (Q_B (t)) (Q_B (t) = Q_α + Q_β·sin (ωt), where Q_α is the mean flow rate, Q_β is the alternating flow rate, and ω is the angular frequency of syringe pump) [18]. While the blood sample is infused periodically, the viscoelasticity of the blood sample is obtained by monitoring the interface in coflowing streams and by calculating the pulsatility index (PI) (PI = 0.5 × (Q_{max} - Q_{min})/Q_{ave}, where Q_{max} is the maximum flow rate, Q_{min} is the minimum flow rate, and Q_{ave} is the average flow rate). A first-order differential equation for coflowing streams is derived by constructing a simple discrete fluidic circuit. Here, using a conventional microelectromechanical system technique, a microfluidic device has rectangular shape with an extremely low aspect ratio (aspect ratio = depth/width = 4/250) which is devised to compensate for the boundary condition difference between a real physical model and a mathematical condition. First, the viscosity of the blood sample is calculated by averaging the equation over a single period. Second, instead of an analytical solution of the equation, the time constant is obtained from the expression of PI. Variations of velocity and interface are required simultaneously to find out time constant of interface. The elasticity is then obtained with a linear Maxwell model. However, the differential equation does not include a correction factor (CF), which makes it necessary to compensate for the boundary condition difference between the real model and mathematical model under coflowing streams [19]. Additionally, the previous study did not use the analytical expression to obtain the viscoelasticity of a blood sample. At last, the method required variations of blood velocity over time. Nonetheless, the previous method shows promise for quantifying the viscoelasticity of blood samples under a periodic blood flow-rate pattern. It is extremely difficult to obtain the viscoelasticity of a blood sample circulated under an ex vivo or in vivo condition (i.e., a real and complex situation). As a preliminary study, it is necessary to develop a simple method for measuring viscoelasticity under a single sinusoidal flow patterns with a syringe pump.

In this study, to resolve these issues, a CF is inserted while deriving a differential equation for coflowing streams. Because the differential equation includes nonlinear terms, it is difficult to find an analytical solution. Conducting computational fluid dynamics (CFD) simulation enables an approximate expression of the CF to be obtained. Then, two approximation factors (F_1, F_2) are suggested and calculated to convert nonlinear terms into linear terms. Analytical expressions of the viscoelasticity of blood samples are obtained by solving the differential equation. Here, viscosity and compliance are derived analytically. To demonstrate the present method, a T-shaped microfluidic channel is used. When measuring velocity fields of blood sample, a T-shaped microfluidic channel is not required to align a microscopic image in the horizontal or vertical direction. It consists two inlets, one outlet, two guiding channels (blood sample channel, reference fluid channel), and one coflowing channel. Using two syringe pumps, a blood sample is infused into the blood sample channel with a sinusoidal flow-rate pattern. A reference fluid is supplied into the reference fluid channel at a constant flow rate. By monitoring the interface of both fluids in the coflowing channel, the viscosity and compliance are obtained at an interval of a specific period. As a performance demonstration, the present method was used to evaluate the contributions of period (T), diluents (plasma, 1x phosphate-buffered saline (PBS), and hematocrit (Hct) to viscoelasticity. The present method was then employed to quantify the viscoelasticity of a fixed blood sample prepared by adding fixed RBCs into plasma.

2. Materials and Methods

2.1. Blood Sample Preparation

According to the ethics committee of Chosun University Hospital (CHOSUN 2018-05-11), all experiments were conducted after ensuring that the experimental protocols were appropriate and humane.

Human concentrated RBCs and fresh frozen plasma (FFP) were purchased from the Gwangju–Chonnam blood bank (Gwangju, Korea) and were stored at 4 °C and −20 °C, respectively. Because the RBCs were preserved in citrate phosphate dextrose adenine (CPDA) as an anticoagulant solution, it was necessary to remove CPDA from the concentrated RBCs. The concentrated RBCs (~7 mL) were added into 1x PBS (pH 7.4, Gibco, Life Technologies, Carlsbad, CA, USA) (~7 mL) in a 15-mL tube. After the tube was inserted into a centrifugal separator (Allegra X-30R benchtop, Beckman Coulter, Brea, CA, USA), it was set to 4000 rpm and operated for 10 min. The diluted blood was separated into two layers: an upper layer (plasma), and a lower layer (RBCs). Pure RBCs were collected after removing liquid in the upper layer. Additionally, FFP was thawed at room temperature (25 °C). Plasma was filtered to remove cellular debris and unwanted white blood cells with a syringe filter (mesh size = 5 μm, Minisart, Sartorius, Göttingen, Germany). The RBCs and plasma were stored at 4 °C in a refrigerator before the blood test [20].

First, to evaluate the effect of the contribution of Hct and diluents (1x PBS, plasma) on the viscoelasticity of blood samples, blood samples with Hct = 30%, 40%, 50%, and 60% were prepared by adding normal RBCs into 1x PBS or plasma. Except in the experiment for evaluating the contribution of Hct, all blood samples were adjusted to Hct = 50%. Second, to fix normal RBCs chemically, three different concentrations of glutaraldehyde (GA) solution (C_{GA} = 4, 8, and 12 μL/mL) were diluted by mixing GA solution (Grade II, 25% in H_2O, Sigma-Aldrich, St. Louis, MO, USA) into 1x PBS. Normal RBCs were fixed for consistent measurement because RBCs needed to be unchanged over experimental time. To fix normal RBCs, normal RBCs were mixed with each concentration of GA solution for 10 min prior to washing them. Fixed RBCs were collected after a washing procedure. The fixed blood sample (Hct = 50%) was then prepared by adding the fixed RBCs into plasma. Here, to evaluate the contribution of fixed RBCs to viscoelasticity effectively, it was necessary to remain constant at a level of hematocrit (i.e., Hct = 50%).

2.2. Fabrication on a Microfluidic Device and Experimental Procedure

A T-shaped microfluidic device for measuring blood viscoelasticity consisted of two inlets (a, b), one outlet (a), two guiding channels (blood sample channel (BC), reference fluid channel (RC)), and one coflowing channel (CC), as shown in Figure 1A-a and Figure S1 (Supplementary Materials). The blood sample channel (width = 250 μm, length = 7500 μm) and reference fluid channel (width = 250 μm, length = 7500 μm) were connected to the coflowing channel (width = 250 μm, length = 9200 μm). Here, dimensions of a microfluidic channel were selected to measure velocity fields and blood viscosity accurately. First, velocity fields of blood flows were obtained accurately with microscopic images captured with at least 10× objective lens. Based on fields of view, channel width and length were selected suitably. Second, a rectangular channel with low aspect to ratio was preferred to measure blood viscosity effectively under coflowing method. The channel depth of the microfluidic device was fixed at 20 μm.

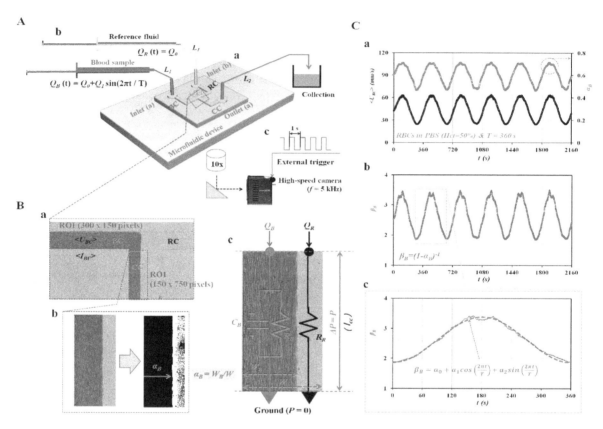

Figure 1. Proposed method for measuring blood viscoelasticity by monitoring the interface of both fluids in coflowing streams under a pulsatile blood flow rate. (**A**) Schematic diagram of the proposed method, including a microfluidic device, two syringe pumps, and an image acquisition system. (**a**) Microfluidic device composed of two inlets (a, b), one outlet (a), two guiding channels (blood sample channel (BC) and reference-fluid channel (RC)), and a coflowing channel (CC). (**b**) Two syringe pumps employed to supply blood sample and reference fluid into the corresponding inlets. (**c**) High-speed camera with a frame rate of 5 kHz employed to capture microscopic images at an interval of 1 s. (**B**) Quantification of interface in coflowing channel and its mathematical model with a discrete fluidic circuit. (**a**) Region of interest (ROI, 150 × 750 pixels) selected in coflowing channel for evaluating interface (α_B) and ROI (300 × 150 pixels) selected in blood sample channel for evaluating averaged blood velocity ($<U_{BC}>$) or averaged image intensity ($<I_{BC}>$). (**b**) Image conversion from gray-scale image to binary-scale image by using digital image processing. Interface (α_B) was obtained as $\alpha_B = W_B/W$. W_B and W represent blood-filled width and channel width, respectively. (**c**) Discrete fluidic circuit for mathematical representation of two fluids flowing in coflowing channel. Ground represented zero value of pressure ($P = 0$). (**C**) As a preliminary demonstration, a blood sample ($Hct = 50\%$, RBCs suspended in 1x PBS) was supplied into inlet (a) at a sinusoidal flow rate ($Q_B(t) = 1 + 0.5 \sin(2\pi t/360)$ mL/h); 1x PBS was supplied into inlet (b) at a constant flow rate of $Q_R(t) = 1$ mL/h. (**a**) Temporal variations of $<U_{BC}>$ and α_B with an elapse of time. (**b**) Temporal variations of $\beta_B = (1 - \alpha_B)^{-1}$ over time. (**c**) Extractions of three constants (a_0, a_1, and a_2) of $\beta_B(t) = a_0 + a_1 \cdot \cos(\omega \cdot t) + a_2 \cdot \sin(\omega \cdot t)$ by conducting a curve-fitting technique for a single period of 360 s.

Conventional microelectromechanical-system fabrication techniques (photolithography and deep reactive ion etching) were used to fabricate a master mold on a 4-inch silicon wafer. polydimethylsiloxane (PDMS) (Sylgard 184, Dow Corning, Midland, MI, USA) prepolymer and a curing agent were mixed at a ratio of 10:1. After the mold was fixed in a Petri dish, the PDMS mixture was poured on the master mold. Air bubbles in the PDMS were removed with a vacuum pump for 1 h. After curing the PDMS mixture in a convective oven (70 °C for 1 h), a PDMS block was peeled from the master mold. It was cut with a razor blade. Three ports (two inlets and one outlet) were punched with a biopsy punch (outer diameter = 1.2 mm). After oxygen–plasma treatment on the PDMS block and a glass slide with an oxygen–plasma system (CUTE-MPR, Femto Science Co., Gyeonggi, Korea), a microfluidic device was finally prepared by bonding the PDMS block on the glass slide.

As shown in Figure 1A-b, two polyethylene tubes (L_1, inner diameter = 500 μm, thickness = 500 μm, and length = 300 mm) were connected from two disposable syringes (~1 mL) to two inlets (a and b). The other polyethylene tube (L_2, inner diameter = 500 μm, thickness = 500 μm, and length = 200 mm) was connected from an outlet (a) to a waste collection unit. To remove air bubbles in the channels and avoid nonspecific binding of plasma proteins to the inner surfaces of the channels, all channels were filled completely with bovine serum albumin (BSA) solution of C_{BSA} = 2 mg/mL through outlet (a) with a disposable syringe. After 10 min, all channels were rinsed then filled with 1x PBS. After two disposable syringes (~1 mL) were filled with blood sample (~1 mL) and 1x PBS (~1 mL), they were installed into two syringe pumps (neMESYS, Cetoni GmbH, Germany). The blood sample was supplied into inlet (a) at a sinusoidal flow rate (Q_B $(t) = Q_0 + Q_1 \cdot \sin(2\pi t/T)$). Q_0 and Q_1 are the average and amplitude of the sinusoidal flow rate. Additionally, T represents the period. Reference fluid (1x PBS) was supplied into inlet (b) at a constant flow rate (Q_R $(t) = Q_0$).

As shown in Figure 1A-c, the microfluidic device was positioned on an optical microscope (BX51, Olympus, Tokyo, Japan) equipped with a 10× objective lens (NA = 0.25). A high-speed camera (FASTCAM MINI, Photron, USA) was used to capture microscopic images of the blood sample and 1x PBS flowing in microfluidic channels. It offered a spatial resolution of 1280 × 1000 pixels. Each pixel corresponded to 10 μm. With a function generator (WF1944B, NF Corporation, Yokohama, Japan), a pulse signal with a period of 1 s triggered the high-speed camera. Microscopic images were sequentially captured at a frame rate of 5 kHz. All experiments and blood sample preparations were conducted at a room temperature of 25 °C.

2.3. Quantification of Interface (α_B), Averaged Blood Velocity ($<U_{BC}>$), and Averaged Image Intensity ($<I_{BC}>$)

Variations of the interface in the coflowing channel were used to quantify the viscoelasticity of the blood sample. Additionally, the image intensity and velocity fields of the blood sample flowing in the blood sample channel were obtained to evaluate the erythrocyte sedimentation rate (ESR) that occurred in the driving syringe while the blood flow rate was controlled by the syringe pump. First, to obtain the interface between the blood sample and 1x PBS in the coflowing channel, a specific ROI of 150 × 750 pixels was selected in the coflowing channel, as shown in Figure 1B-a. To obtain the interface in the coflowing channel effectively, a gray-scale image was converted into a binary-scale image by adopting Otsu's method [21]. As shown in Figure 1B-b, the blood-filled width (W_B) over the ROI was calculated by using a commercial software package (MATLAB 2019, MathWorks, Natick, MA, USA). The interface (α_B) was obtained as $\alpha_B = W_B/W$. Here, W is the channel width of the coflowing channel. Second, to monitor variations of blood flow rate supplied from the syringe pump, velocity fields of the blood sample flowing in the blood sample channel were obtained by conducting a time-resolved micro particle image velocimetry (micro-PIV) technique. A specific ROI of 300 × 150 pixels was selected in the blood sample channel. The size of the interrogation window was 32 × 32 pixels. The window overlap was 50%. The obtained velocity fields were validated with a median filter. The averaged velocity ($<U_{BC}>$) was calculated as an arithmetic average of U_{BC} distributed over the ROI. Third, to evaluate the ESR that occurred in the driving syringe, it was necessary to quantify the microscopic image intensity of the blood sample flowing in the blood sample channel. A specific ROI with 300 × 150 pixels was selected in the blood sample channel. The image intensity of the blood sample flowing in the blood sample channel was obtained by conducting digital image processing with MATLAB. An averaged image intensity ($<I_{BC}>$) was obtained by averaging variations of I_{BC} distributed over the ROI.

2.4. Discrete Fluidic Circuit for Representing Viscoelasticity of Blood Sample

Blood samples were assumed to be Newtonian fluids. To evaluate the viscoelasticity of the blood sample, a simple mathematical model was constructed with discrete fluidic circuit elements. As shown in Figure 1B-c, two fluids flowing in the coflowing channel (i.e., blood sample stream, reference fluid stream) are represented with individual discrete fluidic circuit elements. The fluid circuit model is composed of a flow-rate element (Q_B, Q_R), resistance element (R_B and R_R), and compliance element (C_B). Q_B and Q_R are the flow rates of the blood sample and reference fluid, respectively. Ground represented zero value of pressure ($P = 0$).

The blood stream for representing the viscoelasticity of the blood sample was modeled as a resistance element (R_B) and compliance element (C_B) combined in parallel. The C_B was included to account for the compliance effect of the RBCs, the microfluidic channel, and a connected tube. However, because the reference fluid flowed at a constant flow rate in the coflowing channel, the compliance effect of a microfluidic channel and tube filled with reference fluid was negligible. For this reason, the reference stream was simply modeled only as a single resistance element (R_R). The coflowing channel was partially filled with the blood sample stream (W_B) and reference fluid stream ($W - W_B$). Because ground represented zero value of pressure, both streams had the same pressure drop ($P_B = P_R = \Delta P = P$). Based on mass conservation for the blood sample stream and reference fluid stream in the coflowing channel, two equations were derived:

$$Q_B = \frac{P}{R_B} + C_B \frac{dP}{dt} \tag{1}$$

for the blood sample stream, and

$$Q_R = \frac{P}{R_R} \tag{2}$$

for the reference fluid stream. By inserting Equation (2) into Equation (1), a first-order ordinary differential equation was derived:

$$\frac{Q_B}{Q_R} = \frac{R_R}{R_B} + C_B \frac{d}{dt}(R_R) \tag{3}$$

Because a rectangular-shaped channel (width = w, depth = h, and length = l) with a lower aspect ratio (AR) (i.e., AR = depth/width = 20/250) was filled with fluid (viscosity = μ), the resistance element was modeled approximately as [21]:

$$R = \frac{12 \, \mu \, L}{w \, h^3} \tag{4}$$

Based on the analytical expression of a rectangular channel, the corresponding resistance element for each stream was derived as

$$R_B = \frac{12\mu_B l_{cc}}{W \alpha_B \, h^3} \tag{5}$$

for the blood sample stream and

$$R_R = CF \times \frac{12\mu_R l_{cc}}{W(1 - \alpha_B) \, h^3} \tag{6}$$

for the reference fluid stream. In Equation (6), the CF was included to compensate for the boundary condition difference between the real physical model and approximate circuit model [17]. When inserting Equations (5) and (6) into Equation (4), the following equation was derived.

$$\frac{Q_B}{Q_R} = C_B \frac{d}{dt}\left(CF \frac{12\mu_R l_{cc}}{W(1 - \alpha_B)h^3}\right) + CF\left(\frac{\mu_R}{\mu_B}\right)\left(\frac{\alpha_B}{1 - \alpha_B}\right) \tag{7}$$

The first part in the right side of Equation (7) was expressed again in a different form.

$$C_B \frac{d}{dt}\left(CF \frac{12\mu_R l_{cc}}{W(1-\alpha_B)h^3}\right) = C_B \frac{d}{dt}\left(CF \times R_{WB} \times \frac{1}{(1-\alpha_B)} \times \frac{\mu_R}{\mu_B}\right) \tag{8}$$

In Equation (8), R_{WB}, which assumed that the coflowing channel was filled with the blood sample, was given as $R_{WB} = \frac{12\mu_B l_{cc}}{Wh^3}$. According to a previous study, blood viscosity remained constant with respect to the interface [18]. Because R_{WB} and $\frac{\mu_R}{\mu_B}$ were independent of time, Equation (8) became a simple expression of Equation (9).

$$C_B \frac{d}{dt}\left(CF \frac{12\mu_R l_{cc}}{W(1-\alpha_B)h^3}\right) = C_B \times R_{WB} \times \left(\frac{\mu_R}{\mu_B}\right) \times \frac{d}{dt}\left(CF \times \frac{1}{(1-\alpha_B)}\right) \tag{9}$$

When Equation (9) was inserted into Equation (7), Equation (7) was then expressed as Equation (10).

$$\left(\frac{Q_B}{Q_R}\right)\left(\frac{\mu_B}{\mu_R}\right) = C_B R_{WB} \frac{d}{dt}\left(CF \times \frac{1}{1-\alpha_B}\right) + CF \times \left(\frac{\alpha_B}{1-\alpha_B}\right) \tag{10}$$

In Equation (10), CF was varied depending on the interface (α_B) (i.e., $CF = CF(\alpha_B)$). Here, the CF was obtained by conducting numerical simulation. Because Equation (10) had nonlinear terms, it was substantially difficult to find an analytical solution. For this reason, it was necessary to approximate the nonlinear Equation (10) as a simple linear equation. Equation (10) was modified as a simple form.

$$\left(\frac{Q_B}{Q_R}\right)\left(\frac{\mu_B}{\mu_R}\right) = F_1 C_B R_{WB} \frac{d}{dt}\left(\frac{1}{1-\alpha_B}\right) + F_2\left(\frac{\alpha_B}{1-\alpha_B}\right) \tag{11}$$

In Equation (11), F_1 and F_2 were obtained by obtaining the weighted average of CF (i.e., $CF \times (1 - \alpha_B)^{-1}$ or $CF \times \alpha_B \times (1 - \alpha_B)^{-1}$) within a specific value of the interface. As the interface was relocated periodically within a specific range ($0.1 < \alpha_B < 0.9$), two approximate factors (F_1 and F_2) with constant values were calculated from Equations (12) and (13).

$$\sum_{i=1}^{i=n} CF(\alpha_B[i]) \times \frac{1}{1-\alpha_B(i)} = F_1 \sum_{i=1}^{i=n} \frac{1}{1-\alpha_B(i)} \tag{12}$$

and

$$\sum_{i=1}^{i=n} CF(\alpha_B[i]) \times \frac{\alpha_B(i)}{1-\alpha_B(i)} = F_2 \sum_{i=1}^{i=n} \frac{\alpha_B(i)}{1-\alpha_B(i)} \tag{13}$$

By dividing Equation (11) with F_2, Equation (11) was changed to a simple linear differential equation.

$$\lambda_B \frac{d}{dt}(\beta_B) + \beta_B = 1 + \left(\frac{1}{F_2}\right)\left(\frac{Q_B}{Q_R}\right)\left(\frac{\mu_B}{\mu_R}\right) \tag{14}$$

In Equation (14), β_B and time constant (τ_B) were derived as $\beta_B = (1 - \alpha_B)^{-1}$ and $\lambda_B = C_B R_{WB}\left(\frac{F_1}{F_2}\right)$, respectively. In this study, the flow rates of the blood sample and reference fluid were controlled as $Q_B(t) = Q_0 + Q_1 \sin(\omega t)$ and $Q_R(t) = Q_0$, respectively. Here, ω was given as $\omega = \frac{2\pi}{T}$. The particular solution of Equation (14) was then derived as

$$\beta_B = \beta_0 + \beta_1 \sin(\omega t - \varphi) \tag{15}$$

In Equation (15), β_0 and β_1 were given as Equations (16) and (17).

$$\beta_0 = 1 + \frac{1}{F_2}\left(\frac{\mu_B}{\mu_R}\right) \tag{16}$$

and

$$\beta_1 = \frac{1}{F_2}\left(\frac{\mu_B}{\mu_R}\right)\left(\frac{Q_1}{Q_0}\right)\frac{1}{\sqrt{1+\omega^2\lambda_B^2}} \tag{17}$$

Additionally, time delay (φ) was given as $\varphi = \omega\lambda_B$. From Equation (16), the blood viscosity (μ_B) was given as

$$\mu_B = \mu_R F_2(\beta_0 - 1) \tag{18}$$

Additionally, from Equation (17), the time constant (λ_B) was derived as

$$\lambda_B = \frac{T}{2\pi}\sqrt{\left(\frac{1}{\beta_1 F_2}\right)^2\left(\frac{Q_1}{Q_0}\right)^2\left(\frac{\mu_B}{\mu_R}\right)^2 - 1} \tag{19}$$

According to $\lambda_B = R_{WB}C_B\left(\frac{F_1}{F_2}\right)$, the analytical expression of compliance (C_B) was derived as

$$C_B = \left(\frac{F_2}{F_1}\right)\left(\frac{1}{R_{WB}}\right)\left(\frac{T}{2\pi}\right)\sqrt{\left(\frac{1}{\beta_1 F_2}\right)^2\left(\frac{Q_1}{Q_0}\right)^2\left(\frac{\mu_B}{\mu_R}\right)^2 - 1} \tag{20}$$

In other words, if β_0 and β_1 could be obtained from periodic variations of the interface (α_B) in the coflowing channel, μ_B and C_B as blood viscoelasticity could be evaluated from Equations (18) and (20), respectively.

As shown in Figure 1C, as a preliminary study, a blood sample ($Hct = 50\%$) was prepared by adding normal RBCs into 1x PBS. The blood sample was supplied into inlet (a) at a sinusoidal flow rate (Q_B (t) = 1 + 0.5 sin ($2\pi t/360$) mL/h). Simultaneously, 1x PBS was supplied into inlet (b) at a constant flow rate of Q_R (t) = 1 mL/h. Figure 1C-a showed temporal variations of $<U_{BC}>$ and α_B over time. In addition, $<U_{BC}>$ and α_B exhibited periodic variations over time. Figure 1C-b showed temporal variations of $\beta_B = (1 - \alpha_B)^{-1}$ over time. Figure 1C-c showed temporal variations of β_B selected for a single period ($T = 360$ s). The expression of β_B (t) was assumed to be β_B (t) = $a_0 + a_1$·cos (ωt) + a_2·sin (ωt). Using the orthogonal property of the sinusoidal function (sin (ωt) and cos (ωt)), three unknown constants (a_0, a_1, and a_2) were obtained from Equations (21)–(23).

$$a_0 = \frac{1}{T}\int_{t=0}^{t=T}\beta_B(t)dt \tag{21}$$

$$a_1 = \frac{2}{T}\int_{t=0}^{t=T}\beta_B(t)\cos(\omega t)dt \tag{22}$$

and

$$a_2 = \frac{2}{T}\int_{t=0}^{t=T}\beta_B(t)\sin(\omega t)dt \tag{23}$$

According to Equations (21)–(23), three unknown constants (a_0, a_1, and a_2) were obtained as $a_0 = 2.61, a_1 = -0.758,$ and $a_2 = -0.017$. In Equation (15), β_0 and β_1 were obtained as $\beta_0 = a_0 = 2.61$ and $\beta_1 = \sqrt{a_1^2 + a_2^2} = 0.785$, respectively. Using Equations (18)–(20), blood viscosity, time constant, and blood compliance were estimated to be $\mu_B = 1.785$ cP, $\lambda_B = 20.491$ s, and $C_B = 208.492 \frac{\mu m^3}{mPa}$, respectively.

3. Results and Discussion

3.1. Correction Factor (CF) and Approximate Factors (F_1 and F_2) via Numerical Simulation

To find two approximate factors (F_1, F_2) in Equation (11), it was necessary to obtain the CF by conducting numerical simulation with CFD software (CFD-ACE+, ESI Group, Paris, France). For convenience, the flow rate of the blood sample was assumed to be $Q_B = 1$ mL/h. The viscosities of both fluids (blood sample, reference fluid) were assumed as $\mu_B = 1$ cP and $\mu_R = 1$ cP, respectively.

Figure 2A showed variations of the interface (α_B) through numerical simulation with respect to the flow-rate ratio (Q_R/Q_B) ((a) $Q_R/Q_B = 1$, (b) $Q_R/Q_B = 0.8$, (c) $Q_R/Q_B = 0.6$, (d) $Q_R/Q_B = 0.4$, (e) $Q_R/Q_B = 0.2$, and (f) $Q_R/Q_B = 0.1$). The interfaces (α_B) for the corresponding flow-rate ratio (Q_R/Q_B) were obtained as (a) $\alpha_B = 0.5$ for $Q_R/Q_B = 1$, (b) $\alpha_B = 0.553$ for $Q_R/Q_B = 0.8$, (c) $\alpha_B = 0.619$ for $Q_R/Q_B = 0.6$, (d) $\alpha_B = 0.704$ for $Q_R/Q_B = 0.4$, (e) $\alpha_B = 0.818$ for $Q_R/Q_B = 0.2$, and (f) $\alpha_B = 0.891$ for $Q_R/Q_B = 0.1$.

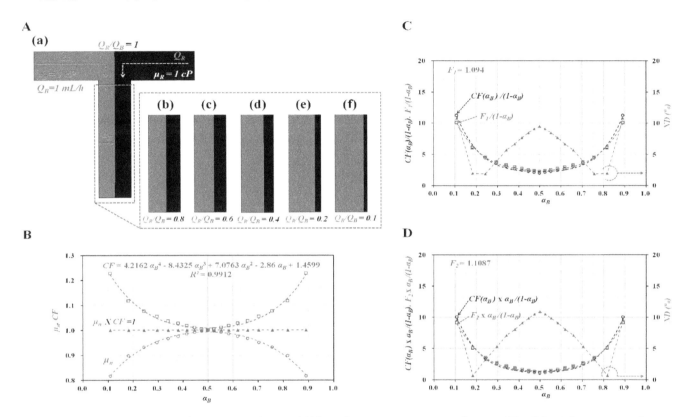

Figure 2. Estimation of correction factor (CF) and two approximate factors (F_1, F_2) with numerical simulation. (**A**) Variations of interface (α_B) through numerical simulation with respect to flow-rate ratio (Q_R/Q_B): (**a**) $Q_R/Q_B = 1$, (**b**) $Q_R/Q_B = 0.8$, (**c**) $Q_R/Q_B = 0.6$, (**d**) $Q_R/Q_B = 0.4$, (**e**) $Q_R/Q_B = 0.2$, and (**f**) $Q_R/Q_B = 0.1$. For convenience, the flow rate of the blood sample was assumed to be $Q_B = 1$ mL/h. The viscosities of both fluids were given as $\mu_B = 1$ cP and $\mu_R = 1$ cP, respectively. (**B**) Variations of estimated normalized viscosity (μ_n) of blood sample and CF with respect to interface ($0.1 < \alpha_B < 0.9$). The CF was obtained as $CF = 4.2162\,\alpha_B^4 - 8.4325\,\alpha_B^3 + 7.0763\,\alpha_B^2 - 2.86\,\alpha_B^2 + 1.4599$ ($R^2 = 0.9912$). (**C**) Variations of CF (α_B)/$(1 - \alpha_B)$, $F_1/(1 - \alpha_B)$, and normalized difference (ND) over α_B. (**D**) Variations of CF (α_B) $\times \alpha_B/(1 - \alpha_B)$, $F_2 \times \alpha_B/(1 - \alpha_B)$, and ND over α_B.

According to the coflowing-streams method [22,23], the viscosity ratio of the blood sample to the reference fluid (μ_B/μ_R) was obtained as $\frac{\mu_B}{\mu_R} = \frac{\alpha_B}{1-\alpha_B}$ by quantifying the interface (α_B) in coflowing streams at the same flow-rate condition ($Q_B = Q_R$). The normalized viscosity of the blood sample was obtained by dividing the estimated viscosity ($\mu_{est} = \mu_R \cdot \alpha_B/(1 - \alpha_B)$) by the given viscosity ($\mu_{given} = 1$ cP) ($\mu_n = \mu_{est}/\mu_{given}$). As shown in Figure 2B, variations of μ_n were obtained by varying the interface ($0.1 < \alpha_B < 0.9$). When the interface was located at the center line ($\alpha_B = 0.5$), μ_n was given as $\mu_n = 1$. In other words, the blood viscosity could be measured accurately when the interface was located at the center line [24]. However, when α_B was relocated from the center line to both walls, μ_n tended to decrease by approximately 0.8. Because the viscosity of the blood sample was given as $\mu_B = 1$ cP, the coflowing-streams method exhibited a large measurement error of approximately 20% when compared with the given viscosity of the blood sample. The reason could be explained by the boundary condition difference between the real physical model and simple mathematical model. Instead of a real and complex model, to construct a simple model of coflowing streams, the coflowing-streams method assumed that the interface of two streams was a virtual wall. In other words, it assumed that the interface was a virtual-wall boundary. Because the CF varied by channel dimensions (width and depth), the CF was calculated by referring to the general procedure discussed in previous studies [17,19]. The CF was then estimated by the reciprocating μ_n obtained at a specific interface ($CF \cdot (\alpha_n) = \mu_n^{-1}$ for α_n). As shown in Figure 2B, the CF was obtained as $CF = 1$ at the center line ($\alpha_B = 0.5$). However, the CF tended to increase gradually when the interface moved to both walls. According to regression analysis, the CF was obtained as $CF = 4.2162\,\alpha_B{}^4 - 8.4325\,\alpha_B{}^3 + 7.0763\,\alpha_B{}^2 - 2.86\,\alpha_B + 1.4599$ ($R^2 = 0.9912$). By inserting the correction factor into the coflowing-streams method, the viscosity of the blood sample was estimated with $\mu_B = \mu_R CF(\alpha_B) \frac{\alpha_B}{1-\alpha_B}$. The coflowing method with correction factor could be used to measure the viscosity of blood with a specific hematocrit. Based on Equation (12), the approximate factor (F_1) was obtained as $F_1 = 1.094$. As shown in Figure 2C, variations of $CF(\alpha_B)\frac{1}{1-\alpha_B}$ and $F_1\frac{1}{1-\alpha_B}$ were obtained with respect to α_B. The normalized difference (ND) between both terms exhibited its maximum value at the center and both walls. The normalized difference was less than 10%. Additionally, according to Equation (13), the approximate factor (F_2) was obtained as $F_2 = 1.1087$. As shown in Figure 2D, variations of $CF(\alpha_B)\frac{\alpha_B}{1-\alpha_B}$ and $F_2\frac{\alpha_B}{1-\alpha_B}$ were obtained with respect to α_B. The maximum value of normalized difference was estimated to be approximately 11%. The simulation study showed that the two approximate factors ($F_1 = 1.094$, $F_2 = 1.1087$) could give consistent results when compared with the original expression. Using F_1 and F_2, the nonlinear Equation (10) was converted into the simple linear Equation (11) for consistency.

3.2. Effect of Period (T) on Viscoelasticity of Blood Sample

To verify the contribution of the period (T) to the viscoelasticity of the blood sample (Equations [18] and [20]), the viscosity and compliance were evaluated by varying the period ($T = 120, 240, 360,$ and 480 s). The blood sample ($Hct = 50\%$) was prepared by adding normal RBCs into 1x PBS. Q_0 and Q_1 of the two syringe pumps were controlled at $Q_0 = 1$ and $Q_1 = 0.5$ mL/h, respectively. For a rectangular channel with a lower aspect ratio, the shear rate ($\dot{\gamma}$) was derived as $\dot{\gamma} = \frac{6Q}{wh^2}$ [19]. Based on the shear rate formula, the shear rates of the corresponding flow rate were estimated as $\dot{\gamma} = 8333$ s^{-1} for $Q_B = 0.5$ mL/h and $\dot{\gamma} = 25{,}000$ s^{-1} for $Q_B = 1.5$ mL/h. Because the shear rate ($\dot{\gamma}$) was much greater than 1000 s^{-1}, it was reasonable that the blood sample behaves as a Newtonian fluid. In other words, the blood viscosity (μ_B) remained constant within the specific flow rates of the blood sample.

As shown in Figure 3A, temporal variations of α_B and $\beta_B = (1 - \alpha_B)^{-1}$ were obtained with respect to the period ((a) $T = 120$ s, (b) $T = 240$ s, (c) $T = 360$ s, and (d) $T = 480$ s). Based on Equations (21)–(23), β_0 and β_1 were obtained at an interval of the corresponding period. Figure 3B-a showed variations of β_0 and β_1 with respect to T, where β_0 and β_1 fluctuated at a shorter period ($T = 120, 360$ s). However, they remained stable at a longer period ($T = 360, 480$ s). Figure 3B-b showed variations of λ_B with respect to T. The λ_B tended to increase linearly for up to $T = 360$ s. However, the slope of λ_B tended to decrease between $T = 360$ and $T = 480$ s. According to Equation (19), the λ_B was linearly proportional to the period (i.e., $\lambda_B \sim T$). The experimental results showed appropriately consistent variations of λ_B with respect to T. Using Equations (18) and (20), the blood viscosity (μ_B) and compliance (C_B) were obtained with respect to T. As shown in Figure 3B-c, μ_B did not exhibit a linear dependency of T. It fluctuated at a shorter period. However, it remained constant at a longer period ($T = 360, 480$ s). The results agreed with Equation (18), which did not relate to the period. It was necessary, however, to set a longer period for consistently measuring the viscosity of the blood sample. Compliance (C_B) tended to increase linearly for up to $T = 360$ s. The slope of C_B tended to decrease between $T = 360$ and $T = 480$ s. According to the mathematical relation, C_B was linearly proportional to λ_B. The experimental results indicated that blood viscosity was independent of period. However, compliance varied linearly depending on the period.

From the results, for consistent measurement of viscoelasticity (blood viscosity and compliance), the period of the syringe pump was set to a longer period of $T = 360$ s throughout all experiments for convenience.

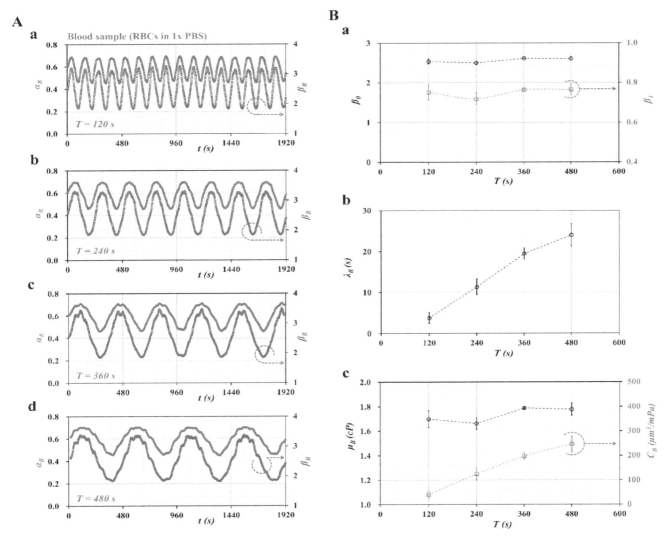

Figure 3. Evaluation of the effect of period (T) on viscoelasticity (blood viscosity and compliance). (**A**) Temporal variations of α_B and β_B with respect to period (T) ((**a**) $T = 120$ s, (**b**) $T = 240$ s, (**c**) $T = 360$ s, and (**d**) $T = 480$ s). (**B**) Quantification of viscosity (μ_B) and compliance (C_B) with respect to period. (**a**) variations of β_0 and β_1 with respect to T, (**b**) variations of λ_B with respect to T, and (**c**) variations of μ_B and C_B with respect to T.

3.3. Quantification of the Effect of Hematocrit on Blood Viscoelasticity

According to a previous study, hematocrit caused an increase in blood viscosity and elasticity [16]. In addition, a blood sample with a low hematocrit ($Hct = 30\%$) exhibited a continuous ESR occurring in a driving syringe [25]. According to the previous study, to increase the ESR significantly, a blood sample was prepared by adding normal RBCs into various concentrations of dextran solution ($C_{dex} = 2$, 5, 8, and 10 mg/mL). Because the hematocrit of the blood sample flowing in the microfluidic channel varied continuously over time, RBC aggregation or blood viscosity tended to vary continuously [19]. In this study, under blood perfusion with a sinusoidal flow-rate pattern, the contribution of hematocrit to blood viscoelasticity and ESR was quantified by varying the hematocrit. To induce the ESR in a driving syringe, plasma was used as the diluent. In other words, blood samples ($Hct = 30\%$, 40%, 50%, and 60%) were prepared by adding normal RBCs into the plasma.

Figure 4A showed temporal variations of β_B with respect to hematocrit ((**a**) $Hct = 30\%$, (b) $Hct = 40\%$, (c) $Hct = 50\%$, and (d) $Hct = 60\%$). Using temporal variations of β_B, blood viscosity and compliance were obtained at an interval of a specific period. As shown in Figure 4B, temporal variations of μ_B and C_B were obtained with respect to hematocrit ((a) $Hct = 30\%$, (b) $Hct = 40\%$,

(c) Hct = 50%, and (d) Hct = 60%). Both parameters were obtained as mean ± standard deviation at a specific time (t = 290, 650, 1010, 1370, and 1730 s).

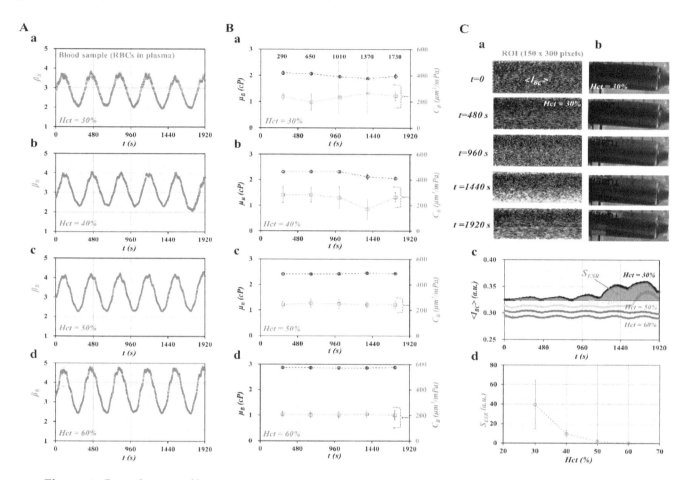

Figure 4. Contribution of hematocrit (Hct) to viscoelasticity and ESR. Blood samples (Hct = 30%, 40%, 50%, and 60%) were prepared by adding normal RBCs into plasma. (**A**) Temporal variations of β_B with respect to hematocrit ((**a**) Hct = 30%, (**b**) Hct = 40%, (**c**) Hct = 50%, and (**d**) Hct = 60%). (**B**) Temporal variations of μ_B and C_B with respect to hematocrit ((**a**) Hct = 30%, (**b**) Hct = 40%, (**c**) Hct = 50%, and (**d**) Hct = 60%). (**C**) Evaluation of ESR occurring in driving syringe. (**a**) Microscopic images of blood sample (Hct = 30%) flowing in blood channels over time (t = 0, 480, 960, 1440, and 1920 s). (**b**) Side view of a driving syringe over time (t = 0, 480, 960, 1440, and 1920 s). (**c**) Temporal variations of $<I_{BC}>$ with respect to Hct. (**d**) Variations of S_{ESR} with respect to Hct.

For the blood sample with Hct = 30%, compliance (C_B) fluctuated greatly over time. It tended to decrease after t = 290 s, but it tended to increase between t = 650 and t = 1370 s. After t = 1370 s, it remained constant over time. Blood viscosity tended to decrease after t = 650 s. In other words, the ESR of RBCs in a driving syringe accelerated over time. In other words, after a certain time, the hematocrit of the blood sample tended to decrease. Thus, μ_B tended to decrease, and C_B tended to increase with an elapse of time. For the blood sample with Hct = 40%, blood viscosity tended to decrease after t = 1010 s. Compliance remained constant for up to t = 1010 s. After that, it fluctuated over time. When the hematocrit increased from Hct = 30% to Hct = 40%, the time when C_B had the minimum value tended to increase substantially. However, for the blood samples with high hematocrit (Hct = 50%, 60%), blood viscosity and compliance remained constant over time. The blood viscosity tended to increase at a higher hematocrit. The compliance tended to decrease at a higher hematocrit. According to a previous study, blood elasticity tended to increase with respect to hematocrit [16]. When compared with the previous result, compliance tended to decrease with respect to the hematocrit. The experimental results can be considered reasonable, because compliance had the reciprocal of elasticity (i.e., compliance ~ 1/elasticity).

To quantify the ESR that occurred in a driving syringe, the microscopic image intensities of the blood sample were obtained over time. A driving syringe was installed horizontally. Because of the ESR in the driving syringe, the hematocrit of the blood sample flowing in a microfluidic channel tended to decrease over time. Here, variations of hematocrit were used by monitoring the image intensity of the blood sample [26]. Figure 4C-a showed microscopic images of the blood sample ($Hct = 30\%$) flowing in the blood sample channel over time ($t = 0$, 480, 960, 1440, and 1920 s). After $t = 960$ s, the number of RBCs tended to decrease significantly. The image intensity tended to increase. At $t = 1920$ s, the image intensity tended to decrease as RBCs tended to increase significantly. The contrast of each image was enhanced by conducting image processing with the software Image-J (NIH, Maryland, USA). A specific ROI (300 x 150 pixels) in the blood sample channel was selected to quantify the image intensity ($<I_{BC}>$). To visualize the ESR in a driving syringe, a side view of a syringe filled with a blood sample ($Hct = 30\%$) was captured sequentially with a smartphone camera (Galaxy A5, Samsung, Korea). As lower level of hematocrit exhibited higher value of $<I_{BC}>$, the results of blood sample ($Hct = 30\%$) was selected and summarized at a specific time. Figure 4C-b showed snapshots of a driving syringe over time (t) ($t = 0$, 480, 960, 1440, and 1920 s). Before $t = 480$ s, there was no indication of the ESR occurring in a driving syringe, because the RBCs were distributed uniformly. After $t = 960$ s, because of the continuous ESR, the blood sample inside the syringe was separated into two regions: an RBC-rich region (i.e., lower layer) and an RBC-free region (i.e., upper layer). As shown in Figure 4C-a, the ESR in the driving syringe caused a reduced number of RBCs in the microfluidic channel. To quantify the decrease in hematocrit resulting from ESR in the driving syringe, the image intensity of the blood sample ($<I_{BC}>$) was obtained over time. Figure 4C-c showed temporal variations of $<I_{BC}>$ with respect to $Hct = 30\%$, 40%, 50%, and 60%. For a blood sample with $Hct = 30\%$, $<I_{BC}>$ tended to increase after $t = 1190$ s. For a blood sample with $Hct = 40\%$, image intensity tended to increase after $t = 1570$ s. For blood samples with a high hematocrit ($Hct = 50\%$, 60%), the image intensity remained constant over time. This result showed that a lower hematocrit contributed to varying image intensity (or numbers of RBCs) of blood samples flowing in a microfluidic channel. According to a specific parameter (S_{ESR}) suggested in a previous study [20], variations of ESR were quantified with respect to Hct. The S_{ESR} was obtained as $S_{ESR} = \int_{t=0}^{t=1920}(\langle I_{BC}\rangle - I_{min})dt$. Here, I_{min} represents the minimum value of $<I_{BC}>$ within a specific duration, $t = 1920$ s. Figure 4C-d showed variations of S_{ESR} with respect to Hct. The S_{ESR} tended to decrease substantially with respect to Hct. The blood sample with $Hct = 30\%$ showed the maximum value of S_{ESR}. This result indicated that S_{ESR} varied significantly depending on the hematocrit.

From the result, one can conclude that the viscoelasticity of the blood sample suggested by the present method can be varied with the hematocrit. In addition, it can be employed to quantify variations of the ESR occurring in the driving syringe by monitoring temporal variations of viscoelasticity.

3.4. Quantification of the Contribution of Hardened RBCs to Blood Viscoelasticity

Finally, the method was employed to quantify the contribution of hardened RBCs to the viscoelasticity of blood samples. According to previous studies [27,28], normal RBCs were hardened chemically with GA solution. The degree in rigidity increased gradually by varying concentrations of the GA solution. Normal RBCs were hardened chemically with three different concentrations of GA solution (C_{GA}) (C_{GA} = 4, 8, and 12 μL/mL). The hardened blood sample ($Hct = 50\%$) was then prepared by adding hardened RBCs into plasma.

Figure 5A showed temporal variations of β_B with respect to C_{GA}. As the concentration of GA solution increased, β_B tended to increase gradually. In addition, the β_B exhibited steady and periodic variations over time. Figure 5B showed temporal variations of $<I_{BC}>$ with respect to C_{GA}. The inset showed a microscopic image of the fixed blood sample (i.e., fixed RBCs with $C_{GA} = 12$ μL/mL) captured at $t = 480$ s. The $<I_{BC}>$ tended to decrease slightly at a higher concentration of GA solution. However, it exhibited steady and periodic variations over time. The result indicated that the fixed blood sample with $Hct = 50\%$ did not induce the ESR in the driving syringe as shown in Figure 4.

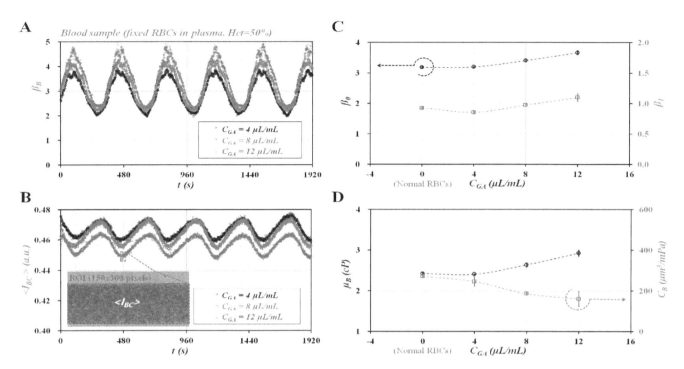

Figure 5. Contribution of fixed blood sample to viscoelasticity of blood sample. Fixed RBCs were prepared chemically with GA solution (C_{GA}) (C_{GA} = 4, 8, and 12 μL/mL). A fixed blood sample (Hct = 50%) was then prepared by adding fixed RBCs into plasma: (**A**) temporal variations of β_B with respect to C_{GA}, (**B**) temporal variations of $<I_{BC}>$ with respect to C_{GA}, (**C**) variations of β_0 and β_1 with respect to C_{GA}, and (**D**) variations of μ_B and C_B with respect to C_{GA}.

Figure 5C showed variations of β_0 and β_1 with respect to C_{GA}. Both parameters (β_0 and β_1) tended to increase substantially at a higher concentration of GA solution. Because the GA solution was employed to increase the rigidity of RBCs, both parameters presented distinctive variations of hardness. Based on Equations (18)–(20), variations of μ_B and C_B were obtained at an interval of T = 360 s. As β_B and $<I_{BC}>$ showed stable variations over time, μ_B and C_B remained constant over the specific duration of the test as shown in Figure 5A,B. Thus, μ_B and C_B were represented as average ± standard deviation (n = 5). Figure 5D showed variations of μ_B and C_B with respect to C_{GA}. According to previous studies [17,18], blood viscosity and elasticity tended to increase at a higher concentration of GA solution. When compared with the previous results, blood viscosity exhibited consistent variations with respect to the concentration of GA solution. Because compliance was defined as the reciprocal of elasticity, the compliance also showed consistent variations with respect to the concentration of GA solution.

The results lead to the conclusion that the present method could be employed to monitor variations of the viscoelasticity of blood samples while the syringe pump was set to a pulsatile flow-rate pattern.

3.5. Quantificative Comparison of Viscoelasticty Obtained with Preesent Method and Conventional Viscometer

Using a conventional viscometer, viscoelasticity of cells was modeled with the linear Maxwell model. As shown in Figure 6A-a, the viscoelasticity of each blood sample was modeled as a solid element and a fluid element connected in series. The corresponding constitutive expression of each element was given as $\tau = G\gamma$ (solid element) and $\tau = \mu\dot{\gamma}$ (fluid element), respectively. Here, G and μ represented elasticity and viscosity, respectively. τ and γ denoted shear stress and shear strain. External shear strain was excited periodically as $\gamma(t) = \gamma_0 e^{j\omega t}$. The governing equation was then derived as $\dot{\tau} + \frac{1}{\lambda_{cv}}\tau = G\dot{\gamma}$. Here, the time constant of viscometry (l_{cv}) was expressed as $l_{cv} = \mu/G$.

The viscous effect of the viscometer was considered as negligible since the viscometer did not have an influence on relaxation time of the cells. The viscometer had operated at a wider range of frequency from ω = 0.3 rad/s to ω = 700 rad/s [29]. The previous study indicated that the time constant of whole blood was obtained as λ_{cv} = 1.5–13.4 ms for shear flow [29], and λ_{cv} = 114–259 ms for extensional flow [30].

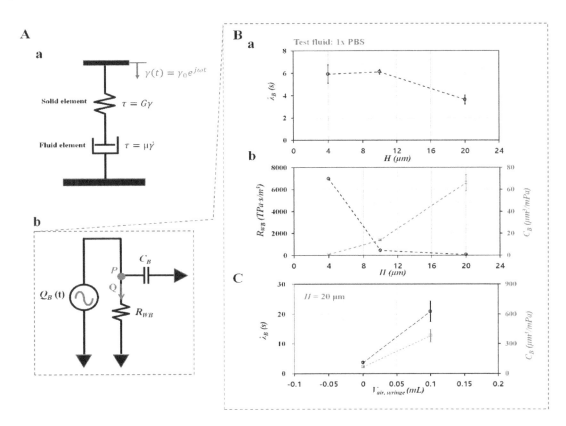

Figure 6. Mathematical representation and quantification of contributions of channel depth and air cavity to compliance. (**A**) Mathematical representation of conventional viscometer and microfluidic system. (**a**) Mathematical representation of conventional viscometer. (**b**) Mathematical representation of microfluidic system. (**B**) Evaluation of channel depth (H) on compliance. Here, 1x PBS as test fluid was infused into a microfluidic system. (**a**) Variations of λ_B with respect to H. (**b**) Variations of R_{WB} and C_B with respect to H. (**C**) Evaluation of air cavity on compliance.

On the other hand, under periodic blood flow in the microfluidic system, Figure 6A-b showed the simple fluidic circuit model of the microfluidic system. Based on electric circuit analysis, the governing equation of fluidic system was derived as $\lambda_B \dot{Q} + Q = Q_B(t)$. Here, Q represented the flow rate which passed through resistance element. Time constant (λ_B) was derived as $\lambda_B = R_{WB} \cdot C_B$. R_{WB} and C_B represented fluidic resistance of the coflowing channel filled with only blood sample and compliance, respectively. As shown in Figure 6A-b, a microfluidic system behaved as an R-C low pass filer. To effectively infuse alternating components in the periodic flow rate into a microfluidic system, the period of the excitation flow rate should be much longer than the time constant of the microfluidic system (i.e., $T > \lambda_B$). In addition, the syringe pump used in this study did not infuse blood samples during short periods. From the experimental results as shown in Figure 3B, period (T) of the sinusoidal flow rate was fixed as T = 360 s.

The λ_B was determined by R_{WB} and C_B. Flexible tubing and the PDMS channels tended to vary the time constant substantially [11]. A microfluidic channel with different channel depths (H) (H = 4, 10, and 20 µm) was prepared to change R_{WB}. Here, 1x PBS was infused into a microfluidic channel to reduce or remove the viscoelastic effects. As shown in Figure 6B-a, the corresponding time constant for each channel depth was obtained as λ_B = 5.92 ± 0.81 s (H = 4 µm), λ_B = 6.11 ± 0.20 s (H = 10 µm), and

$l_B = 3.64 \pm 0.40$ s ($H = 20$ μm). In addition, Figure 6B-b showed variations of R_{WB} and C_B with respect to H. A lower channel depth contributed to increasing R_{WB}, and decreasing C_B. The result indicated that fluidic resistance (R_{WB}) had a strong influence on C_B. To find out the contribution of compliance element (C_B), the compliance of the microfluidic system increased intentionally by securing the air cavity inside the driving syringe. As shown in Figure 6C, variations of λ_B and C_B were obtained with respect to $V_{air} = 0$ and 0.1 mL. When the air cavity of 0.1 mL existed inside the driving syringe, λ_B and C_B increased considerably as $\lambda_B = 20.84 \pm 3.42$ s and $C_B = 378.59 \pm 62.11$ s. From the result, the air cavity tended to increase λ_B and C_B substantially. When compared with viscometry data, the time constant (λ_B) increased about O (10^2) significantly because of the compliance effect of the microfluidic system (i.e., flexible tubing, PDMS channels, and the air cavities existing in the driving syringe). In addition, minimum threshold of C_B (i.e., detection limit) was estimated as 66.05 ± 7.30 μm^3/mPa at a specific condition (i.e., $V_{air} = 0$, $H = 20$ μm). According to a previous study [17], time constants obtained with two different systems (i.e., λ_{PM}: microfluidic system, λ_{CPV}: conventional viscometer) were obtained and compared with respect to $C_{glycerin} = 10\%$, 20%, 30% and 40%. As glycerin solution did not include viscoelasticity, both time constants remained unchanged with respect to different concentrations of glycerin solution. However, the microfluidic system had a longer time constant with O (10^0). The ratio of time constant between λ_{CPV} and λ_{PM} was obtained as $\lambda_{CPV}/\lambda_{PM} =$ O (10^2). To quantitatively determine elasticity obtained with both methods, a scatter plot was employed by plotting G_{PM} on the vertical axis and G_{CPV} on the horizontal axis. According to linear regression analysis, regression coefficient (R^2) had a higher value ($R^2 = 0.9617$). This result indicated that the elasticity obtained with microfluidic system exhibited consistent variations with respect to $C_{glycrin}$ when compared with elasticity obtained with conventional viscometer. Thus, the microfluidic system could be employed to measure viscoelasticity effectively. The slope of 0.0022 indicated that elasticity obtained with the microfluidic system was much less than that obtained with the conventional viscometer.

According to order analysis, C_B had an order of O (10^{-13}) from the analytical expression of time constant. Here, O represented order. According to experimental results as shown in Figure 5, the blood sample (normal RBCs suspended in plasma, $Hct = 50\%$) had $\lambda_B = 36.084 \pm 0.713$ s, $\mu_B = 2.422 \pm 0.028$ cP, and $R_{WB} = 135.148 \pm 2.03$ TPa·s/m^3. The compliance (C_B) was then obtained as $C_B = 270.598 \pm 4.63$ μm^3/mPa. The corresponding order of each parameter was calculated as (1) O (10^1) for λ_B, (2) O (10^0) for μ_B, and O (10^{12}) for R_{WB}. As the unit of C_B was expressed as μm^3/mPa, the order of C_B was calculated as O (10^{-18})/O (10^{-3}) = O (10^{-15}). Thus, C_B obtained for the blood sample had an order of O (10^{-13}). In order words, both approaches (i.e., analytical expression, and experimental data) exhibited the same order of O (10^{-13}). Thus, the present method could be used to monitor C_B of blood samples sufficiently.

To compare the relationship between G_B and C_B, it was assumed that λ_{cv} of the conventional viscometer had the same λ_B as the microfluidic system (i.e., $\lambda_{cv} = \lambda_B$). The time constant obtained by the microfluidic system was used to evaluate G_B and C_B simultaneously. The following relation was given as $\frac{\mu}{G} = R_{WB} \times C_B$. The analytical expression indicated that G_B and C_B had a reciprocal relationship (i.e., $G \sim 1/C_B$). Using experimental results as shown in Figure 4, G_B and C_B were obtained with respect to $Hct = 30\%$, 40%, 50%, and 60%. Additionally, by referring to the previous study [18], variations of G_B were represented with respect to $Hct = 30\%$, 40%, and 50%. Here, blood samples were prepared by adding normal RBCs into plasma. As shown in Figure 7A, at $Hct > 40\%$, G_B tended to increase with respect to Hct. Inversely, C_B tended to decrease with respect to Hct. When compared with the previous study, the trend of G_B increased similarly with respect to Hct. It can be inferred that different microfluidic systems contributed to differences of G_B between both studies. Additionally, variations of C_B and G_B were summarized with respect to C_{GA} as shown in Figure 7B. Here, in the previous study [4], fixed blood samples were prepared by adding fixed RBCs into 1x PBS instead of plasma. G_B of both studies tended to increase gradually with respect to C_{GA}. From quantitative comparisons between the previous study and the present study, elasticity (G_B) and compliance (C_G) had a reciprocal relationship. Additionally, they varied significantly when the rigidity of RBCs increased substantially.

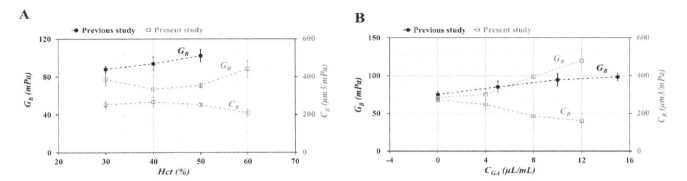

Figure 7. Quantitative compliance of G_B and C_B with respect to previous study [18] and present study. (**A**) Variation of G_B and C_B with respect to *Hct*. (**B**) Variations of G_B and C_B with respect to C_{GA}.

Viscoelasticity (G) was represented as $G = G_1 + j\, G_2$. Here, G_1 (storing modulus) and G_2 (loss modulus) were expressed as $G_1 = G\left(\frac{\lambda_B^2 \omega^2}{1+\lambda_B^2 \omega^2}\right)$ and $G_2 = G\left(\frac{\lambda_B \omega}{1+\lambda_B^2 \omega^2}\right)$. Variations of G_1 and G_2 were represented with respect to radial frequency (ω). G_1 and G_2 tended to vary depending on $\lambda_B \cdot \omega$. However, as $\lambda_B \cdot \omega$ showed a significant difference for both systems, it was apparent that both systems exhibited different variations of G_1 and G_2 with respect to ω. The microfluidic system and conventional viscometer showed different characteristics in terms of angular frequency (or period) and time constants. However, according to experimental results, the microfluidic system could be used effectively to evaluate the viscoelasticity of human blood when compared with conventional viscometers.

4. Conclusions

In this study, a viscoelasticity measurement method for human blood samples (normal blood sample, fixed blood sample) was suggested by quantifying the interface in coflowing streams when a blood sample was infused at a sinusoidal flow rate. Using a discrete fluidic circuit model, a first-order nonlinear differential equation for the interface (α_B) in coflowing streams was derived. Two approximation factors (F_1, F_2) were applied to convert a nonlinear term into a linear term. The viscosity and compliance (as viscoelasticity) were derived analytically from the linear differential equation. From numerical simulation, two approximate factors were obtained: $F_1 = 1.094$ and $F_2 = 1.1087$. The normalized difference between the nonlinear term and linear term was less than 10%. The experimental results showed that compliance varied linearly by period ($T = 120, 240, 360$, and 480 s). However, the blood viscosity remained constant with respect to period. The hematocrit and diluent contributed to varying viscoelasticity. Finally, viscoelasticity varied substantially depending on the degree in rigidity of RBCs. From the experimental results, it was found that the present method had the ability to monitor variations of viscoelasticity while the syringe pump was set to a pulsatile flow-rate pattern. As a limitation, the microfluidic device used in this study had microfluidic channels that were rectangular shape. However, human or animal blood vessels are not rigid and possess circular shape. When compared with live blood vessels, the rectangular shape of microfluidic device might contribute to varying viscoelasticity of the microfluidic channels within the blood sample. Microfluidic channels with 90° turns can cause live mammalian cells to lyse and aggregate in corners, causing fluid flow disruptions. In our next design, we will evaluate the contributions of channel shape and dimensions to viscoelasticity characteristics of the blood samples. In the near future, the present method will be employed to obtain the viscoelasticity of a blood sample circulated under ex vivo and in vivo conditions. In other words, to measure biomechanical properties of blood circulating under an extracorporeal bypass loop or hemodialysis, the blood sample will be collected from the fluidic circuit at periodic intervals. Biomechanical properties are then evaluated with individual conventional viscometers. However, the repetitive collection tends to reduce blood volume in the circuit substantially. If the present method will be integrated into the future fluidic circuit, viscoelasticity of the blood sample will be obtained at various intervals of time, even without periodic collection of blood samples.

Blood volume loss might be reduced considerably in our microfluidic device when compared with the conventional method. Finally, the data obtained by the novel microfluidic system could be employed effectively to monitor vascular diseases and human health.

Figure S1: Mask drawing of silicon mold.

References

1. Benjamin, E.J.; Muntner, P.; Alonso, A.; Bittencourt, M.S.; Callaway, C.W.; Carson, A.P.; Chamberlain, A.M.; Chang, A.R.; Cheng, S.; Das, S.R.; et al. Heart disease and stroke statistics—2019 update. *Circulation* **2019**, *139*, e56–e528. [CrossRef] [PubMed]

2. Upadhyay, R.K. Emerging risk biomarkers in cardiovascular diseases and disorders. *J. Liqids* **2015**, *2015*, 971453. [CrossRef] [PubMed]

3. Melander, O.; Modrego, J.; Zamorano-Leon, J.J.; Santos-Sancho, J.M.; Lahera, I.; Lopez-Farre, A.J. New circulating biomarkers for predicting cardiovascular death in healthy population. *J. Cell. Mol. Med.* **2015**, *19*, 2489–2499. [CrossRef] [PubMed]

4. Mikeska, T.; Craig, J.M. DNA methylation biomarkers: Cancer and beyond. *Genes* **2014**, *5*, 821–864. [CrossRef] [PubMed]

5. Agrawal, R.; Smart, T.; Nobre-Cardoso, J.; Richards, C.; Bhatnagar, R.; Tufail, A.; Shima, D.; Jones, P.H.; Pavesio, C. Assessment of red blood cell deformability in type 2 diabetes mellitus and diabetic retinopathy by dual optical tweezers stretching technique. *Sci. Rep.* **2016**, *6*, 15873. [CrossRef] [PubMed]

6. Yeom, E.; Byeon, H.; Lee, S.J. Effect of diabetic duration on hemorheological properties and platelet aggregation in streptozotocin-induced diabetic rats. *Sci. Rep.* **2016**, *6*, 21913. [CrossRef]

7. Lygirou, V.; Latosinska, A.; Makridakis, M.; Mullen, W.; Delles, C.; Schanstra, J.P.; Zoidakis, J.; Pieske, B.; Mischak, H.; Vlahou, A. Plasma proteomic analysis reveals altered protein abundances in cardiovascular disease. *J. Transl. Med.* **2018**, *16*, 104. [CrossRef]

8. Lowe, G.; Rumley, A.; Norrie, J.; Ford, I.; Shepherd, J.; Cobbe, S.; Macfarlane, P.; Packard, C. Blood rheology, cardiovascular risk factors, and cardiovascular disease: The west of scotland coronary prevention study. *Thromb. Haemost.* **2000**, *84*, 553–558.

9. Koenig, W.; Sund, M.; Filipiak, B.; Doring, A.; Lowel, H.; Ernst, E. Plasma viscosity and the risk of coronary heart disease results from the MONICA-Augsburg cohort study, 1984 to 1992. *Aeterior. Thromb. Vasc. Biol.* **1998**, *18*, 768–772. [CrossRef]

10. Tomaiuolo, G.; Carciati, A.; Caserta, S.; Guido, S. Blood linear viscoelasticity by small amplitude oscillatory flow. *Rheol. Acta* **2016**, *55*, 485–495. [CrossRef]

11. Kang, Y.J.; Yang, S. Fluidic low pass filter for hydrodynamic flow stabilization in microfluidic environments. *Lab Chip* **2012**, *12*, 1881–1889. [CrossRef] [PubMed]

12. Hong, H.; Song, J.M.; Yeom, E. 3D printed microfluidic viscometer based on the co-flowing stream. *Biomicrofluidics* **2019**, *13*, 014104. [CrossRef] [PubMed]

13. Yeom, E.; Kim, H.M.; Park, J.H.; Choi, W.; Doh, J.; Lee, S.-J. Microfluidic system for monitoring temporal variations of hemorheological properties and platelet adhesion in LPS-injected rats. *Sci. Rep.* **2017**, *7*, 1801. [CrossRef] [PubMed]

14. Tomaiuolo, G.; Barra, M.; Preziosi, V.; Cassinese, A.; Rotoli, B.; Guido, S. Microfluidics analysis of red blood cell membrane viscoelasticity. *Lab Chip* **2011**, *11*, 449–454. [CrossRef] [PubMed]

15. Cha, S.; Shin, T.; Lee, S.S.; Shim, W.; Lee, G.; Lee, S.J.; Kim, Y.; Kim, J.M. Cell stretching measurement utilizing viscoelastic particle focusing. *Anal. Chem.* **2012**, *84*, 10471–10477. [CrossRef] [PubMed]

16. Kang, Y.J.; Lee, S.-J. Blood viscoelasticity measurement using steady and transient flow controls of blood in a microfluidic analogue of Wheastone-bridge channel. *Biomicrofluidics* **2013**, *7*, 054122. [CrossRef] [PubMed]

17. Kang, Y.J. Continuous and simultaneous measurement of the biophysical properties of blood in a microfluidic environment. *Analyst* **2016**, *141*, 6583–6597. [CrossRef]

18. Kang, Y.J. Simultaneous measurement of erythrocyte deformability and blood viscoelasticity using micropillars and co-flowing streams under pulsatile blood flows. *Biomicrofluidics* **2017**, *11*, 014102. [CrossRef]

19. Kang, Y.J. Periodic and simultaneous quantification of blood viscosity and red blood cell aggregation using a microfluidic platform under in-vitro closed-loop circulation. *Biomicrofluidics* **2018**, *12*, 024116. [CrossRef]

20. Kang, Y.J. Microfluidic-based biosensor for sequential measurement of blood pressure and RBC aggregation over continuously varying blood flows. *Micromachines* **2019**, *10*, 577. [CrossRef]

21. Otsu, N. A threshold selection method from gray-level histograms. *IEEE Trans. Syst. Man. Cybern.* **1979**, *9*, 62–66. [CrossRef]

22. Lee, J.; Tripathi, A. Intrinsic Viscosity of Polymers and Biopolymers Measured by Microchip. *Anal. Chem.* **2005**, *77*, 7137–7147. [CrossRef]

23. Solomon, D.E.; Vanapalli, S.A. Multiplexed microfluidic viscometer for high-throughput complex fluid rheology. *Microfluid. Nanofluid.* **2014**, *16*, 677–690. [CrossRef]

24. Choi, S.; Park, J.-K. Microfluidic Rheometer for Characterization of Protein Unfolding and Aggregation in Microflows. *Small* **2010**, *6*, 1306–1310. [CrossRef] [PubMed]

25. Kang, Y.J. Microfluidic-based measurement of RBC aggregation and the ESR using a driving syringe system. *Anal. Methods* **2018**, *10*, 1805–1816. [CrossRef]

26. Jalal, U.M.; Kim, S.C.; Shim, J.S. Histogram analysis for smartphone-based rapid hematocrit determination. *Biomed. Opt. Express* **2017**, *8*, 3317–3328. [CrossRef]

27. Kim, B.J.; Lee, Y.S.; Zhbanov, A.; Yang, S. A physiometer for simultaneous measurement of whole blood viscosity and its determinants: Hematocrit and red blood cell deformability. *Analyst* **2019**, *144*, 3144–3157. [CrossRef]

28. Kang, Y.J. Simultaneous measurement of blood pressure and RBC aggregation by monitoring on–off blood flows supplied from a disposable air-compressed pump. *Analyst* **2019**, *144*, 3556–3566. [CrossRef]

29. Campo-Deano, L.; Dullens, R.P.A.; Aarts, D.G.A.L.; Pinho, F.T.; Oliveira, M.S.N. Viscoelasticity of blood and viscoelastic blood analogues for use in polydymethylsiloxane in vitro models of the circulatory system. *Biomicrofluidics* **2013**, *7*, 034102. [CrossRef]

30. Sousa, P.C.; Vaz, R.; Cerejo, A.; Oliveira, M.S.N.; Alves, M.A.; Pinho, F.T. Rheological behavior of human blood in uniaxial extensional flow. *J. Rheol.* **2018**, *62*, 447–456. [CrossRef]

8

Fabrication and Hydrodynamic Characterization of a Microfluidic Device for Cell Adhesion Tests in Polymeric Surfaces

J. Ponmozhi [1], J. M. R. Moreira [2], F. J. Mergulhão [2], J. B. L. M. Campos [1] and J. M. Miranda [1,*]

[1]   Transport Phenomena Research Center (CEFT), Department of Chemical Engineering,
      Faculty of Engineering, University of Porto, Rua Dr. Roberto Frias s/n, 4200-465 Porto, Portugal;
      jponmozhi@gmail.com (J.P.); jmc@fe.up.pt (J.B.L.M.C.)
[2]   Laboratory for Process Engineering, Environment (LEPABE), Biotechnology and Energy,
      Department of Chemical Engineering, Faculty of Engineering, University of Porto, Rua Dr. Roberto Frias
      s/n, 4200-465 Porto, Portugal; joanarm@fe.up.pt (J.M.R.M.); filipem@fe.up.pt (F.J.M.)
*   Correspondence: jmiranda@fe.up.pt

Abstract: A fabrication method is developed to produce a microfluidic device to test cell adhesion to polymeric materials. The process is able to produce channels with walls of any spin coatable polymer. The method is a modification of the existing poly-dimethylsiloxane soft lithography method and, therefore, it is compatible with sealing methods and equipment of most microfluidic laboratories. The molds are produced by xurography, simplifying the fabrication in laboratories without sophisticated equipment for photolithography. The fabrication method is tested by determining the effective differences in bacterial adhesion in five different materials. These materials have different surface hydrophobicities and charges. The major drawback of the method is the location of the region of interest in a lowered surface. It is demonstrated by bacterial adhesion experiments that this drawback has a negligible effect on adhesion. The flow in the device was characterized by computational fluid dynamics and it was shown that shear stress in the region of interest can be calculated by numerical methods and by an analytical equation for rectangular channels. The device is therefore validated for adhesion tests.

Keywords: cell adhesion; biomedical coatings; microfabrication; computational fluid dynamics; microfluidics

1. Introduction

The term 'biofilm' was coined in 1981 [1] and refers to a community of microbial cells that is attached to a surface and enclosed in a self-produced exopolymeric matrix mainly composed by polysaccharide material [2]. Biofilm formation is due to the onset of adhesion of cells to a surface. The development of biofilms in medical devices is a common problem, which can lead to hospitalization, revision surgery due to microbiological implant colonization or mortality.

Recent reviews provide a source of evidence to the undesirable biofilm formation in medical devices [3–9]. These biofilms pose a challenge to the health care community. Currently, to reduce biofouling, there is a spurring development of smart polymers that are used for coating biomedical implants, artificial organs, lab on chip surfaces, implantable drug delivery systems [10], giving way to the development of next generation biomedical devices with reduced fouling.

Many types of measures were proposed to combat biofilms, like conventional usage of antibiotics or surfaces designed to inhibit initial adhesion of cells, for the first stage of biofilm formation [11]. A clear understanding of the initial adhesion mechanisms can lead to the development of ideal biomaterials in which cells are unable to attach and growth of biofilms would be hindered [12]. Consequently, there arises a need to quantify and understand the initial adhesion phenomenon over diverse materials.

Different types of biomaterials were used throughout the past 30 years, for different types of biomedical applications. Ramakrishna, et al. [13] have given a brief introduction of different biocompatible polymers used for different types of implants. For example, poly-l-lactide acid (PLLA) is a biodegradable polymer, which degrades over time without harmful consequences to the body [14,15]. Different types of pins and screws, coated with PLLA, are used to fix the implants. Autografts, namely suspensory fixation, hamstring fixation [16] are used as fixing agents for femoral implants to reduce operation failures.

Recently, researchers started taking advantage of microfluidic devices for biofilm research [17–19] due to several benefits:

- The different biological cells can be monitored in real time with microscopy visualization techniques;
- Low-cost assays and reagents can be used in the microliter range helping in cost cutting;
- Leak-proof inlet and outlet connections can be made easily as the poly-dimethylsiloxane (PDMS) microfluidic channels are deformable;
- The surface can be easily modified and the geometry can be designed according to the application;
- The flow is always laminar, even at a high shear stress range.

In the particular case of adhesion tests, tests can be conducted in a simpler and smaller setup. The pumps required have lower power, the amount of fluid is smaller, and the setup is more flexible. Multiple tests can be conducted in parallel in a single chip and new geometries are easy to produce. Additionally, by using microfluidic devices, researchers can easily mimic the dynamical conditions of biomedical settings. It has been shown that adhesion is influenced by the flow patterns near the wall, the wall shear stress being the most important parameter used to characterize the flow influence on adhesion. For this reason, microdevices to study the wall adhesion must have well characterized hydrodynamic conditions. It is crucial that the wall shear stress is predictable given the flow rate used in the experiments. Additionally, geometrical features of the device should not interfere with the flow or with adhesion in the regions of interest. For this reason, straight channels are the preferred configuration for dynamic adhesion tests. New cells need to be validated to assure they are adequate for routine adhesion tests. Computational fluid dynamics (CFD) is usually used to characterize the flow and calculate the wall shear stress.

To aid the vast developing applications based on microfluidics, there are many conventional rapid prototyping techniques developed for microchannels fabrication. Duffy, et al. [20] demonstrated a method to produce PDMS channels for microfluidic applications. First, the channel is designed in Computer-Aided Design (CAD) software. The design is printed in a transparency and used as a mask for making a positive relief master mold. The master mold is produced in SU-8 polymer epoxy photoresist, step described in detail by Blanco, et al. [21] and Che-Hsin, et al. [22]. The PDMS channels are then casted with this mold and baked to obtain irreversibly sealed channels. Other conventional methods are commercially used for micromolding such as: micromilling [23], micropowder blasting [24], hot embossing [25], laser ablation [26] and stereo lithography [27].

Xurography is a technique developed by Bartholomeusz, et al. [28] utilizing a simple cutter plotter. The microchannels can be cut, according to the application, on vinyl films or other types of films. Positive relief molds, of thicknesses ranging from 25 to 1000 μm, can be generated in the cutter plotter and made ready for casting microchannels in less than 30 min. These molds can also be used as normal molds to produce PDMS microchannels through soft lithographic technique [29].

The foremost advantages of xurography technique are the reduced capital cost and manufacture time. The alternative to xurography is photolithography, a technique that needs expensive machines and clean rooms. Design modifications using photolithography techniques require more than a day, with procedures with long pre and post bake steps. The main disadvantage of xurography is the low resolution that precludes the production of microchannels with dimensions smaller than 200 µm.

Microfabrication techniques that increase the range of possible materials to be used in microfluidics adhesion tests would contribute significantly to the research progress. The objective of adhesion tests is to evaluate different materials in their original form, and therefore a fabrication procedure that changes the material must be avoided. The new techniques must be compatible with existing equipment and with microfabrication techniques, the PDMS soft lithography being the most used. In PDMS soft lithography, irreversible PDMS-PDMS sealing has some important advantages: the bond between the device and the cover is strong and there is no need to use plasma oxygen that would change the surface properties being tested. With existing techniques, PDMS does not bond easily with any polymer unless a surface treatment is applied that would change the surface properties of the polymer. The techniques must also be inexpensive and with short development cycles.

In this work we introduce a technique to incorporate a small wall patch into a PDMS microchannel produced from molds easily made in-house by xurography. The molds can be produced through any other technique, but xurography has low costs and large accessibility. The wall patch can be made of different polymers. The technique is useful to produce channels for adhesion tests, by adapting a standard PDMS soft-lithography. The procedure is compatible with irreversible PDMS-PDMS sealing and does not require plasma oxygen or any other surface treatment. Care was taken to validate the device for adhesion tests performing adhesion experiments and flow numerical simulations. Since one of the key factors influencing cell adhesion is the wall shear stress, the flow in the device was characterized by computational fluid dynamics and the wall shear stress was calculated for the conditions studied.

2. Materials and Methods

2.1. Mold Preparation

The molds of the microchannels were produced by xurography [28], a technique that uses a cutter-plotter to produce molds by removing excess material from adhesive films. The design of the models was made in CorelDRAW. Afterwards, the design was copied to GreatCut software, which instructed an Expert24 GCC plotter (GCC, New Taipei City, Taiwan) to cut the microchannels.

Four different polymer films were tested to check compatibility with PDMS soft lithography [29]. Adhesive film obtained from Sadipal (Girona, Spain) showed to be the most suitable and was selected for mold production. The thickness of the Sadipal adhesive films used was 100 µm and this was the height of the microchannel.

2.2. PDMS Soft Lithography

Microchannels were made from poly-dimethylsiloxane (PDMS) using soft lithography techniques [29]. The microchannels were prepared with a homogenous mixture of PDMS and curing agent (Sylgard 184, Dow Corning, Midland, MI, USA) at a ratio of 5:1. A desiccator connected to the vacuum pump was used to remove the air bubbles formed during the PDMS mixing process. The PDMS mixture was poured over a mold and kept in the oven for 20 min at 80 °C. After curing, the PDMS microchannel was peeled off from the mold. Holes of 1 mm in diameter were punched through the PDMS replicas, at both ends of the channel, to provide inlet and outlet flow with the help of a syringe tip. The PDMS microchannels were sealed with a PDMS coated thin slab (usually a glass slide, see next section) and kept in the oven for approximately 12 h at 80 °C. The sealing method is based on partial curing PDMS-PDMS bonding without plasma treatment described in the literature [30].

2.3. Insertion of Polymer Wall Patches in the Channels

To test the adhesion of cells in a given material, a patch of the material must be inserted in one of the walls of the channel (usually the bottom wall). With this in mind, channels comprising 5 different wall materials were fabricated by modifying the sealing slides. In one case, polystyrene cover was used as substrate to fabricate microchannels with polystyrene wall surfaces, while in the other 4 cases different polymers were spincoated over the sealing glass slide to insert a patch of polymer in the wall of the channel.

The coated glass slides, used to seal the channels, were prepared by a two-layer spin coating technique (Figure 1) using a WS-650S-6NPP-Lite Laurell Technologies spin coater (North Wales, PA, USA). Different volatile polymers and solvents were mixed in appropriate volume percentages (Table 1). The polymer solution was spincoated over the substrate (Figure 1b). After the formation of a polymeric film, by evaporation of the solvent, a scotch tape was pasted over the polymer surface (Figure 1c) and the PDMS was spincoated for 50 s at 5000 rpm over both the polymer and the scotch tape (Figure 1d). The scotch tape was carefully peeled off (Figure 1e) and the slide was baked for 5 min in the oven at 80 °C. A lowered surface (3×3 mm^2) was left on the slide. The level of the lowered surface was determined from the experimental relation between thickness, coating speed and time [31,32] and found to be approximately 10 μm. The PDMS slab with the channel imprinted on it was sealed over the slide. The PDMS slab and the slide were aligned to ensure that the microchannel crossed the lowered surface.

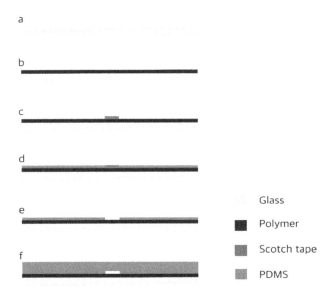

Figure 1. Fabrication procedure: (**a**) Substrate; (**b**) Polymer coating; (**c**) Scotch tape pasted over the polymer layer; (**d**) poly-dimethylsiloxane (PDMS) coating; (**e**) Removal of the Scotch tape; (**f**) Sealing with PDMS slab with the microchannel imprinted in it.

Table 1. Polymers and solvents used to prepare polymeric solutions.

Polymer	Solvent	Polymer Concentration (w/w)
Polyethylene oxide (PEO)	Dichloromethane (DCM)	1.14%
Poly-l-lactide acid (PLLA)	Dichloromethane (DCM)	5.00%
Polyamide (PA)	Trichloroethanol	0.49%
Polydimethylsiloxane (PDMS)	Curing agent (Sylgard 184)	10.0%

The procedure can also be used to test the adhesion to the substrate (e.g., polystyrene surfaces) and in this case the first layer spin coating step (Figure 1b) is skipped. This alternative procedure can be used to produce microchannels with other surfaces, such as glass, provided that a transparent thin slab is available.

The method described above produces microchannels with PDMS surface along most of its length and a small patch of a different material located in a lowered surface half-length from the inlet (see Figure 2). The lowered surface is an unavoidable side effect of the method. To allow for

PDMS-PDMS bonding, a layer of PDMS must be added above the polymer layer, with the exception of a small region that is not covered with PDMS and corresponds to the lowered surface of polymer. To test the effect of the lowered surface on bacterial cell adhesion, microchannels with PDMS walls along the full length of the microchannel were produced following the double layer technique, in which both layers are made of PDMS.

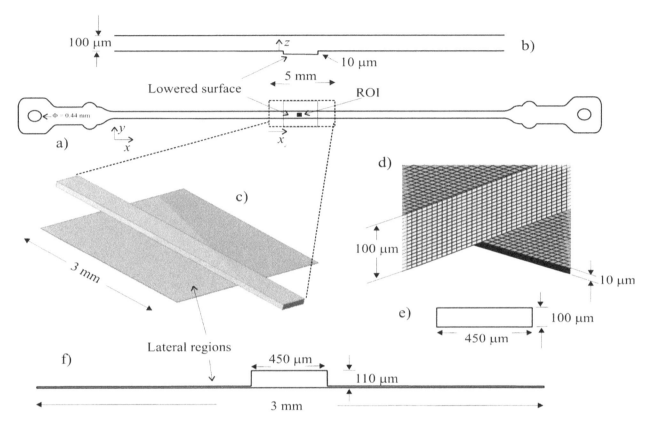

Figure 2. Microchannel representation and mesh details: (**a**) Microchannel, showing the lowered surface in grey, the region of interest in black and domain limits; (**b**) Profile representing the level of the upper and lower surfaces of the channel; (**c**) 3D representation of the numerical domain; (**d**) Lowered surface detail; (**e**) Microchannel cross-section outside the lowered region; (**f**) Cross-section available to the flow in the lowered surface region.

2.4. Bacteria and Culture Conditions

Escherichia coli JM109(DE3) was used, since this strain had already demonstrated a good adhesion capacity [33]. A starter culture was prepared as described by Teodosio, et al. [34] and incubated overnight. A volume of 60 mL from this culture was centrifuged (for 10 min at 3202× g) and the cells were washed twice with citrate buffer 0.05 M [35], pH 5.0. The pellet was then resuspended and diluted in the same buffer to obtain a cell concentration of 7.6×10^7 cell mL^{-1}.

2.5. Cell Adhesion Test

Cell adhesion tests with *E. coli* were performed with different polymer channels. Three trials were conducted for each material. The cell suspension was pumped using a syringe pump (Cetoni, neMESYS syringe pump, Korbussen, Germany) through a tygon® tube to the microfluidic channel. Adhesion was followed using a fluorescence inverted microscope (DMI 5000M, Leica Microsystems GmbH, Wetzlar, Germany) with a 40× objective. Microscopic images were captured with a CCD camera (Leica DFC350FX, Leica Microsystems GmbH, Wetzlar, Germany) with a time interval of 60 s. The image sequence obtained is in tiff format as recorded by Leica Application Suite software. The area of the region of interest was 312 × 233 μm^2. Initial adhesion experiments lasted for 1800 s.

2.6. Flow Conditions

The flow conditions studied are indicated in Table 2. With these conditions, the shear stress range is from 0.01 Pa to 1 Pa, covering the majority of shear stresses that can be found in the human body [36,37].

Table 2. Hydrodynamic conditions.

Flow Rate (μL/min)	Mean Velocity (m/s)	Reynolds Number	Nominal Wall Shear Stress (Equation (6)) (Pa)
0.667	2.50×10^{-4}	0.06	0.01
1.35	5.00×10^{-4}	0.12	0.02
15	5.56×10^{-3}	1.30	0.2
65.1	2.41×10^{-2}	5.65	1

2.7. Image Analysis

All the 30 images were imported to Image J software [38]. A low noise region was selected in the images using the crop tool. The images were converted from 8 bit to 32 bit to improve contrast. To set the scale for processing, the pixel aspect ratio was set to one. Depending on the images, they can be smoothed using the mean filter with 1 pixel as radius. Then, the background was subtracted with rolling ball radius ranging from 1 to 18 pixels. A light background was obtained with the *E. coli* cells bright and visible. The brightness and contrast were fine-tuned to get more accurate cell count. The threshold was adjusted, for the stack of images, to generate a black and white image containing black cells over a white background. Cells have a characteristic size range (from about 0.5 μm to 3 μm) and particles and noise outside the size range were filtered out. Then the cells were automatically counted. The image for $t = 0$ already shows some cells, since the first image is taken some minutes after the flow starts. The number of cells for $t = 0$ was subtract from the total of cells counted.

By observation of the images obtained it was possible to distinguish cells from other particles due the characteristic shape of *E. coli* and the progressive increase of the number of cells throughout the experiments. The automatic counting method was compared with manual counting and this comparison showed that the automatic counting was accurate.

2.8. Hydrophobicity Test

The surface hydrophobicity can be determined by the contact angle formed between a surface and a polar and apolar liquid drop [39]. In this work, the contact angles were determined automatically by the sessile drop method in a contact angle meter (OCA 15 Plus; Dataphysics, Filderstadt, Germany) using water, formamide and α-bromonaphtalene (Sigma-Aldrich Corporation, St. Louis, MI, USA) as reference liquids [40]. For each surface, at least 10 measurements with each liquid were performed at $25 \pm 2\,°C$.

According to van Oss [39], the total surface energy (γ^{TOT}) of a pure substance is the sum of the apolar Lifshitz-van der Waals components of the surface free energy (γ^{LW}) with the polar Lewis acid-base component (γ^{AB}):

$$\gamma^{TOT} = \gamma^{LW} + \gamma^{AB} \tag{1}$$

The polar AB component comprises the electron acceptor γ^{+} and electron donor γ^{-} parameters, and is given by:

$$\gamma^{AB} = 2\sqrt{\gamma^{+}\gamma^{-}} \tag{2}$$

The surface energy components of a solid surface (s) are obtained by measuring the contact angles (θ) with the three different liquids (l), with known surface tension components, followed by the simultaneous resolution of three equations of the type:

$$(1 + \cos\theta)\gamma_1 = 2\left(\sqrt{\gamma_s^{LW}\gamma_1^{LW}} + \sqrt{\gamma_s^+\gamma_1^-} + \sqrt{\gamma_s^-\gamma_1^+}\right) \tag{3}$$

The degree of surface hydrophobicity is expressed as the free energy of interaction (ΔG mJ·m^{-2}) between two entities of that surface immersed in a polar liquid (such as water (w) as a reference solvent). ΔG was calculated from the surface tension components of the interacting entities, using the equation:

$$\Delta G = -2\left(\sqrt{\gamma_s^{LW}} - \sqrt{\gamma_w^{LW}}\right)^2 + 4\left(\sqrt{\gamma_s^+\gamma_w^-} + \sqrt{\gamma_s^-\gamma_w^+} - \sqrt{\gamma_s^+\gamma_s^-} - \sqrt{\gamma_w^+\gamma_w^-}\right) \tag{4}$$

If the interaction between the two entities is stronger than the interaction of each entity with water, $\Delta G < 0$, the material is hydrophobic and if $\Delta G > 0$, the material is hydrophilic.

Additionally, the surface charge of each polymer was characterized through the zeta potential. Particle suspensions of each material [41] were prepared in order to measure the electrophoretic mobility, using a Nano Zetasizer (Malvern Instruments, Malvern, Worcestershire, UK).

2.9. Numerical Simulations

The flow in the cell was simulated by numerical methods to clarify the stability and the predictability of the flow patterns near the observation region. The microchannel used has a rectangular cross section of 450 × 100 µm and a length of 15 mm. The channel is represented in Figure 2a. In Figure 2a it is possible to observe the lowered surface represented in grey, the region of interest in black and the limits of the numerical domain. The inlet and outlet have a diameter (D_{in}) of 0.44 mm (represented in Figure 2a). A profile along the channel, showing the level of the lower and upper walls, is represented in Figure 2b.

A section of the microchannel, around the visualization region, was selected for simulation domain (Figure 2c). This region includes the lowered surface, which results from the fabrication method, where the region of interest is located. The length of the domain is 5 mm. The lowered surface has a length of 3 mm and a width of 3 mm. The lowered surface level is approximately 10 µm. The cross section available for flow in the lowered surface region is shown in Figure 2f. Outside the lowered region the cross section available for the flow is rectangular (Figure 2e). A detail of the mesh used is shown in Figure 2d.

The flow regime was determined by the Reynolds number based on the equivalent diameter of the channel:

$$Re = \frac{2\rho Q}{(W + H)\mu} \tag{5}$$

where ρ and μ are the density and viscosity of the fluid, respectively, Q the flow rate, W the width of the channel and H the depth of the channel.

Numerical values of the wall shear stress (WSS) are compared with data from the analytical solution for the flow in a parallel plate channel [42]:

$$\tau = \mu\frac{3Q}{2\left(\frac{H}{2}\right)^2 W} \tag{6}$$

Nominal wall shear stress, used to distinguish the experiments, was calculated through the analytical Equation (6). The real wall shear stress, as given by the numerical simulation, is slightly different.

The equation for the lowered surface can be corrected by the following equation:

$$\tau_{ls} = \tau \left(\frac{H}{H_{ls}} \right)^2 \tag{7}$$

where τ is the wall shear stress in the straight channel (outside the lowered surface) and H_{ls} the depth of the channel in the lowered surface section.

Numerical simulations were made with the commercial code Ansys Fluent CFD package (version 14.5) by solving Navier–Stokes equations. A model of the microchannel was built in Design Modeler 14.5 and was discretized into a grid of 278,000 cells by Meshing 14.5. The QUICK scheme [43] was used for the discretization of the momentum equations and the PRESTO! scheme for the discretization of the pressure terms. The velocity–pressure coupled equations were solved by the PISO algorithm [44]. The no slip boundary condition was considered for all the walls. Simulations were made in steady state mode until convergence. The properties of water (density and viscosity) at 37 °C were used.

Corrected numerical results were calculated by applying Equation (7). The value of τ used was the wall shear stress of a straight channel (without a lowered surface) previously obtained numerically.

3. Results

3.1. Hydrophobicity

The surface properties of the different materials fabricated are presented in Table 3. Results showed that PLLA, PDMS, PA and PS are hydrophobic surfaces ($\Delta G < 0$ mJ·m^{-2}) whereas PEO is hydrophilic ($\Delta G > 0$ mJ·m^{-2}). For illustration, water droplets are shown in Figure 3 for different materials. Additionally, the zeta potential results showed that all the polymers' surfaces have a negative charge. The range of surface characteristics assures that the procedure can be used to study a large range of surface parameters, a very important factor for bacterial adhesion studies, wherein it is desirable to cover the characteristics of all available materials used in medical or industrial applications.

Table 3. Surface properties of different materials.

Polymer Surface	Hydrophobicity ΔG (mJ·m^{-2})	Zeta Potential (mV)
PLLA	−65.32	−27.9
PDMS	−61.82	−29.3
PA	−37.58	−28.0
PEO	0.350	−11.0
PS	−49.56	−29.8

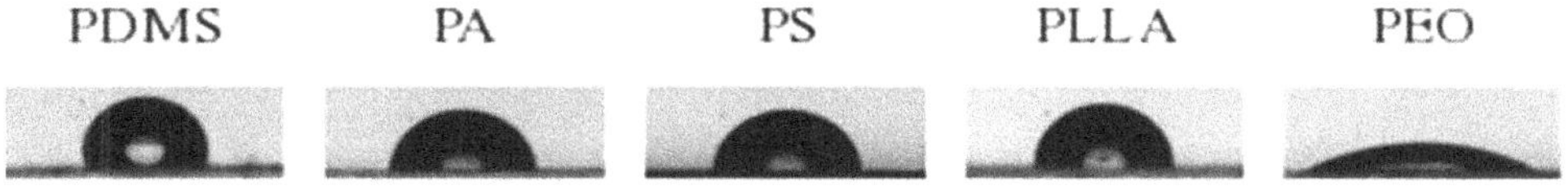

Figure 3. Water droplet over the surfaces of PDMS, PA, PS, poly-l-lactide acid (PLLA) and Polyethylene oxide (PEO) illustrating the hydrophobicity of the materials.

3.2. Adhesion

Adhesion tests were performed for all 5 materials cited in Table 3. A subset of the results obtained (for PS, PLLA and PDMS) is represented in Figure 4. The images show the surface after 1800 s assays and the processed images. Cells are visible in all three surfaces studied and so the images can be processed to obtain a clean image for cell counting. Adhesion data for the 1800 s of test are shown in Figure 5. The data show that different materials have distinct adhesion behaviour. A higher bacterial adhesion was observed on the PDMS surface during the 1800 s assay while a lower bacterial adhesion was observed on the PS surface. Additionally, it was observed that bacterial adhesion increases linearly with time. Additional results are shown for PA and PEO in Figures 6 and 7.

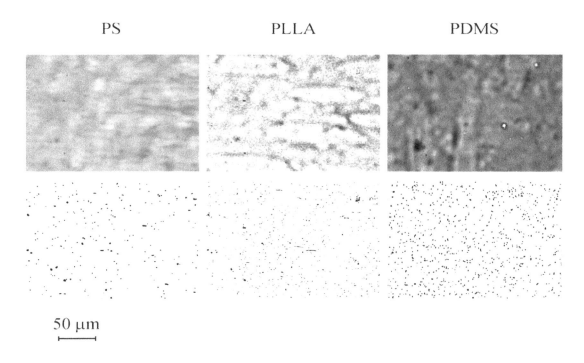

Figure 4. Images for adhesion in different materials for t = 1800 s: PS, PLLA and PDMS. Top row is before and bottom row after image processing. Results obtained for nominal wall shear stress of 0.02 Pa.

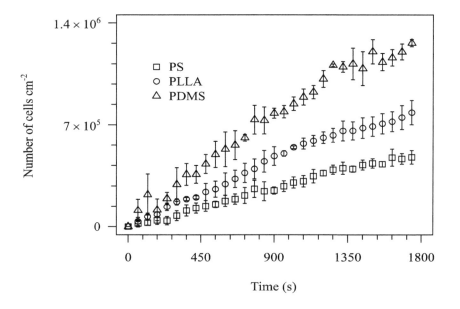

Figure 5. Number of adhered cells per cm^2 for PS, PLLA and PDMS for nominal wall shear stress of 0.02 Pa.

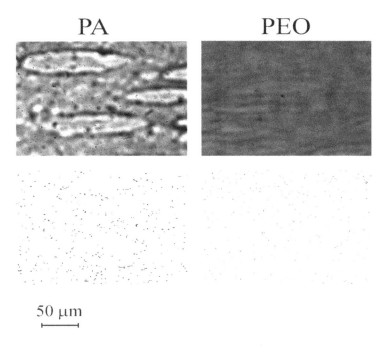

Figure 6. Images for adhesion in different materials for t = 1800 s: PA and PEO. Top row is before and bottom row after image processing. Results obtained for nominal wall shear stress of 0.01 Pa.

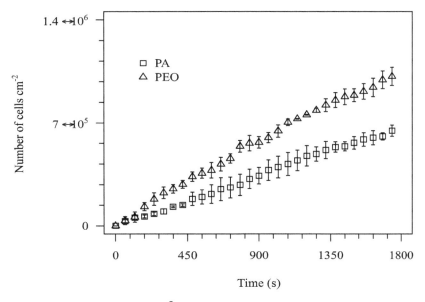

Figure 7. Number of adhered cells per cm^2 for PA and PEO for nominal wall shear stress of 0.01 Pa.

An experiment was performed to test if the unevenness of the channel can change significantly the adhesion rate. To achieve this goal, experiments were performed in a PDMS channel produced by the same fabrication method. First, a layer of PDMS was spincoated over a glass slide. Then, a scotch tape was used to protect a small region, as described in the methods section. Then, a second layer of PDMS was spincoated over the first one. The slide was then used to produce the channels. Figure 8 shows the bacterial cell density along the channel after 1800 s for three different shear stresses. As can be seen in the figure, the presence of a lowered surface in the scotch tape location is not perceptible. The variability of adhesion along the channel is much higher than any possible effect produced by the lowered surface.

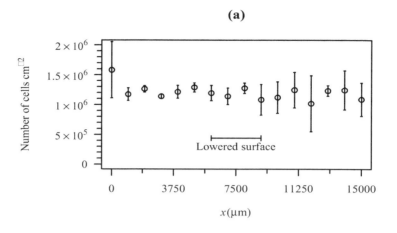

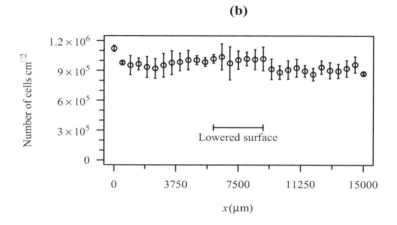

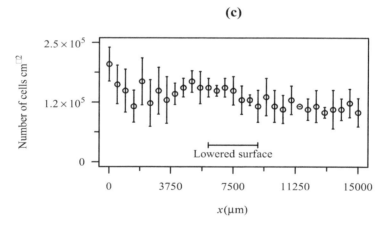

Figure 8. Cell density after 1800 s of adhesion on PDMS for three different nominal wall shear stresses. (**a**) WSS = 0.02 Pa; (**b**) WSS = 0.2 Pa; (**c**) WSS = 1 Pa.

3.3. Numerical Simulation

Wall shear stress (WSS) at the bottom wall and velocity fields at the midplan are represented in Figures 9 and 10, respectively. These figures show a small velocity decrease in the region of the channel crossing the lowered surface. Lateral regions (see Figure 2) of the lowered surface have an almost zero velocity. The wall shear stress is also smaller in the part of the channel that crosses the lowered surface region, where the region of interest is located.

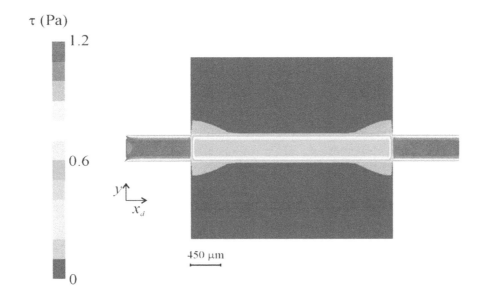

Figure 9. Wall shear stress (WSS) in the lowered surface region for a nominal wall shear stress of 1 Pa.

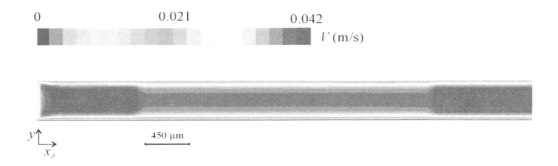

Figure 10. Velocity magnitude in the midplan in the lowered surface region for a nominal wall shear stress of 1 Pa.

Figure 11 shows the wall shear stress along the centreline of the bottom wall of the channel. The figure is for the higher nominal WSS studied (1 Pa), but results for the other wall shear stresses, not shown here, are similar. Some edge effects are observable, mainly due to the influence of the inlet and outlet boundary conditions. At the inlet, the edge effects are small, revealing that the flow develops in a short length, and enters fully developed in the lowered surface region. In this lowered region, the wall shear stress is smaller. A small transition region exists of about 300 μm.

The analytical Equation (6) underpredicts the numerical WSS data in the channel outside the lowered region. This result is expected since the analytical equation is exact only for channels with an infinite width. In the present case the ratio between the width and the height of the channel is 4.5, which implies that the velocity is higher than what would be in a channel with infinite width.

The correction—Equation (7)—made on the analytical equation underpredicts the WSS in the lowered surface, while the correction made to the numerical results predicts correctly the WSS in the lowered surface.

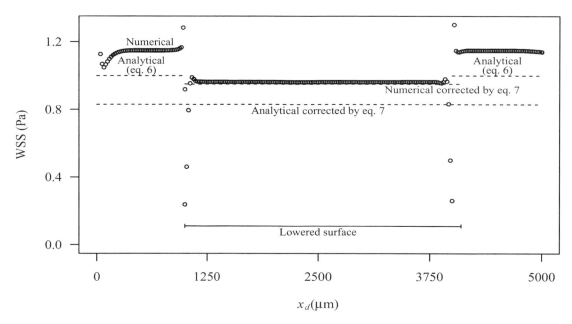

Figure 11. Wall shear stress along the centreline at the bottom surface in the lowered region for a nominal wall shear stress of 1 Pa. Figure shows numerical predictions (symbols), predictions based on analytical Equation (6) and predictions with corrections based on Equation (7). Local domain coordinates are used to represent the distance from the domain inlet.

4. Discussion

A technique developed to create microchannels with polymeric patches for adhesion tests allows the fabrication of patches with several different materials. Surface hydrophobicities of the materials used in this work, range from -65.32 to 0.350 mJ m^{-2} and zeta potential from -11.0 to -29.8 mV. From the bacterial adhesion results on five selected materials (PLLA, PDMS, PA, PEO and PS), it was verified that these different materials led to different adhesion behaviours. According to the thermodynamic theory, a higher bacterial adhesion would be expected on the most hydrophobic surface and a decrease would be expected with decreasing hydrophobicity [45]. A lower bacterial adhesion was in fact obtained in PS, the less hydrophobic surface. However, a higher number of adhered bacteria was observed in PDMS and not in the most hydrophobic surface, PLLA and PEO, which is hydrophilic, has a higher adhesion that PA, which is hydrophobic. Additionally, no correlation between bacterial adhesion and surface charge was found. Although it was verified that bacterial adhesion was not controlled by surface hydrophobicity or charge, other specific parameters of each surface, such as chemical composition, may have affected bacterial adhesion. The effect of surface properties may also be concealed by the flow conditions. The results presented in this paper are for WSS of 0.01–0.02 Pa and low Reynolds number, for which cell sedimentation has relevant contribution to cell adhesion. These results show that different materials, with different properties, were in fact placed in a specific position in the microchannel and induce different bacterial adhesion.

One of the inherent weaknesses of the method is the fact that a region of the microchannel is lowered, i.e., there is a small gap of about 10 μm in the edges of this region. The tests performed with PDMS surfaces (Figure 8) for wall shear stresses between 0.02 Pa and 1 Pa show that the lowered surface does not influence adhesion. Hydrodynamic consequences of this lowered surface were studied in detail by CFD. The CFD study shows that the region has a smaller WSS. Nevertheless, the WSS in this region is stable and calculable by Equation (7). Overall, the results obtained showed that the device performs predictably in adhesion tests and can be adopted for general use in routine tests.

The accuracy of the channels obtained by the current procedure is limited by the accuracy of the underlying microfabrication technique. In the current work the channels were fabricated by xurography, which has an error of approximately 5% to produce channels of 450 μm width [46].

5. Conclusions

A new low-cost device for adhesion tests in polymeric surfaces, which can be fabricated in a laboratory with low resources, was developed and characterized. The most expensive equipment used in the fabrication procedure is a spin coater. The fabrication method is suitable to produce microchannels to test bacterial adhesion in different materials, provided that the material is available as a transparent substrate or that the material is a spincoatable transparent polymer that can be casted by solvent evaporation.

The section of the channel containing the region of interest is lowered. However, this lowered surface has a predictable effect on wall shear stress and a negligible one on bacterial adhesion, as shown by adhesion tests and CFD.

The device was validated to be used to perform bacterial adhesion tests under relevant shear stresses. This work contributes to increase the options for experimenters to perform adhesion tests in microfluidic devices, with advantages related to reactant consumption and parallelization.

Author Contributions: J.P. conducted the experimental work and data processing and wrote the first draft of the paper. J.M.R.M. prepared the cell suspensions and contributed to the hydrophobicity tests. F.J.M. supervised the biological component of the work. J.B.L.M.C. contributed to computational fluid dynamics component of the work. J.M.M. conducted the numerical simulations and supervised the microfluidics component of the work. All authors read the paper and added contributions for improvements.

References

1. McCoy, W.F.; Bryers, J.D.; Robbins, J.; Costerton, J.W. Observations of Fouling Biofilm Formation. *Can. J. Microbiol.* **1981**, *27*, 910–917. [CrossRef]

2. Donlan, R.M. Biofilms: Microbial Life on Surfaces. *Emerg. Infect. Dis.* **2002**, *8*, 881–890. [CrossRef] [PubMed]

3. Costerton, J.W.; Stewart, P.S.; Greenberg, E.P. Bacterial Biofilms: A Common Cause of Persistent Infections. *Science* **1999**, *284*, 1318–1322. [CrossRef]

4. Harris, L.G.; Richards, R.G. Staphylococci and Implant Surfaces: A Review. *Injury* **2006**, *37* (Suppl. 2), S3–S14. [CrossRef] [PubMed]

5. Kong, K.F.; Vuong, C.; Otto, M. Staphylococcus Quorum Sensing in Biofilm Formation and Infection. *Int. J. Med. Microbiol. IJMM* **2006**, *296*, 133–139. [CrossRef] [PubMed]

6. Arciola, C.R.; Campoccia, D.; Speziale, P.; Montanaro, L.; Costerton, J.W. Biofilm Formation in Staphylococcus Implant Infections. A Review of Molecular Mechanisms and Implications for Biofilm-Resistant Materials. *Biomaterials* **2012**, *33*, 5967–5982. [CrossRef]

7. Bjarnsholt, T.; Alhede, M.; Alhede, M.; Eickhardt-Sorensen, S.R.; Moser, C.; Kuhl, M.; Jensen, P.O.; Hoiby, N. The in Vivo Biofilm. *Trends Microbiol.* **2013**, *21*, 466–474. [CrossRef] [PubMed]

8. Seth, A.K.; Geringer, M.R.; Hong, S.J.; Leung, K.P.; Mustoe, T.A.; Galiano, R.D. In Vivo Modeling of Biofilm-Infected Wounds: A Review. *J. Surg. Res.* **2012**, *178*, 330–338. [CrossRef] [PubMed]

9. Esposito, S.; Purrello, S.M.; Bonnet, E.; Novelli, A.; Tripodi, F.; Pascale, R.; Unal, S.; Milkovich, G. Central Venous Catheter-Related Biofilm Infections: An Up-To-Date Focus on Meticillin-Resistant Staphylococcus Aureus. *J. Glob. Antimicrob. Resist.* **2013**, *1*, 71–78. [CrossRef] [PubMed]

10. Middleton, J.C.; Tipton, A.J. Synthetic Biodegradable Polymers as Orthopedic Devices. *Biomaterials* **2000**, *21*, 2335–2346. [CrossRef]

11. Abu-Lail, N.I.; Beyenal, H. Chapter 5.2—Characterization of Bacteria–Biomaterial Interactions, from a Single Cell to Biofilms. In *Characterization of Biomaterials*; Bandyopadhyay, A., Bose, S., Eds.; Academic Press: Oxford, OH, USA, 2013; pp. 207–253.

12. Dillow, A.K.; Tirrell, M. Targeted Cellular Adhesion at Biomaterial Interfaces. *Curr. Opin. Solid State Mater. Sci.* **1998**, *3*, 252–259. [CrossRef]

13. Ramakrishna, S.; Mayer, J.; Wintermantel, E.; Leong, K.W. Biomedical Applications of Polymer-Composite Materials: A Review. *Compos. Sci. Technol.* **2001**, *61*, 1189–1224. [CrossRef]

14. Meng, B.; Wang, J.; Zhu, N.; Meng, Q.Y.; Cui, F.Z.; Xu, Y.X. Study of Biodegradable and Self-Expandable Plla Helical Biliary Stent in Vivo and in Vitro. *J. Mater. Sci. Mater. Med.* **2006**, *17*, 611–617. [CrossRef] [PubMed]

15. Tamai, H.; Igaki, K.; Kyo, E.; Kosuga, K.; Kawashima, A.; Matsui, S.; Komori, H.; Tsuji, T.; Motohara, S.; Uehata, H. Initial and 6-Month Results of Biodegradable Poly-l-Lactic Acid Coronary Stents in Humans. *Circulation* **2000**, *102*, 399–404. [CrossRef]

16. Colvin, A.; Sharma, C.; Parides, M.; Glashow, J. What is the Best Femoral Fixation of Hamstring Autografts in Anterior Cruciate Ligament Reconstruction?: A Meta-Analysis. *Clin. Orthop. Relat. Res.* **2011**, *469*, 1075–1081. [CrossRef] [PubMed]

17. Beebe, D.J.; Mensing, G.A.; Walker, G.M. Physics and Applications of Microfluidics in Biology. *Annu. Rev. Biomed. Eng.* **2002**, *4*, 261–286. [CrossRef]

18. Jain, K.K. *Biochips and Microarrays: Technology and Commercial Potential*; Urch Publishing: London, UK, 2000.

19. Stone, H.A.; Stroock, A.D.; Ajdari, A. Engineering Flows in Small Devices Microfluidics Towards Lab-On-A-Chip. *Annu. Rev. Fluid Mech.* **2004**, *36*, 381–411. [CrossRef]

20. Duffy, D.C.; McDonald, J.C.; Schueller, O.J.; Whitesides, G.M. Rapid Prototyping of Microfluidic Systems in Poly (Dimethylsiloxane). *Anal. Chem.* **1998**, *70*, 4974–4984. [CrossRef] [PubMed]

21. Blanco, F.J.; Agirregabiria, M.; Garcia, J.; Berganzo, J.; Tijero, M.; Arroyo, M.T.; Ruano, J.M.; Aramburu, I.; Mayora, K. Novel Three-Dimensional Embedded Su-8 Microchannels Fabricated Using a Low Temperature Full Wafer Adhesive Bonding. *J. Micromech. Microeng.* **2004**, *14*, 1047–1056. [CrossRef]

22. Che-Hsin, L.; Gwo-Bin, L.; Bao-Wen, C.; Guan-Liang, C. A New Fabrication Process for Ultra-Thick Microfluidic Microstructures Utilizing Su-8 Photoresist. *J. Micromech. Microeng.* **2002**, *12*, 590.

23. Tseng, A.A. Recent Developments in Micromilling Using Focused Ion Beam Technology. *J. Micromech. Microeng.* **2004**, *14*, R15–R34. [CrossRef]

24. Schlautmann, S.; Wensink, H.; Schasfoort, R.; Elwenspoek, M.; Van Den Berg, A. Powder-Blasting Technology as an Alternative Tool for Microfabrication of Capillary Electrophoresis Chips with Integrated Conductivity Sensors. *J. Micromech. Microeng.* **2001**, *11*, 386–389. [CrossRef]

25. Becker, H.; Heim, U. Hot Embossing as a Method for the Fabrication of Polymer High Aspect Ratio Structures. *Sens. Actuators A Phys.* **2000**, *83*, 130–135. [CrossRef]

26. Morales, A.M.; Lieber, C.M. A Laser Ablation Method for the Synthesis of Crystalline Semiconductor Nanowires. *Science* **1998**, *279*, 208–211. [CrossRef]

27. Ikuta, K.; Hirowatari, K. In Real Three Dimensional Micro Fabrication Using Stereo Lithography and Metal Molding. In Proceedings of the IEEE Micro Electro Mechanical Systems, Fort Lauderdale, FL, USA, 7–10 February 1993; pp. 42–47.

28. Bartholomeusz, D.A.; Boutte, R.W.; Andrade, J.D. Xurography: Rapid Prototyping of Microstructures Using a Cutting Plotter. *J. Microelectromech. Syst.* **2005**, *14*, 1364–1374. [CrossRef]

29. Xia, Y.; Whitesides, G.M. Soft Lithography. *Annu. Rev. Mater. Sci.* **1998**, *28*, 153–184. [CrossRef]

30. Eddings, M.A.; Johnson, M.A.; Gale, B.K. Determining the Optimal Pdms–Pdms Bonding Technique for Microfluidic Devices. *J. Micromech. Microeng.* **2008**, *18*, 067001. [CrossRef]

31. Zhang, W.; Ferguson, G.; Tatic-Lucic, S. Elastomer-Supported Cold Welding for Room Temperature Wafer-Level Bonding. In Proceedings of the 17th IEEE International Conference on MEMS, Maastricht, The Netherlands, 25–29 January 2004; pp. 741–744.

32. Koschwanez, J.H.; Carlson, R.H.; Meldrum, D.R. Thin Pdms Films Using Long Spin Times or Tert-Butyl Alcohol as a Solvent. *PLoS ONE* **2009**, *4*, e4572. [CrossRef] [PubMed]

33. Moreira, J.M.; Araujo, J.D.; Miranda, J.M.; Simoes, M.; Melo, L.F.; Mergulhao, F.J. The Effects of Surface Properties on Escherichia Coli Adhesion are Modulated by Shear Stress. *Coll. Surf. B Biointerfaces* **2014**, *123*, 1–7. [CrossRef] [PubMed]

34. Teodosio, J.S.; Simoes, M.; Melo, L.F.; Mergulhao, F.J. Flow Cell Hydrodynamics and Their Effects on E. Coli Biofilm Formation under Different Nutrient Conditions and Turbulent Flow. *Biofouling* **2011**, *27*, 1–11. [CrossRef] [PubMed]

35. Simoes, M.; Simoes, L.C.; Cleto, S.; Pereira, M.O.; Vieira, M.J. The Effects of a Biocide and a Surfactant on the Detachment of Pseudomonas Fluorescens from Glass Surfaces. *Int. J. Food Microbiol.* **2008**, *121*, 335–341. [CrossRef] [PubMed]

36. Ronald, L.S. *Analysis of Pathoadaptive Mutations in Escherichia Coli*; ProQuest: Michigan, MI, USA, 2008.

37. Michelson, A. *Platelets*, 2nd ed.; Academic Press: Cambridge, MA, USA, 2002.

38. Schneider, C.A.; Rasband, W.S.; Eliceiri, K.W. Nih Image to Imagej: 25 Years of Image Analysis. *Nat. Methods* **2012**, *9*, 671–675. [CrossRef]

39. Van Oss, C. *Interfacial Forces in Aqueous Media*; Marcel Dekker Inc.: New York, NY, USA, 1994.

40. Janczuk, B.; Chibowski, E.; Bruque, J.M.; Kerkeb, M.L.; Caballero, F.G. On the Consistency of Surface Free-Energy Components as Calculated from Contact Angles of Different Liquids—An Application to the Cholesterol Surface. *J. Colloid Interface Sci.* **1993**, *159*, 421–428. [CrossRef]

41. Simoes, L.C.; Simoes, M.; Vieira, M.J. Adhesion and Biofilm Formation on Polystyrene by Drinking Water-Isolated Bacteria. *Antonie Van Leeuwenhoek* **2010**, *98*, 317–329. [CrossRef]

42. Busscher, H.J.; Van Der Mei, H.C. Microbial Adhesion in Flow Displacement Systems. *Clin. Microbiol. Rev.* **2006**, *19*, 127–141. [CrossRef]

43. Leonard, B.P. A Stable and Accurate Convective Modelling Procedure Based on Quadratic Upstream Interpolation. *Comput. Methods Appl. Mech. Eng.* **1979**, *19*, 59–98. [CrossRef]

44. Issa, R.I. Solution of the Implicitly Discutised Fluid Flow Equations by Operating-Splitting. *J. Comput. Phys.* **1986**, *62*, 40–65. [CrossRef]

45. Absolom, D.R.; Lamberti, F.V.; Policova, Z.; Zingg, W.; Van Oss, C.J.; Neumann, A.W. Surface Thermodynamics of Bacterial Adhesion. *Appl. Environ. Microbiol.* **1983**, *46*, 90–97.

46. Pinto, E.; Faustino, V.; Rodrigues, R.; Pinho, D.; Garcia, V.; Miranda, J.; Lima, R. A Rapid and Low-Cost Nonlithographic Method to Fabricate Biomedical Microdevices for Blood Flow Analysis. *Micromachines* **2015**, *6*, 121–135. [CrossRef]

9

Experimental Investigation of Air Compliance Effect on Measurement of Mechanical Properties of Blood Sample Flowing in Microfluidic Channels

Yang Jun Kang[ORCID]

Department of Mechanical Engineering, Chosun University, 309 Pilmun-daero, Dong-gu, Gwangju 61452, Korea; yjkang2011@chosun.ac.kr

Abstract: Air compliance has been used effectively to stabilize fluidic instability resulting from a syringe pump. It has also been employed to measure blood viscosity under constant shearing flows. However, due to a longer time delay, it is difficult to quantify the aggregation of red blood cells (RBCs) or blood viscoelasticity. To quantify the mechanical properties of blood samples (blood viscosity, RBC aggregation, and viscoelasticity) effectively, it is necessary to quantify contributions of air compliance to dynamic blood flows in microfluidic channels. In this study, the effect of air compliance on measurement of blood mechanical properties was experimentally quantified with respect to the air cavity in two driving syringes. Under periodic on–off blood flows, three mechanical properties of blood samples were sequentially obtained by quantifying microscopic image intensity ($<I>$) and interface (α) in a co-flowing channel. Based on a differential equation derived with a fluid circuit model, the time constant was obtained by analyzing the temporal variations of $\beta = 1/(1-\alpha)$. According to experimental results, the time constant significantly decreased by securing the air cavity in a reference fluid syringe (~0.1 mL). However, the time constant increased substantially by securing the air cavity in a blood sample syringe (~0.1 mL). Given that the air cavity in the blood sample syringe significantly contributed to delaying transient behaviors of blood flows, it hindered the quantification of RBC aggregation and blood viscoelasticity. In addition, it was impossible to obtain the viscosity and time constant when the blood flow rate was not available. Thus, to measure the three aforementioned mechanical properties of blood samples effectively, the air cavity in the blood sample syringe must be minimized ($V_{air, R} = 0$). Concerning the air cavity in the reference fluid syringe, it must be sufficiently secured about $V_{air, R} = 0.1$ mL for regulating fluidic instability because it does not affect dynamic blood flows.

Keywords: air compliance effect; RBC aggregation; blood viscosity; blood viscoelasticity; blood velocity fields; interface in co-flowing streams; microfluidic device

1. Introduction

A blood sample is composed of cells (i.e., red blood cells (RBCs), white blood cells, and platelets) and plasma. Given that the number of RBCs is much larger than that of the other cells, RBCs have a significant role in determining mechanical properties of blood samples (viscosity, deformability, and aggregation). In addition, plasma proteins substantially contribute to increasing aggregation. Since a strong relationship between cardiovascular diseases and mechanical properties of blood samples was reported [1–4], mechanical properties of blood samples have been suggested as label-free biomarkers for early detection of cardiovascular diseases.

In contrast with bulky viscometers [5,6], a microfluidic-based device can provide numerous advantages including fast response, small volume consumption, and disposability. Currently, such devices are widely employed for quantifying mechanical properties of blood samples (viscosity [7–10], RBC aggregation [11–14], RBC deformability [3,15], and hematocrit (Hct) [16–18]). A microfluidic device has been also employed to separate RBCs or tumor cells from whole blood sample [19–21].

In microfluidic environments, blood flows must remain unchanged over time to measure blood viscosity accurately. However, during the process of supplying a blood sample into a microfluidic device, the syringe pump causes fluidic instability at low flow rates [22]. To stabilize unstable flows resulting from the syringe pump, several techniques including air cavity in a driving syringe [23] or microfluidic channel [24,25], portable air cavity unit [22,26], and flexible compliance unit [27–32], were demonstrated in microfluidic systems. These methods act on the compliance element in the fluidic circuit model. The compliance was defined as $C = \Delta V/\Delta P$. Here, ΔV and ΔP represents variations of volume and pressure, respectively. This contributes to regulating alternating components and increasing the time constant. Thus, they contribute to removing alternating components of blood flows. Owing to the compliance effect, the fluidic flow remains constant over time. Additionally, the compliance effect tends to delay transient blood flows significantly. Among the aforementioned methods, an air cavity secured inside the syringe is simple and effective because it does not require additional devices. In other words, a disposable syringe (~1 mL) is partially filled with a blood sample (~lower layer) and an air cavity (~upper layer), respectively. Then, the syringe is placed into a syringe pump. Given that the air cavity secured inside the syringe contributes to damping out fluidic fluctuations resulting from the syringe pump [22], the blood flows remain constant over time in the microfluidic channel.

Blood viscosity is measured with a microfluidic device under constant shearing flow condition. After a blood sample and a reference fluid are infused into the microfluidic device at the same flow rate, blood viscosity can be quantified by monitoring the interface in co-flowing streams [8,10]. RBC aggregation is obtained by quantifying the microscopic image intensity of the blood sample under periodic on-off fashion or transient fluidic flows [33,34]. Owing to RBC aggregation in blood samples, the image intensity tends to increase after the blood flow stops suddenly. However, the air cavity secured inside the disposable syringe (i.e., air compliance) has an influence on transient behaviors of blood flows. When turning the syringe pump off suddenly, it takes a longer time to stop blood flows because of the air-compliance effect. Within a specific duration, the blood flow rate does not decrease to sufficiently lower shear rates where RBC aggregation occurs. Thus, it is impossible to quantify RBC aggregation. A simple method to resolve this issue is a pinch valve to stop blood flows immediately [35]. A time constant defining blood viscoelasticity can be obtained by monitoring the interface in co-flowing streams under periodic transient blood flows [33,36]. In other words, after turning the syringe pump off, a time constant is obtained by analyzing the transient behavior of blood flows (i.e., blood velocity). However, when a pinch valve is used to stop blood flows immediately, it is impossible to obtain the time constant throughout transient variations of blood flows. Although air compliance is used effectively for measuring blood viscosity, it hinders the quantification of RBC aggregation or blood viscoelasticity. To quantify the mechanical properties of blood samples (i.e., blood viscosity, RBC aggregation, and viscoelasticity) effectively, it is necessary to quantify contributions of air compliance to dynamic blood flows in microfluidic channels.

In this study, the air compliance effect on measurement of blood mechanical properties was quantified experimentally with respect to the air cavity in two driving syringes. To measure the three aforementioned mechanical properties of the blood sample (i.e., blood viscosity, RBC aggregation, and viscoelasticity), both the blood sample and the reference fluid were filled with individual syringes. The air cavity inside each syringe set a certain volume ranging from 0 to 0.2 mL. After placing them into syringe pumps, the blood sample and reference fluid were infused into a microfluidic channel. The flow rate of the reference fluid remained constant over time. The flow rate of the blood sample was controlled by turning the syringe pump on or off periodically. Three mechanical properties of the blood sample were obtained sequentially by quantifying the microscopic image intensity of the blood sample and the interface between the two fluids flowing in a co-flowing channel, respectively.

As a demonstration, the time constants of test fluids (i.e., blood sample and glycerin (20%)) were first obtained by varying the air cavity in the reference fluid syringe for up to 0.2 mL. Second, variations of the time constant were obtained with respect to Hct = 30%, 40%, and 50%. Finally, to stimulate RBC aggregation, a blood sample (Hct = 50%) was prepared by adding normal RBCs into different diluents (i.e., 1× PBS (phosphate-buffered saline), plasma, and two dextran solutions). The effect of air compliance on the three mechanical properties of blood samples considered was evaluated by varying the air cavity secured in each syringe (~0.1 mL).

2. Materials and Methods

2.1. Blood Sample Preparation

The Ethics Committee of Chosun University Hospital (CHOSUN 2018-05-11) approved all experimental protocols conducted for this study. Such protocols were deemed appropriate and humane. Gwangju–Chonnam blood bank (Gwangju, Korea) provided concentrated RBCs and fresh frozen plasma (FFP). After conducting washing procedures with a centrifuge twice, pure RBCs were collected from the concentrated RBCs. Additionally, plasma was prepared by thawing FFP at a room temperature of 25 °C. To evaluate the three considered mechanical properties of blood sample with respect to air cavity, various blood samples were prepared by changing hematocrit or diluent. First, to evaluate the contributions of hematocrit or diluent to the time constant (or viscoelasticity), the hematocrit of blood sample was adjusted to Hct = 30%, 40%, and 50% by adding normal RBCs into the diluent (i.e., 1× phosphate-buffered saline (PBS), and plasma). Second, to stimulate RBC aggregation in blood samples, a specific concentration of dextran solution was added into 1× PBS. Dextran powder (*Leuconostoc* spp., MW = 450–650 kDa, Sigma–Aldrich, St. Louis, MO, USA) was diluted with 1× PBS. A blood sample (Hct = 50%) was prepared by adding normal RBCs into two dextran solutions (5, and 10 mg/mL).

2.2. Microfluidic Device and Experimental Setup

As shown in Figure 1A-a, a microfluidic device consisted of two inlets (a, b), one outlet, and two guiding channels (test fluid channel (TC, width (W) = 1000 μm), reference fluid channel (RC, width (W) = 100 μm)), and co-flowing channel (CC, width (W) = 1000 μm). To increase blood volume flowing in test channel, channel depth was set to h = 100 μm if available under micro-electromechanical-system technique (MEMS) fabrication. A four-inch sized silicon mold was fabricated using the MEMS techniques (i.e., photolithography and deep reactive ion etching). Polymer PDMS (polydimethylsiloxane) (Sylgard 184, Dow Corning, Midland, MI, USA) and a curing agent were mixed at a ratio of 10:1. Mixed PDMS was poured onto the silicon mold. After letting it solidify into a convective oven (70 °C for 1 h), the cured PDMS was peeled off from the mold. Two inlets (a, b) and one outlet were punched with a biopsy punch (outer diameter = 0.5 mm). Using an oxygen plasma system (CUTE-MPR, Femto Science Co., Hwaseong-si, South Korea), the PDMS block was strongly bonded to the glass slide.

To squeeze out the air bubble inside the microfluidic channels and avoid adherence of RBCs to the channels, microfluidic channels were filled with a bovine serum albumin of 2 mg/mL through the outlet. After an elapse of 10 min, the microfluidic channels were filled again with 1× PBS. As shown in Figure 1A-b, a reference fluid syringe was filled with 1× PBS (~0.5 mL) and air cavity ($V_{air, R}$), respectively. Likewise, a test fluid syringe was filled with a test fluid (~0.5 mL) and air cavity ($V_{air, T}$), respectively. To supply the reference fluid into the reference fluid channel, a polyethylene tubing (length = 300 mm, inner diameter = 0.25 mm, and thickness= 0.25 mm) was connected from a syringe needle to inlet (a). To infuse the test fluid into the blood sample channel, a polyethylene tubing (length = 300 mm, inner diameter = 0.25 mm, and thickness = 0.25 mm) was connected from a syringe needle to inlet (b). To collect both samples from the co-flowing channel, a polyethylene tubing (length = 200 mm, inner diameter = 0.25 mm, and thickness = 0.25 mm) was fitted tightly into the outlet. Using two syringe pumps (neMESYS, Cetoni Gmbh, Korbussen, Germany), the reference fluid was infused at a constant flow rate of $Q_R = Q_0$. The test fluid was supplied at periodic on-off fashion (period (T) = 240 s, duty ratio = 0.5, and $Q_T = Q_0$). A microfluidic device was placed on an optical inverted microscope (BX51, Olympus, Tokyo, Japan) equipped with a 10× objective lens (NA = 0.25). A high-speed camera (FASTCAM MINI, Photron, Tokyo, Japan) captured two microscopic images sequentially at a frame rate of 500 fps. The image acquisition continued at an interval of 0.5 s with a function generator. All experiments were conducted at a temperature of 25 °C.

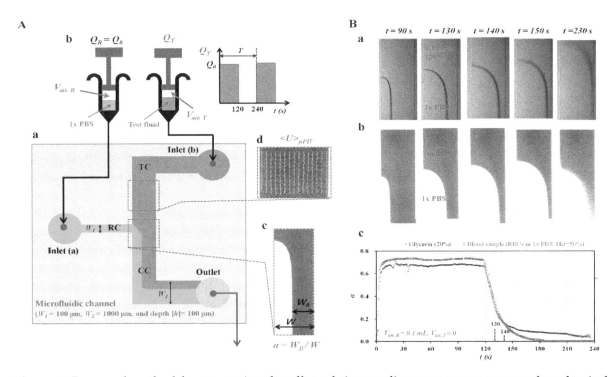

Figure 1. Proposed method for measuring the effect of air compliance on measurement of mechanical properties of blood samples flowing in microfluidic channels. (**A**) Schematic diagram of experimental setup including a microfluidic device, two syringe pumps, and an image acquisition system. (a) A microfluidic device comprising two inlets (a, b), one outlet, two guiding channels for two fluids (reference channel (RC), test channel (TC)), and a co-flowing channel (CC). (b) Two syringe pumps for delivering reference fluid and test fluid. (c) The interface in the co-flowing channel was quantified as $\alpha = W_B/W$. (d) Velocity fields of blood flows obtained with a micro-particle image velocimetry (PIV) technique. (**B**) As a preliminary demonstration, a blood sample (normal red blood cells (RBCs) in 1× phosphate-buffered saline (PBS), hematocrit (Hct) = 50%) and glycerin (20%) as a test fluid were prepared to show temporal variations of α. (a) Microscopic images of a blood sample and 1× PBS flowing in the co-flowing channel at specific time instants (t = 90, 130, 140, 150, and 230 s). (b) Microscopic images of glycerin (20%) and 1× PBS flowing in the co-flowing channel at specific time instants (t = 90, 130, 140, 150, and 230 s). (c) Temporal variations of α with respect to the blood sample and glycerin (20%).

2.3. Quantification of Interface, Velocity Fields, and Image Intensity

The right side panel in Figure 1A-c shows a microscopic image taken for estimating the interface in a co-flowing channel. A specific region-of-interest (ROI, 240 × 200 pixels) was selected within a straight region of the co-flowing channel. Using MATLAB 2019 (MathWorks, Natick, MA, USA), the blood-filled width (W_B) over the ROI was estimated with Otsu's method [37]. The interface in the co-flowing channel (α) was defined as $\alpha = W_B/W$. As shown in Figure 1A-d, the velocity fields of the blood sample in the test fluid channel were obtained with a micro-particle image velocimetry (PIV) technique [38]. A specific ROI (240×200 pixels) was selected within the test fluid channel. The size of the interrogation window was 32×32 pixels. The window overlap was 50%. The velocity fields within ROI were validated with a local median filter. The average velocity ($<U>_{\mu PIV}$) was obtained by averaging the velocity fields over the ROI. To evaluate the RBC aggregation of the blood sample, the microscopic image intensity of the blood sample flowing in the test fluid channel was quantified with digital image processing. As shown on the right side channel, a specific ROI (240×200 pixels) was selected within the test fluid channel. An average image intensity ($<I>$) was obtained by averaging the image intensities distributed over the ROI.

As a preliminary demonstration, three properties of blood sample (i.e., blood viscosity, RBC aggregation, and viscoelasticity) were quantified by analyzing interface in coflowing channel (α) and image intensity of blood flows in test channel ($<I>$), respectively. A blood sample (normal RBCs suspended in 1× PBS, Hct = 50%) and glycerin (20%) as the test fluid were prepared to show temporal variations of the interface (α) depending on the air cavity in a syringe. Two syringes were filled with the test fluid (~0.5 mL) and reference fluid (~0.5 mL), respectively. Then, the air cavity in the reference fluid syringe was set to 0.1 mL. The air cavity in the test fluid syringe was set to zero. Furthermore, 1× PBS as reference fluid was injected at a constant flow rate of Q_0 =1 mL/h. The test fluid was injected in a periodic on-off fashion (T = 240 s, duty ratio = 0.5, and Q_0 =1 mL/h). Figure 1B-a,b show microscopic images of two test fluids (i.e., blood sample and glycerin (20%)) at specific time instants (t = 90, 130, 140, 150, and 230 s). When capturing microscopic images as shown in Figure 1B-b, light intensity increases significantly in order to clearly see RBCs flowing in the test channel. After turning off the syringe pump of the test fluid at t =120 s, the blood-filled width (W_B) tended to decrease over time. Figure 1B-c shows temporal variations of the obtained α with respect to blood sample and glycerin (20%), respectively. Under the constant blood flow condition (i.e., $t < 120$ s), the value of α of the blood sample was higher than that of glycerin (20%). Under the transient flow condition (i.e., 120 s < $t < 240$ s), the value of α of the blood sample took longer to reach a constant value compared with glycerin (20%). After turning on the syringe pump for the blood sample, the blood flow rate and interface (α) remained constant after an elapse of time constant. Blood viscosity was then quantified with the information of the interface. After an elapse of a half period, the syringe pump for the blood sample was set to turn off. The interface decreased substantially over time. After an elapse of the time constant, RBC aggregation occurred and contributed to increasing image intensity of the blood sample. RBC aggregation was then obtained by analyzing temporal variations of image intensity. In other words, blood viscosity and RBC aggregation were obtained at a constant flow rate and extremely low flow rate, respectively. Thus, to measure both properties effectively, it was necessary to secure sufficient duration of constant flow rate and stationary flow rate under periodic on–off operation of the syringe pump. In other words, time constant should remain much smaller than half period. Air compliance was used widely to eliminate fluidic instability resulting from the syringe pump. However, the air compliance tended to increase time constant substantially. When turning on syringe pump (i.e., $0 < t < 0.5\ T$), the air cavity (~0.1 mL) inside syringe did not arrive at a constant value of β. When turning off the syringe pump (i.e., $0.5\ T < t < T$), β decreased gradually over time. The longer time constant made it difficult to quantify both properties of blood samples. As air compliance hindered in quantifying blood viscosity and RBC aggregation, it is necessary to minimize the time constant by removing the air cavity in the blood syringe pump and securing the air cavity in reference syringe. Thus, the dynamic behavior of two fluids (i.e., time constant) should be considered as a significant factor for effectively quantifying blood viscosity and RBC aggregation under periodic on–off blood flow condition.

3. Results and Discussion

3.1. Variations of Time Constant with Respect to Air Cavity in Reference Fluid Syringe

According to previous studies [22,23,26,29], air compliance was widely used to stabilize fluidic instability resulting from syringe pumps. In this study, a reference fluid was injected at a constant flow rate with a syringe pump. However, the air cavity in the reference fluid syringe might have an influence on the dynamic variation of the interface in co-flowing channels. For this reason, it was necessary to evaluate the contributions of the air cavity in the reference fluid syringe to time constants of the interface in co-flowing channels. The air cavity in the reference fluid syringe was set to $V_{air,\,R} = 0$, 0.1, and 0.2 mL. To separate the effect of the air cavity in the test fluid syringe, such a cavity was set to zero ($V_{air,\,T} = 0$). Blood samples (normal RBCs suspended in 1× PBS, Hct = 50%) and glycerin (20%) were prepared as test fluids.

To model the contribution of the air cavity in the syringe to interface, it was required to derive a governing equation for two fluids flowing in a co-flowing channel. As shown in Figure 2A, a fluidic circuit model for two fluids (reference fluid and test fluid) flowing in a co-flowing channel was constructed with discrete circuit elements (i.e., flow rate elements: Q_R, Q_T, resistance elements: R_R, R_T, and compliance element: C_T). Here, C_T denotes the compliance element that was combined with flexible tubing, a microfluidic channel, and an air cavity in the syringe. Additionally, ground (▼) represents pressure set to zero. To keep the mathematical model simple, the interface in the co-flowing channel was modeled as a virtual wall. Different boundary conditions between the real physical model and the mathematical model were compensated by adding a correction factor (C_f) into the governing equation [39]. Thus, both fluids in the co-flowing channel were modeled independently with discrete circuit elements. The governing equation on interface (α) for both fluids flowing in the co-flowing channel is expressed as follows:

$$C_T R_{WT} \frac{d}{dt}\left(\frac{C_f}{1-\alpha}\right) + \frac{C_f\,\alpha}{1-\alpha} = \left(\frac{Q_T}{Q_R}\right)\left(\frac{\mu_T}{\mu_R}\right) \tag{1}$$

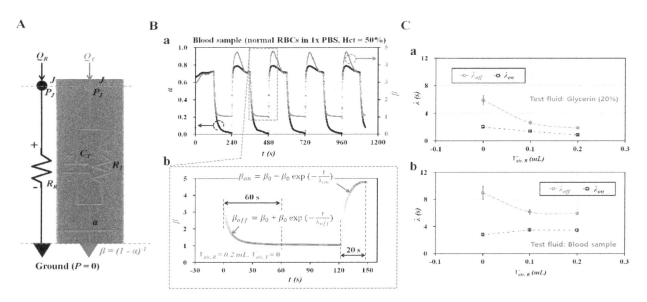

Figure 2. Quantitative evaluations of time constant with respect to the air cavity in the reference fluid syringe ($V_{air,\,R} = 0$, 0.1, and 0.2 mL). Here, the air cavity in the test fluid syringe was set to zero. (**A**) Fluidic circuit model for two fluids (reference fluid, test fluid) flowing in a co-flowing channel. (**B**) Quantifications of time constants (λ_{off}, λ_{on}) during each period. (a) Temporal variations of α and β with respect to $V_{air,\,R} = 0.2$ mL. (b) Quantifications of λ_{off} and λ_{on} during turn-on and turn-off operation of the syringe pump. (**C**) Variations of λ_{off} and λ_{on} with respect to the test fluids (blood sample and glycerin (20%)) and air cavity in the reference syringe ($V_{air,\,R} = 0$, 0.1 and 0.2 mL). (a) Variations of λ_{off} and λ_{on} with respect to $V_{air,\,R}$ and glycerin (20%). (b) Variations of λ_{off} and λ_{on} with respect to $V_{air,\,R}$ and blood sample.

Here, R_{WT} is given by $R_{WT} = 12\mu_T L_{cc}/(W_T h^3)$, where L_{cc} denotes the channel length of the co-flowing channel. Subscript T means test fluid. Instead of subscript T, subscript B is also used for representing blood sample. According to a numerical simulation using CFD-ACE+ (Ver. 2019, ESI Group, Paris, France), the correction factor could be approximately expressed as $C_f = 6.6908\,\alpha^4 - 13.382\,\alpha^3 + 10.81\,\alpha^2 - 4.1196\,\alpha + 1.6206$ ($R^2 = 0.9922$, $0.1 < \alpha < 0.9$) (Figure A1, Appendix A). Because of the nonlinear terms in the left member of Equation (1), the differential equation was difficult to solve substantially. Based on an approximate procedure [39], two approximate coefficients (F_1, F_2) were obtained as $F_1 = 1.112$, $F_2 = 1.129$, respectively. Consequently, $1/(1-\alpha)$ was converted into β and Equation (1) was transformed into a linear differential equation as follows:

$$\lambda \frac{d}{dt}(\beta) + \beta = 1 + \frac{1}{F_2}\left(\frac{Q_T}{Q_R}\right)\left(\frac{\mu_T}{\mu_R}\right) \tag{2}$$

In Equation (2), the time constant (λ) is expressed as $\lambda = \frac{F_1}{F_2}C_T R_{WT} \cong C_T R_{WT}$. The compliance element (C_T) presents a linear relation with the time constant (λ) and includes the effect of the air cavity in the syringe. Thus, the contribution of the air cavity could be obtained quantitatively by measuring the time constant (λ) with transient behaviors of β.

As shown in Figure 2B-a, temporal variations of α and β were obtained with respect to the blood sample (normal RBCs suspended in 1× PBS, Hct = 50%). Here, the air cavity in the reference fluid syringe was set to 0.2 mL ($V_{air, R} = 0.2$ mL). Based on Equation (2), the temporal variations of β were represented as shown in Figure 2B-b. When sequentially turning syringe pumps on and off, two time constants (λ_{off}, λ_{on}) could be obtained by analyzing transient variations of β. First, under the turn-off operation of a syringe pump, temporal variations of β_{off} were extracted for 60 s. Based on an exponential model (i.e., $\beta_{off} = \beta_0 + \beta_1 \exp(-t/\lambda_{off})$), λ_{off} was obtained by conducting nonlinear regression analysis with Matlab 2019. Second, under the turn-on operation of a syringe pump, β_{on} converged in a shorter time interval than for β_{off}. Temporal variations of β_{on} were extracted for 20 s. Similarly, based on an exponential model (i.e., $\beta_{on} = \beta_0 + \beta_1 \exp(-t/\lambda_{on})$), λ_{on} was obtained by conducting non-linear regression analysis. Figure 2C-a shows variations of λ_{off} and λ_{on} with respect to $V_{air, R}$ and glycerin (20%). All experimental data were expressed as mean ± standard deviation. The error bar represented single standard deviation. Note that λ_{off} was much longer than λ_{on} within 0.2 mL of the air cavity. Additionally, λ_{off} decreased substantially when the cavity volume increased from 0 to 0.1 mL. Above $V_{air, R} = 0.1$ mL, it decreased slightly. Figure 2C-b shows variations of λ_{off} and λ_{on} with respect to $V_{air, R}$ and the blood sample. Similar to the glycerin solution, λ_{off} decreased considerably when the air cavity increased from 0 to 0.1 mL. The air cavity in the reference fluid syringe (~0.1 mL) contributed to decreasing the time constant (λ_{off}) significantly. However, λ_{on} did not present distinctive variations with respect to the air cavity in the reference fluid syringe. Additionally, two time constants remained unchanged above $V_{air, R} = 0.1$ mL. According to discrete fluidic circuit analysis, air compliance (C) plays a role in regulating the alternating component of the flow rate. In this study, flow rate of the reference fluid remained unchanged over time. It was modeled as direct component of flow rate. Thus, air cavity secured in reference syringe did not contribute to the changing time constant. However, air cavity with 0.1 mL decreased time constant substantially. Taking into account the fact that air compliance caused the time constant to increase generally, the result showed different trends. Above a 0.1 mL air cavity, the time constant varied slightly. The constant value of the time constant was obtained through fluid viscosity and the compliance effect of the tubing and PDMS device. According to these experimental results, the air cavity in the reference fluid syringe (~0.1 mL) contributed to decreasing λ_{off} greatly. Note that λ_{off} decreased more significantly than λ_{on}. Above an air cavity volume of 0.1 mL, the time constants did not present substantial variation.

3.2. Valuations of Time Constant with Respect to Hematocrit and Air Cavity in Blood Sample Syringe

First, to evaluate the contribution of hematocrit to the time constant, the blood sample (Hct = 30%, 40%, and 50%) was prepared by adding normal RBCs into 1× PBS. As shown in Figure 3A-a, variations of λ_{off} and λ_{on} were obtained with respect to Hct. To evaluate the contribution of the air cavity in the reference fluid syringe, such a cavity was set to $V_{air, R} = 0$ and 0.1 mL. The air cavity in the blood sample syringe was set to $V_{air, B} = 0$. In contrast with λ_{on}, λ_{off} increased largely with respect to Hct. In addition, the air cavity in the reference fluid syringe contributed to decreasing the time constant substantially. As shown in Figure 3A-b, a scatter plot was constructed by plotting λ_{on} on Y-axis and λ_{off} on X-axis. According to linear regression analysis, the following linear regression formula was obtained: $\lambda_{on} = 0.2815 \lambda_{off} + 1.4967$ ($R^2 = 0.8282$). The high regression coefficient (R^2) denotes that λ_{on} and λ_{off} showed a strong linear relationship. From these results, λ_{off} was selected as the representative time constant throughout this study.

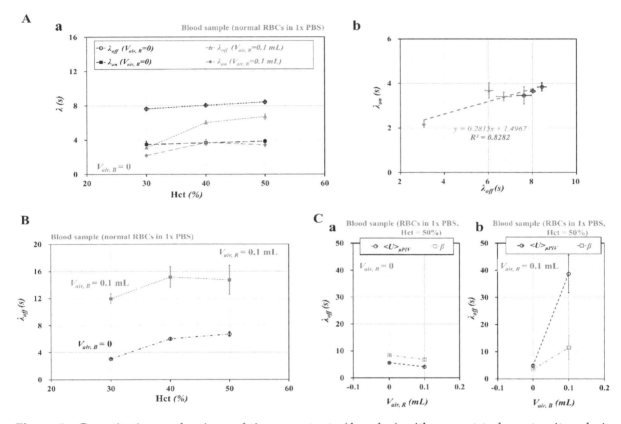

Figure 3. Quantitative evaluations of time constants (λ_{off}, λ_{on}) with respect to hematocrit and air cavity in each syringe. Here, a blood sample was prepared by adding normal RBCs into 1× PBS. (**A**) The comparison of two time constants with respect to hematocrit and air cavity. (a) Variations of λ_{off} and λ_{on} with respect to Hct = 30%, 40%, and 50% and $V_{air, R} = 0$ and 0.1 mL. (b) Linear relationship between λ_{off} and λ_{on}. Here, the air cavity in the blood sample syringe was set to zero. (**B**) Variations of λ_{off} and λ_{on} with respect to Hct = 30%, 40%, and 50% with $V_{air, B} = 0$ and 0.1 mL. Here, the air cavity in the reference fluid syringe was set to 0.1 mL. (**C**) Quantitative comparison of λ_{off} obtained from $<U>_{\mu PIV}$ and β. The hematocrit of the blood sample was adjusted to Hct = 50% by adding normal RBCs into 1× PBS. (a) Comparison of λ_{off} obtained from $<U>_{\mu PIV}$ and β with respect to $V_{air, R} = 0$ and 0.1 mL. Here, the air cavity in the blood sample syringe was set to zero. (b) Comparison of λ_{off} obtained from $<U>_{\mu PIV}$ and β with respect to $V_{air, B} = 0$ and 0.1 mL. Here, the air cavity in the reference fluid syringe was set to 0.1 mL.

Second, to evaluate the effect of the air cavity in the blood sample syringe ($V_{air, B}$) on the time constant (λ_{off}), such cavity was set to $V_{air, B} = 0$, and 0.1 mL. Additionally, to stabilize the fluidic instability resulting from the syringe pump, the air cavity in the reference fluid syringe was set to $V_{air, R} = 0.1$ mL. As shown in Figure 3B, variations of λ_{off} were obtained with respect to Hct = 30%, 40%, and 50% and $V_{air, B} = 0$, and 0.1 mL. The air cavity in the blood sample syringe contributed to increasing the time constant substantially. Theoretically, the size of syringe pump did not contribute to the varying time constant. According to the previous study [22], the time constant tended to increase linearly with respect to air cavity volume. In other words, air cavity secured in each syringe varied dynamic behaviors of β in coflowing channels (i.e., time constant). Thus, it is necessary to fix air cavity secured in each syringe. Note that, interestingly, the air cavity in the reference fluid syringe contributed to decreasing λ_{off}, as shown in Figure 3A-a. From these results, we inferred that the air cavity increased or decreased the time constant depending on whether it existed in the reference fluid syringe or the blood sample syringe.

Third, to compare the time constant with temporal variations of β, the time constant was additionally obtained with temporal variations of the average velocity of the blood flow in the test fluid channel ($<U>_{\mu PIV}$). A blood sample (Hct = 50%) was prepared as the test fluid by adding normal RBCs into 1× PBS. Figure 3C-a shows λ_{off} of $<U>_{\mu PIV}$ and λ_{off} of β with respect to $V_{air, R}$ = 0 and 0.1 mL. Here, the air cavity in the blood sample syringe was set to zero. Consequently, λ_{off} tended to decrease with respect to $V_{air, R}$. Both $<U>_{\mu PIV}$ and β exhibited a similar trend of λ_{off} with respect to $V_{air, R}$. Figure 3C-b shows a comparison of λ_{off} obtained from $<U>_{\mu PIV}$ and β with respect to $V_{air, B}$ = 0 and 0.1 mL. Here, the air cavity in the reference fluid syringe was set to 0.1 mL. Consequently, λ_{off} tended to increase with respect to $V_{air, B}$. Both $<U>_{\mu PIV}$ and β exhibited increase in λ_{off} significantly with respect to $V_{air,B}$. The time constant obtained with β presented a very similar trend with respect to the air cavity compared with the time constant obtained with $<U>_{\mu PIV}$. As quantification of $<U>_{\mu PIV}$ required an expensive high-speed camera and much time for the micro-PIV procedure, the quantification of β could be considered more effective.

Finally, to evaluate the contribution of the air cavity in the blood sample syringe to blood viscosity (μ_B), the value of μ_B was obtained with respect to $V_{air, B}$ = 0 and 0.1 mL. The blood viscosity was quantified under constant flow rate; both fluids were infused at the same flow rate (i.e., $Q_B = Q_R$). By setting $\frac{d\beta}{dt} = 0$ in Equation (2), a formula of blood viscosity was derived as follows:

$$\mu_B = \mu_R \times (\beta - 1) \times F_2 \tag{3}$$

As shown in Figure 4A, μ_B tended to increase with respect to Hct. As expected, the air cavity in the blood sample syringe did not contribute to varying blood viscosity. In addition, it was inferred that the air cavity in the reference fluid syringe (~0.1 mL) was sufficient to maintain a constant flow rate, even at $V_{air, B}$ = 0.

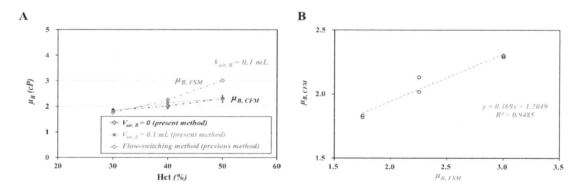

Figure 4. Quantitative comparison of blood viscosity (μ_B) between the co-flowing method (present method) and a flow switching method (previous method). To evaluate the effect of $V_{air, B}$ on μ_B, $V_{air, B}$ was varied from 0 to 0.1 mL. Here, $V_{air, R}$ was set to 0.1 mL. (**A**) Variations of μ_B obtained with two different methods with respect to Hct. (**B**) The inset shows the linear relationship between $\mu_{B, CFM}$ (co-flowing method) and $\mu_{B, FSM}$ (flow switching method).

To compare with the blood viscosity obtained with the present method (i.e., co-flowing method), the blood viscosity of the same blood sample was also obtained with a previous method (i.e., flow-switching method) [40]. The previous method produced a higher value of blood viscosity than the present method. The Fåhræus–Lindqvist effect indicated that blood viscosity varied with respect to channel diameter. In other words, blood viscosity tended to decrease at a smaller channel due to the existence of a cell-free layer. However, blood viscosity remained constant for wider channel with above 300~500 μm. Here, the contribution of a cell-free layer was negligible because it was much smaller than the channel size. As a rectangular channel (width = W, and depth = h) was filled with a blood sample, an equivalent circular diameter (d) was estimated as $d = \sqrt{\frac{4}{\pi} W \cdot h}$ with mass conservation. For the previous method (i.e., switching flow method), a single fluidic channel was filled with blood sample completely when reversal flow in junction occurred. Then, equivalent diameter was estimated as $d = 358$ μm. However, for the present method (i.e., co-flowing method), the corresponding interface of each hematocrit was obtained as $\alpha = 0.65 \pm 0.01$ for Hct = 30%, $\alpha = 0.67 \pm 0.01$ for Hct = 40%, and $\alpha = 0.68 \pm 0.01$ for Hct = 50%. The equivalent diameter was then estimated as $d = 288~294$ μm. According to the previous study [41], for channel diameter with below $d = 400$ μm, blood viscosity tended to decrease gradually with respect to equivalent diameter. Because the present method had smaller equivalent diameter than the previous method, it was reasonable that blood viscosity obtained by the present method was underestimated substantially when compared with blood viscosity obtained by the previous method. To obtain a linear relationship between both methods, as shown in the inset of Figure 4B, a scatter plot was constructed by plotting the viscosity obtained by the present method (i.e., co-flowing method with $\mu_{B, CFM}$) on Y-axis and the viscosity obtained by previous method (i.e., flow-switching method: $\mu_{B, FSM}$) on X-axis. According to regression analysis, a linear regression formula was obtained: $\mu_{B, CFM} = 0.369 \mu_{B, FSM} + 1.2049$ ($R^2 = 0.9485$). The high value of the regression coefficient (R^2) means that the co-flowing method (i.e., the present method) could be used effectively to monitor blood viscosity compared with the flow-switching method (i.e., the previous method).

3.3. Quantitative Evaluations of Image Intensity, Blood Velocity, and Interface with Respect to Diluent

To evaluate variations of mechanical properties of a blood sample at constant blood flow rate, a blood sample (Hct = 50%) was prepared by adding normal RBCs into two different diluents, namely 1× PBS and dextran solution (10 mg/mL). Here, the dextran solution was used as a diluent to enhance the RBC aggregation in the blood sample. The contribution of the dextran solution to the mechanical properties of the blood sample was evaluated by measuring image intensity ($<I>$), average velocity ($<U>_{\mu PIV}$), and interface ($\alpha = 1 - \beta^{-1}$) with respect to the blood flow rate (or shear rate). Using two syringe pumps, both fluids were injected at the same flow rate ($Q_R = Q_B = Q_{sp}$). The air cavity in each syringe was set to 0.1 mL (i.e., $V_{air, R} = V_{air, B} = 0.1$ mL).

As shown in Figure 5A, the variation of image intensity ($<I>$) was obtained with respect to Q_{sp} and the diluent. The right side panel in the figure shows microscopic images captured at specific flow rates (Q_{sp}): (a) $Q_{sp} = 0.075$ mL/h, (b) $Q_{sp} = 0.2$ mL/h, (c) $Q_{sp} = 0.6$ mL/h, (d) $Q_{sp} = 1$ mL/h, and (e) $Q_{sp} = 5$ mL/h. For the dextran solution as diluent, $<I>$ decreased gradually up to $Q_{sp} = 0.4$ mL/h. RBC aggregation caused to increase $<I>$ at a lower flow rate. However, when the flow rate increased, RBCs tended to disaggregate. Above $Q_{sp} = 0.6$ mL/, $<I>$ tended to increase gradually with respect to Q_{sp}. According to a previous study, the orientation and deformability of RBCs contribute to increasing image intensity [42]. Given that RBCs in 1× PBS did not include RBC aggregation, $<I>$ did not increase, even at lower flow rates. The value of $<I>$ tended to increase gradually by increasing the flow rate.

While measuring blood viscosity accurately, it is necessary to evaluate the effect of flow rate on interface ($\alpha = W_B/W$) in the coflowing channel. As shown in Figure 1A-c, blood-filled width (W_B) could be obtained accurately by conducting image processing. However, the channel width was assumed as $W = 1000$ μm. Maximum flow rate was estimated as 2 mL/h when test fluid and reference fluid were set to the same flow rate of 1 mL/h. While infusing the blood sample into single microfluidic channel, the deformed channel width was quantified by increasing flow rate. Variation of W was obtained by varying flow rate ($Q_B = 0.05, 0.1, 0.2, 0.4, 0.6, 0.8, 1, 2, 3, 4$, and 5 mL/h). As shown in Figure A2 (Appendix A), the channel width of the corresponding flow rate was quantified as $W = 1009 \pm 0.2$ μm ($Q_B = 1$ mL/h), $W = 1012.8 \pm 2.1$ μm ($Q_B = 2$ mL/h), and $W = 1017.5 \pm 1.7$ μm ($Q_B = 4$ mL/h). From the results, variation of channel width was estimated as less than 2% under the maximum flow rate of 2 mL/h.

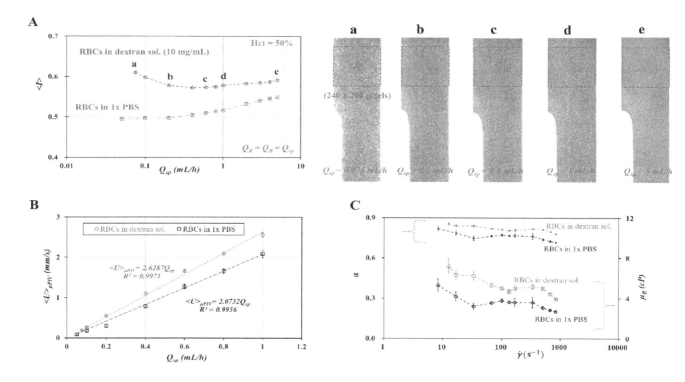

Figure 5. Quantitative evaluations of image intensity ($<I>$), blood velocity ($<U>_{\mu PIV}$), and interface (α) with respect to diluent. Blood samples (Hct = 50%) were prepared by adding normal RBCs into different diluents, namely 1× PBS and dextran solution (10 mg/mL). The flow rate of each fluid was fixed at the same flow rate ($Q_R = Q_B = Q_{sp}$). (**A**) Variations of microscopic image intensity ($<I>$) with respect to Q_{sp} and diluent. The value of $<I>$ was obtained by averaging the image intensity distributed over a specific region-of-interest (ROI) (240 × 200 pixels) selected within the test fluid channel. The right side panel shows microscopic images captured at a specific flow rate ((a) Q_{sp} = 0.075 mL/h, (b) Q_{sp} = 0.2 mL/h, (c) Q_{sp} = 0.6 mL/h, (d) Q_{sp} = 1 mL/h, and (e) Q_{sp} = 5 mL/h). (**B**) Variations of $<U>_{\mu PIV}$ with respect to Q_{sp} and diluent. (**C**) Variations of α and μ_B with respect to γ and diluent.

Variations of $<U>_{\mu PIV}$ with respect to Q_{sp} and diluent were obtained, as shown in Figure 5B. The value of $<U>_{\mu PIV}$ tended to increase linearly with respect to Q_{sp}. According to linear regression analysis, a linear regression formula for each diluent was obtained: $<U>_{\mu PIV}$ = 2.6287 Q_{sp} (R^2 = 0.9971) for dextran solution (10 mg/mL) and $<U>_{\mu PIV}$ = 2.0732 Q_{sp} (R^2 = 0.9956) for 1× PBS. These results indicated that RBCs suspended in dextran solution reached a higher value of $<U>_{\mu PIV}$ (~26.8%) compared with RBCs suspended in 1× PBS.

Finally, to evaluate variations of interface (α) with flow rate and diluent, variations of α and μ_B were obtained with respect to shear rate and diluent. For a rectangular channel (width = W, and depth = h) with low aspect ratio [8], a shear rate for each flow rate (Q_{sp}) is given approximately by $\gamma = \frac{6Q_{sp}}{W\,h^2}$. Using Equation (3), the blood viscosity of the blood sample was obtained in terms of the shear rate. As shown in Figure 5C, the interface (α) of RBCs suspended in the dextran solution reached a higher value of interface compared with RBCs suspended in 1× PBS. The blood viscosity decreased gradually with respect to the shear rate. The blood sample behaved as a non-Newtonian fluid (or shear-thinning fluid). Furthermore, a dextran solution (10 mg/mL) as diluent contributed to increasing the blood viscosity significantly compared with 1× PBS. When compared with previous results [8], our results showed consistent trends with respect to diluents.

3.4. Variations of Red Blood Cells (RBC) Aggregation, Viscosity, and Viscoelasticity with Respect to Diluent and Air Cavity in Syringe

To quantify three mechanical properties of blood sample (RBC aggregation, viscosity, and viscoelasticity) with respect to air cavity (or air compliance), variations of $<I>$, $<U>_{\mu PIV}$, and β were simultaneously obtained with respect to diluent and air cavity in each syringe. A blood sample (Hct = 50%) was prepared by adding normal RBCs into four different diluents, namely 1× PBS, two dextran solutions (5, and 10 mg/mL), and plasma. The air cavity in the reference fluid syringe was fixed at $V_{air, R} = 0.1$ mL. Additionally, the air cavity in the blood sample syringe varied from $V_{air, B} = 0$ to $V_{air, B} = 0.1$ mL. Based on experimental results shown in Figure 5A, the flow rate of each fluid was reset to $Q_0 = 0.5$ mL/h for measuring RBC aggregation effectively.

First, as shown in Figure 6A, temporal variations of $<I>$ and $<U>_{\mu PIV}$ were obtained with respect to diluents. Here, the air cavity in the blood sample syringe was set to $V_{air, R} = 0$. When the syringe pump was turned off periodically, $<U>_{\mu PIV}$ decreased suddenly over time. RBC aggregation increased $<I>$ gradually over time. Given that 1× PBS did not stimulate RBC aggregation, $<I>$ of 1× PBS remain unchanged over time. However, two dextran solutions contributed to increasing $<I>$ over time substantially. Given that plasma proteins contributed to RBC aggregation [43,44], $<I>$ of plasma increased gradually over time.

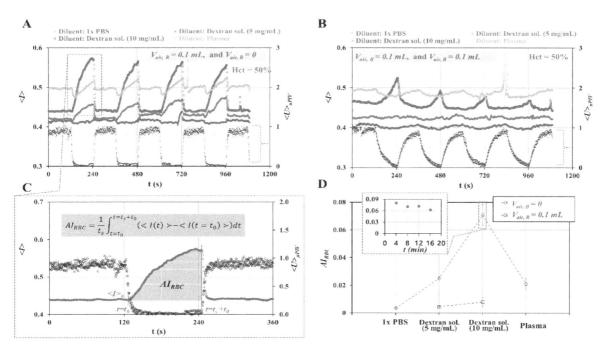

Figure 6. Quantitative evaluations of RBC aggregation with respect to diluent and air cavity in the blood sample syringe. Here, the flow rate of the syringe pump was reset to $Q_0 = 0.5$ mL/h. The air cavity in the reference fluid syringe was set to 0.1 mL. (**A**) Temporal variations of $<I>$ and $<U>_{\mu PIV}$ with respect to diluent, i.e., 1× PBS, two dextran solution (5, and 10 mg/mL), and plasma. The air cavity in the blood sample syringe was set to zero. (**B**) Temporal variations of $<I>$ and $<U>_{\mu PIV}$ with respect to diluent. The air cavity in the blood sample was set to 0.1 mL. (**C**) Quantification of RBC aggregation index (AI_{RBC}). The value of AI_{RBC} was obtained as $AI_{RBC} = \frac{1}{t_s} \int_{t=t_0}^{t=t_0+t_s} (< I(t) > - < I(t = t_0) >) dt$. (**D**) Variations of AI_{RBC} with respect to diluent and $V_{air, B}$. The inset shows temporal variations of AI_{RBC} with respect to dextran solution (10 mg/mL).

To evaluate the effect of air compliance on RBC aggregation, the air cavity in the blood sample syringe was varied from $V_{air, B} = 0$ to $V_{air, B} = 0.1$ mL. As shown in Figure 6B, temporal variations of $<I>$ and $<U>_{\mu PIV}$ were obtained with respect to diluent. Even when turning off the syringe pump, $<U>_{\mu PIV}$ tended to decrease gradually over time. For this reason, except for a higher concentration of dextran solution (10 mg/mL), $<I>$ did not show substantial increase over time. From these results, the air cavity

(~0.1 mL) in the blood sample syringe delayed the transient behaviors of blood velocity considerably. Thus, it was inferred that air compliance hindered the quantification of RBC aggregation. To quantify RBC aggregation with $<I>$, it was necessary to define an RBC aggregation index. From Figure 6A, temporal variations of $<I>$ and $<U>_{\mu PIV}$ were redrawn from $t = 0$ to $t = 360$ s. As shown in Figure 6C, after $t = 120$ s (i.e., turn-off operation of the syringe pump), $<U>_{\mu PIV}$ decreased largely over time. Note also that $<I>$ tended to increase gradually over time. Here, a specific time instant and minimum value of $<I>$ were denoted as $t = t_0$ and $< I (t = t_0) >$, respectively. The RBC aggregation index was then obtained by analyzing $<I>$ from $t = t_0$ to $t = t_0 + t_s$. According to a previous study [45], an RBC aggregation index (AI_{RBC}) can be defined as follows:

$$AI_{RBC} = \frac{1}{t_s} \int_{t=t_0}^{t=t_0+t_s} (< I(t) > - < I(t = t_0) >)dt \tag{4}$$

Based on the temporal variations of $<I>$ shown in Figure 6A,B, AI_{RBC} was quantified at periodic intervals ($T = 240$ s). Figure 6D shows variations of AI_{RBC} with respect to diluent and $V_{air, B}$. The inset of Figure 6D shows temporal variations of AI_{RBC} with respect to dextran solution (10 mg/mL) and $V_{air, B} = 0$. The RBC aggregation index was quantified with repetitive tests (n = 8) and expressed as mean ± standard deviation. Under no air cavity in the blood sample syringe, the RBC aggregation index for each diluent was obtained as $AI_{RBC} = 0.003 ± 0.001$ for 1× PBS, $AI_{RBC} = 0.025 ± 0.001$ for dextran solution (5 mg/mL), $AI_{RBC} = 0.071 ± 0.008$ for dextran solution (10 mg/mL), and $AI_{RBC} = 0.021 ± 0.003$ for plasma. The dextran solutions and plasma contributed to increasing the RBC aggregation index significantly compared with 1× PBS. Additionally, AI_{RBC} tended to increase significantly at higher concentration of dextran solution. When the air cavity in the blood sample syringe was reset to 0.1 mL, the RBC aggregation index for the two dextran solutions was obtained as $AI_{RBC} = 0.004 ± 0.001$ for the first dextran solution (5 mg/mL) and $AI_{RBC} = 0.008 ± 0.003$ for the second dextran solution (10 mg/mL). Given that the air cavity (or air compliance) tended to delay the transient behavior of the blood velocity, AI_{RBC} decreased considerably. From these results, the air cavity (~0.1 mL) in the blood sample syringe hindered the quantification of the RBC aggregation substantially.

Second, as shown in Figure 7A-a, the temporal variations of β were obtained with respect to diluent. Air cavities of each syringe were set to $V_{air, R} = 0.1$ mL and $V_{air, B} = 0$, respectively. Among the values of β obtained in Figure 7A-a, to represent how the blood viscosity (μ_B) and the time constant (λ_{off}) were quantified over a single period, temporal variations of β were redrawn at specific durations ranging from $t = 240$ s to $t = 500$ s.

As shown in Figure 7A-b, the value of μ_B was obtained with the Equation (3) under turn-on operation of the syringe pump ($t < 0.5 T$). Afterward, λ_{off} was estimated with regression analysis ($\beta_{off} = \beta_0 + \beta_1 \exp (-t/\lambda_{off})$ under turn-off operation of the syringe pump ($0.5 T < t < T$). As shown in Figure 7A-c, variations of μ_B were obtained at intervals of 240 s with respect to diluent. The value of μ_B for each diluent was obtained as $\mu_B = 2.95 ± 0.12$ cP for 1× PBS, $\mu_B = 3.53 ± 0.15$ cP for the first dextran solution (5 mg/mL), $\mu_B = 5.89 ± 0.28$ cP for the second dextran solution (10 mg/mL), and $\mu_B = 4.59 ± 0.14$ cP for plasma. Under the turn-off operation of the syringe pump, the time constant (λ_{off}) was obtained with respect to diluent. Using a linear Maxwell model (i.e., $\lambda_{off} = \mu_B/G_B$), G_B was obtained by dividing μ_B by λ_{off}. As shown in Figure 7B-b, variations of λ_{off} were represented with respect to diluent and $V_{air, B} = 0$. Additionally, Figure 7A-d shows variations of elasticity (G_B) with respect to diluent. The value of G_B for each diluent was obtained as $G_B = 0.5 ± 0.02$ mPa for 1× PBS, $G_B = 0.62 ± 0.03$ mPa for the first dextran solution (5 mg/mL), $G_B = 0.79 ± 0.03$ mPa for the second dextran solution (10 mg/mL), and $G_B = 0.76 ± 0.05$ mPa for plasma. From these results, blood viscoelasticity (viscosity, elasticity) was quantified consistently with respect to diluent under the air cavity in each fluid syringe ($V_{air, R} = 0.1$ mL, and $V_{air, B} = 0$). The dextran solution as diluent contributed to increasing viscosity and elasticity substantially compared with 1× PBS. The plasma reached a higher value of viscosity and elasticity compared with 1× PBS. In other words, the plasma proteins led to increased viscosity and elasticity.

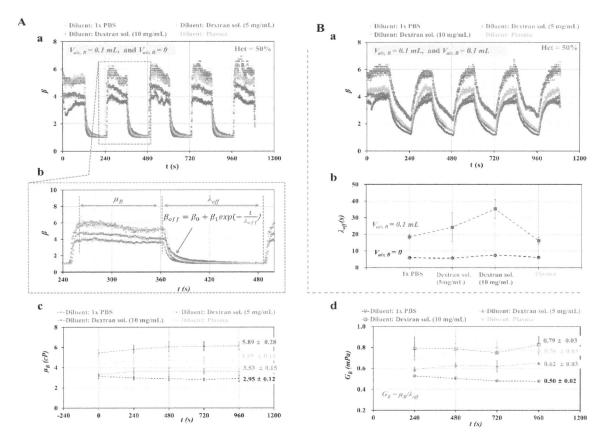

Figure 7. Quantitative evaluations of viscosity (μ_B) and time constant (λ_{off}) with respect to diluent and air cavity in the blood syringe. Here, the flow rate of the individual syringe pump and the air cavity in the reference fluid syringe were fixed at $Q_0 = 0.5$ mL/h and $V_{air, R} = 0.1$ mL, respectively. (**A**) Variations of viscosity (μ_B) and elasticity (G_B) with respect to diluent and $V_{air, B} = 0$. (a) Temporal variations of β with respect to diluent and $V_{air, B} = 0$. (b) Quantification of μ_B and λ_{off} during a single period. Here, μ_B and λ_{off} were obtained sequentially by turning on and off the syringe pump. (c) Variations of μ_B at intervals of 240 s. (d) Variations of G_B with respect to diluent. Here, G_B was obtained by dividing μ_B by λ_{off}. (**B**) Variations of λ_{off} with respect to diluent and $V_{air, B} = 0.1$ mL. (a) Temporal variations of β with respect to diluent. (b) Variations of λ_{off} with respect to diluent and $V_{air, B}$.

To quantify the effect of the air cavity in the blood sample syringe on β, the volume of such air cavities was varied from 0 to 0.1 mL. Additionally, the volume of the air cavity in the reference fluid syringe was set to 0.1 mL. As shown in Figure 7B-a, temporal variations of β were obtained with respect to diluent. The air cavity in the blood sample syringe delayed the transient behavior of β substantially. During turn-on and turn-off operation of the syringe pump, β did not reach a constant value within a specific duration. Given that Equation (3) as blood viscosity was effective for blood viscosity only for constant values of β, it was impossible to obtain the blood viscosity with no information on flow rate (or velocity) at a specific time instant. Figure 7B-b shows variations of λ_{off} with respect to diluent and $V_{air, B}$. Note that the case $V_{air, B} = 0.1$ mL contributed to increasing λ_{off} significantly compared with $V_{air, B} = 0$. When setting $V_{air, B} = 0.1$ mL, λ_{off} was increased largely at a higher concentration of dextran solution.

As shown in Figure 7B-b, while increasing air cavity was secured in the blood syringe from 0 to 0.1 mL, the corresponding time constant of each diluent increased about $\Delta\lambda_{off} = 13.3$ s (1× PBS), $\Delta\lambda_{off} = 18.4$ s (dextran sol. 5 mg/mL), $\Delta\lambda_{off} = 27.8$ s (dextran sol. 10 mg/mL), and $\Delta\lambda_{off} = 10$ s (plasma). As transient time increased largely within a half period, β did not arrive to constant value under periodic on-off operation of syringe pump. As a solution, it is necessary to increase period of blood flow rate. Taking into account the fact that time constant increased about 10~27.8 s for each diluent, half period of blood flow rate should increase at least 27.8 s. When the period of blood flow rate changes from

$T = 240$ s to $T = 300$ s, it will be inferred that β exhibits similar trends as shown in Figure 7A-a. Thus, blood viscosity and RBC aggregation will be obtained without additional information on temporal variations of blood velocity.

To quantify blood viscosity under varying blood flows, it was necessary to obtain β and $<U>_{\mu PIV}$ over time. Figure 8A shows temporal variations of β and $<U>_{\mu PIV}$ with respect to two diluents, namely 1× PBS and dextran solution (10 mg/mL). As shown in Figure 5B, the relationship between $<U>_{\mu PIV}$ and Q_{sp} was obtained in advance as a linear regression formula with respect to each diluent, and the average velocity of the blood sample ($<U>_{\mu PIV}$) was converted into the blood flow rate with a regular formula.

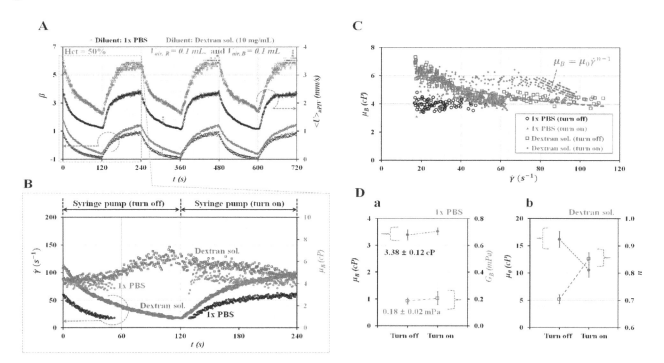

Figure 8. Quantitative evaluation of viscoelasticity with respect to diluent and $V_{air, B} = 0.1$ mL/h. A blood sample (Hct = 50%) was prepared by adding normal RBCs into diluent, i.e., 1× PBS and dextran solution (10 mg/mL). The flow rate of each syringe pump was set to $Q_0 = 0.5$ mL/h. The air cavity of the reference fluid syringe was set to 0.1 mL. (**A**) Temporal variations of β and $<U>_{\mu PIV}$ with respect to diluent. (**B**) Temporal variations of γ and μ_B with respect to diluent during a single period of 240 s. (**C**) Variations of μ_B with respect to diluent and syringe operation (turn-off and turn-on). (**D**) Variations of viscoelasticity with respect to diluent and pump operation. (a) Variations of μ_B and G_B with respect to 1× PBS and syringe operation. (b) Variations of μ_0 and n with respect to dextran solution (10 mg/mL) and syringe operation.

Given that the flow rate of the blood sample varied over time, the formula of blood viscosity was corrected as $\mu_B = \mu_R \times (\beta - 1) \times F_2 \times (Q_R/Q_B)$ by adding a flow rate term into Equation (3). Figure 8B shows temporal variations of γ and μ_B with respect to diluent during a single period of 240 s. Note that μ_B presented large scattering at $Q_{sp} < 0.1$ mL/h. Thus, the minimum value of Q_{sp} was set to 0.1 mL/h. As shown in Figure 8C, variations of μ_B were obtained with respect to γ during the turn-on and turn-off operation of the syringe pump. For 1× PBS as diluent, μ_B remained constant with respect to the shear rate. However, for the dextran solution as diluent, μ_B decreased gradually with respect to the shear rate. As shown in Figure 8D-a, variations of μ_B and G_B were obtained with respect to the syringe operation (i.e., turn-on, turn-off). Given that μ_B remained unchanged over the shear rate, G_B was calculated by dividing μ_B by the time constant (i.e., $G_B = \mu_B/\lambda_{off}$ for turn-off operation, and $G_B = \mu_B/\lambda_{on}$ for turn-on operation). The value of μ_B for each operation was obtained as $\mu_B = 3.38 \pm 0.19$ cP for the turn-off operation, and $\mu_B = 3.52 \pm 0.12$ cP for the turn-on operation. Additionally, the value of G_B for each operation was obtained as $G_B = 0.18 \pm 0.02$ cP for the turn-off operation, and $G_B = 0.21 \pm 0.05$ cP for the turn-on operation. From these results, μ_B and G_B remained unchanged irrespective of the syringe operation. Compared with the results obtained at $V_{air, B} = 0$ as showed in Figure 7A-c, a 0.1-mL air cavity (~0.1 mL) in the blood sample syringe caused to overestimate μ_B. However, it caused G_B to be underestimated. Figure 8D-b shows variations of μ_0 and n with respect to the first dextran solution (10 mg/mL) and syringe operation. The constant μ_0 decreased significantly by switching the syringe pump from turn-off operation to turn-on operation. In addition, the turn-on operation caused to increase the index n substantially compared with the turn-off operation.

In this study, three mechanical properties of blood sample (viscosity, RBC aggregation, and time constant) were quantified with methods suggested in previous studies. First, cone-and-plate viscometer as conventional method has been used to measure blood viscosity. According to the quantitative comparison between conventional viscometer and microfluidic viscometer [40,41,46,47], the previous studies indicated that blood viscosity could be measured consistently in a microfluidic environment. Based on the previous study, as shown in Figure 4A, co-flow method (present method) and flow switching method (previous method) were used to obtain blood viscosity with respect to hematocrit. The present method underestimated blood viscosity when compared with the previous method. However, as shown in Figure 4B, both methods exhibited a high degree of linear relationship (i.e., $R^2 = 0.9485$). Second, RBC aggregation as a conventional method has been quantified by analyzing light intensity [48] or electric impedance [49] of blood sample flowing in slit channel. According to quantitative comparison study [50,51], microscopic image intensity exhibited variations of RBC aggregation in microfluidic channel sufficiently. Thus, without quantitative comparison study, variations of RBC aggregation were quantified by analyzing image intensity of blood flows in the test channel under turn-off blood flows. Finally, under transient flow conditions, time constant has been obtained by analyzing temporal variations of physical parameters including blood velocity, flow rate, and pressure. Based on Equation (2), time constant (l) was obtained by analyzing temporal variations of β. Furthermore, to compare with time constant obtained from information of β, time constant was quantified additionally by analyzing temporal variations of blood velocity ($<U>$). As shown in Figure 3C, both time constants exhibited consistent variations with respect to air cavity in reference syringe.

From these experimental results, it leads to the conclusion that the air cavity in the blood sample syringe made the RBC aggregation and blood viscoelasticity vary substantially. The RBC aggregation index decreased largely, even for a 0.1-mL air cavity in the blood sample syringe because of a longer transient behavior of blood flows. Thus, to measure RBC aggregation and viscoelasticity of blood samples consistently, a 0.1-mL air cavity must be secured in the reference fluid syringe as a minimum condition. Additionally, the air cavity in the blood sample syringe must be minimized as much as possible.

4. Conclusions

In this study, the air compliance effect on measurement of blood mechanical properties was quantified experimentally with respect to the air cavity in two driving syringes. Under periodic on–off blood flows, three mechanical properties of blood samples, namely RBC aggregation, blood viscosity, and time constant, were obtained sequentially by quantifying microscopic image intensity of blood samples ($<I>$) flowing in the test channel and the interface (α) in a co-flowing channel. Based on a differential equation derived with a fluid circuit model, the time constant was obtained by analyzing temporal variations of $\beta = 1/(1-\alpha)$. First, the air cavity in the reference fluid syringe (~0.1 mL) contributed to decreasing λ_{off} greatly. The λ_{off} decreased more significantly than λ_{on}. Above an air cavity volume of 0.1 mL, the time constants did not present substantial variation. The air cavity increased or decreased the time constant depending on whether it existed in the reference fluid syringe or the blood sample syringe. Second, the air cavity did not contribute to varying blood viscosity. From the quantitative comparison study, the co-flowing method (i.e., the present method) could be used effectively to monitor blood viscosity compared with the flow-switching method (i.e., the previous method). Third, given that the air cavity in the blood sample syringe contributed to delaying transient behaviors of blood flows considerably, this hindered the quantification of the RBC aggregation and blood viscosity. As a solution, when the period of blood flow rate increases about twice time constant (i.e., $\Delta T = 2\lambda_{off}$), blood viscosity and RBC aggregation could be obtained without additional information on temporal variations of blood velocity. From these experimental results, to measure the aforementioned three mechanical properties of blood samples effectively, the air cavity in the blood sample syringe must be minimized ($V_{air, B} = 0$). However, it will be necessary to secure the air cavity in the reference fluid syringe ($V_{air, R} = 0.1$ mL) for stabilizing fluidic instability resulting from the syringe pump.

Appendix A

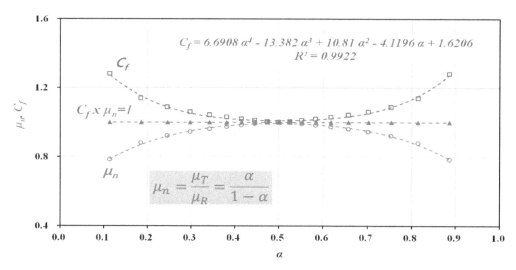

Figure A1. Variations of normalized viscosity (μ_n) with respect to interface (α) in coflowing channel. Based on the principle of parallel streams [47], μ_n was expressed as $\mu_n = \mu_T/\mu_R = \alpha/(1-\alpha)$. μ_T and μ_R represent viscosity of test fluid and reference fluid, respectively. As the viscosity of test fluid is assumed as constant with respect to α, correction factor (C_f) was then obtained as $C_f = 6.6908\,\alpha^4 - 13.382\,\alpha^3 + 10.81\,\alpha^2 - 4.1196\,\alpha + 1.6206$ ($R^2 = 0.9922$) by using the following relationship (i.e., $C_f \times \mu_n = 1$).

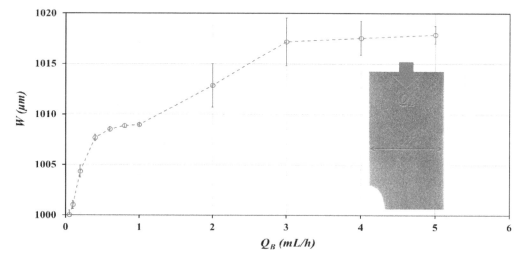

Figure A2. Variations of channel width under blood flow rate (Q_B).

References

1. Danesh, J.; Collins, R.; Peto, R.; Lowe, G.D.O. Haematocrit, viscosity, erythrocyte sedimentation rate: Meta-analyses of prospective studies of coronary heart disease. *Eur. Heart J.* **2000**, *21*, 515–520. [CrossRef] [PubMed]

2. Cho, Y.I.; Mooney, M.P.; Cho, D.J. Hemorheological disorders in diabetes mellitus. *J. Diabetest Sci. Technol.* **2008**, *2*, 1130–1138. [CrossRef] [PubMed]

3. Zeng, N.F.; Mancuso, J.E.; Zivkovic, A.M.; Smilowitz, J.T.; Ristenpart, W.D. Red blood cells from individuals with abdominal obesity or metabolic abnormalities exhibit less deformability upon entering a constriction. *PLoS ONE* **2016**, *11*, e0156070. [CrossRef] [PubMed]

4. Agrawal, R.; Smart, T.; Nobre-Cardoso, J.; Richards, C.; Bhatnagar, R.; Tufail, A.; Shima, D.; Jones, P.H.; Pavesio, C. Assessment of red blood cell deformability in type 2 diabetes mellitus and diabetic retinopathy by dual optical tweezers stretching technique. *Sci. Rep.* **2016**, *6*, 15873. [CrossRef] [PubMed]

5. Kim, H.; Cho, Y.I.; Lee, D.-H.; Park, C.-M.; Moon, H.-W.; Hur, M.; Kim, J.Q.; Yun, Y.-M. Analycal performance evaluation of the scanning tube viscometer for measurement of whole blood viscosity. *Clin. Biochem.* **2013**, *46*, 139–142. [CrossRef]

6. Sousa, P.C.; Vaz, R.; Cerejo, A.; Oliveira, M.S.N.; Alves, M.A.; Pinho, F.T. Rheological behavior of human blood in uniaxial extensional flow. *J. Rheol.* **2018**, *62*, 447–456. [CrossRef]

7. Kim, B.J.; Lee, Y.S.; Zhbanov, A.; Yang, S. A physiometer for simultaneous measurement of whole blood viscosity and its determinants: Hematocrit and red blood cell deformability. *Analyst* **2019**, *144*, 3144–3157. [CrossRef] [PubMed]

8. Kang, Y.J. Microfluidic-based effective monitoring of bloods by measuring RBC aggregation and blood viscosity under stepwise varying shear rates. *Korea-Aust. Rheol. J.* **2020**, *32*, 15–27. [CrossRef]

9. Khnouf, R.; Karasneh, D.; Abdulhay, E.; Abdelhay, A.; Sheng, W.; Fan, Z.H. Microfluidics-based device for the measurement of blood viscosity and its modeling based on shear rate, temperature, and heparin concentration. *Biomed. Microdevices* **2019**, *21*, 80. [CrossRef]

10. Hong, H.; Song, J.M.; Yeom, E. 3D printed microfluidic viscometer based on the co-flowing stream. *Biomicrofluidics* **2019**, *13*, 014104. [CrossRef]

11. Wen, J.; Wan, N.; Bao, H.; Li, J. Quantitative measurement and evaluation of red blood cell aggregation in normal blood based on a modified hanai equation. *Sensors* **2019**, *19*, 1095. [CrossRef] [PubMed]

12. Sherwood, J.M.; Dusting, J.; Kaliviotis, E.; Balabani, S. The effect of red blood cell aggregation on velocity and cell-depleted layer characteristics of blood in a bifurcating microchannel. *Biomicrofluidics* **2012**, *6*, 024119. [CrossRef] [PubMed]

13. Shin, S.; Jang, J.H.; Park, M.S.; Ku, Y.H.; Suh, J.S. A noble RBC aggregometer with vibration-induced disaggregation mechanism. *Korea-Aust. Rheol. J.* **2005**, *17*, 9–13.

14. Zhbanov, A.; Yang, S. Effects of aggregation on blood sedimentation and conductivity. *PLoS ONE* **2015**, *10*, e0129337. [CrossRef] [PubMed]

15. Boas, L.V.; Faustino, V.; Lima, R.; Miranda, J.M.; Minas, G.; Fernandes, C.S.V.; Catarino, S.O. Assessment of the deformability and velocity of healthy and artificially impaired red blood cells in narrow polydimethylsiloxane (PDMS) microchannels. *Micromachines* **2018**, *9*, 384. [CrossRef] [PubMed]

16. Berry, S.B.; Fernandes, S.C.; Rajaratnam, A.; DeChiara, N.S.; Mace, C.R. Measurement of the hematocrit using paper-based microfluidic devices. *Lab Chip* **2016**, *16*, 3689–3694. [CrossRef]

17. Lee, H.Y.; Barber, C.; Rogers, J.A.; Minerick, A.R. Electrochemical hematocrit determination in a direct current microfluidic device. *Electrophoresis* **2015**, *36*, 978–985. [CrossRef]

18. Kim, M.; Yang, S. Improvement of the accuracy of continuous hematocrit measurement under various blood flow conditions. *Appl. Phys. Lett.* **2014**, *104*, 153508. [CrossRef]

19. Zhou, J.; Tu, C.; Liang, Y.; Huang, B.; Fang, Y.; Liang, X.; Ye, X. The label-free separation and culture of tumor cells in a microfluidic biochip. *Analyst* **2020**, *145*, 1706–1715. [CrossRef]

20. Zhou, J.; Papautsky, I. Size-dependent enrichment of leukocytes from undiluted whole blood using shear-induced diffusion. *Lab Chip* **2019**, *19*, 3416–3426. [CrossRef]

21. Zhou, J.; Tu, C.; Liang, Y.; Huang, B.; Fang, Y.; Liang, X.; Papautsky, I.; Ye, X. Isolation of cells from whole blood using shear-induced diffusion. *Sci. Rep.* **2018**, *8*, 9411. [CrossRef] [PubMed]

22. Kang, Y.J.; Yang, S. Fluidic low pass filter for hydrodynamic flow stabilization in microfluidic environments. *Lab Chip* **2012**, *12*, 1881–1889. [CrossRef] [PubMed]

23. Lee, J.; Rahman, F.; Laoui, T.; Karnik, R. Bubble-induced damping in displacement-driven microfluidic flows. *Phys. Rev. E* **2012**, *86*, 026301. [CrossRef] [PubMed]

24. Kasukurti, A.; Eggleton, C.D.; Desai, S.A.; Disharoon, D.I.; Marr, D.W.M. A simple microfluidic dispenser for singlemicroparticle and cell samples. *Lab Chip* **2014**, *14*, 4673–4679. [CrossRef]

25. Araci, I.E.; Agaoglu, S.; Lee, J.Y.; Yepes, L.R.; Diep, P.; Martini, M.; Schmidt, A. Flow stabilization in wearable microfluidic sensors enables noise suppression. *Lab Chip* **2019**, *19*, 3899–3908. [CrossRef]

26. Jiao, Z.; Zhao, J.; Chao, Z.; You, Z.; Zhao, J. An air-chamber-based microfluidic stabilizer for attenuating syringepump-induced fluctuations. *Microfluid. Nanofluid.* **2019**, *23*, 26. [CrossRef]

27. Zhang, X.; Xiang, N.; Tang, W.; Huang, D.; Wang, X.; Yi, H.; Ni, Z. A passive flow regulator with low threshold pressure for high-throughput inertial isolation of microbeads. *Lab Chip* **2015**, *15*, 3473–3480. [CrossRef]

28. Doh, I.; Cho, Y.-H. Passive flow-rate regulators using pressure-dependent autonomous deflection of parallel membrane valves. *Lab Chip* **2009**, *9*, 2070–2075. [CrossRef]

29. Kalantarifard, A.; Haghighi, E.A.; Elbuken, C. Damping hydrodynamic fluctuations in microfluidic systems. *Chem. Eng. Sci.* **2018**, *178*, 238–247. [CrossRef]

30. Zhang, X.; Wang, X.; Chen, K.; Cheng, J.; Xiang, N.; Ni, Z. Passive flow regulator for precise high-throughput flow rate control in microfluidic environment. *RSC Adv.* **2016**, *6*, 31639–31646. [CrossRef]

31. Park, Y.-J.; Yu, T.; Yim, S.-J.; You, D.; Kim, D.-P. A 3D-printed flow distributor with uniform flow rate control for multi-stacked microfluidic systems. *Lab Chip* **2018**, *18*, 1250–1258. [CrossRef] [PubMed]

32. Serra, M.; Gontran, E.; Hajji, I.; Malaquin, L.; Viovy, J.-L.; Descroix, S.; Ferraro, D. Development of a Droplet Microfluidics Device Based on Integrated Soft Magnets and Fluidic Capacitor for Passive Extraction and Redispersion of Functionalized Magnetic Particles. *Adv. Mater. Technol.* **2020**, *5*, 1901088. [CrossRef]

33. Kang, Y.J. Continuous and simultaneous measurement of the biophysical properties of blood in a microfluidic environment. *Analyst* **2016**, *141*, 6583–6597. [CrossRef] [PubMed]

34. Nam, J.-H.; Yang, Y.; Chung, S.; Shin, S. Comparison of light-transmission and -backscattering methods in the measurement of red blood cell aggregation. *J. Biomed. Opt.* **2010**, *15*, 027003. [CrossRef] [PubMed]

35. Kang, Y.J. Simultaneous measurement of blood pressure and RBC aggregation by monitoring on–off blood flows supplied from a disposable air-compressed pump. *Analyst* **2019**, *144*, 3556–3566. [CrossRef]

36. Kang, Y.J. Simultaneous measurement of erythrocyte deformability and blood viscoelasticity using micropillars and co-flowing streams under pulsatile blood flows. *Biomicrofluidics* **2017**, *11*, 014102. [CrossRef]

37. Otsu, N. A threshold selection method from gray-level histograms. *IEEE Trans. Syst. Man. Cybern.* **1979**, *9*, 62–66. [CrossRef]

38. Thielicke, W.; Stamhuis, E.J. PIVlab—Towards user-friendly, affordable and accurate digital particle image velocimetry in MATLAB. *J. Open Res. Softw.* **2014**, *2*, e30. [CrossRef]

39. Kang, Y.J. Blood Viscoelasticity Measurement Using Interface Variations in Coflowing Streams under Pulsatile Blood Flows. *Micromachines* **2020**, *11*, 245. [CrossRef]

40. Kang, Y.J.; Ryu, J.; Lee, S.-J. Label-free viscosity measurement of complex fluids using reversal flow switching manipulation in a microfluidic channel. *Biomicrofluidics* **2013**, *7*, 044106. [CrossRef] [PubMed]

41. Kang, Y.J.; Yang, S. Integrated microfluidic viscometer equipped with fluid temperature controller for measurement of viscosity in complex fluids. *Microfluid. Nanofluid.* **2013**, *14*, 657–668. [CrossRef]

42. Lindberg, L.-G.; Oberg, P.A. Optical properties of blood in motion. *Opt. Eng.* **1993**, *32*, 253–257. [CrossRef]

43. Brust, M.; Aouane, O.; Thie'baud, M.; Flormann, D.; Verdier, C.; Kaestner, L.; Laschke, M.W.; Selmi, H.; Benyoussef, A.; Podgorski, T.; et al. The plasma protein fibrinogen stabilizes clusters of red blood cells in microcapillary flows. *Sci. Rep.* **2014**, *4*, 4348. [CrossRef]

44. Lee, K.; Kinnunen, M.; Khokhlova, M.D.; Lyubin, E.V.; Priezzhev, A.V.; Meglinski, I.; Fedyanin, A.A. Optical tweezers study of red blood cell aggregation and disaggregation in plasma and protein solutions. *J. Biomed. Opt.* **2016**, *21*, 035001. [CrossRef] [PubMed]

45. Kang, Y.J. Microfluidic-based biosensor for sequential measurement of blood pressure and RBC aggregation over continuously varying blood flows. *Micromachines* **2019**, *10*, 577. [CrossRef]

46. Kim, B.J.; Lee, S.Y.; Jee, S.; Atajanov, A.; Yang, S. Micro-viscometer for measuring shear-varying blood viscosity over a wide-ranging shear rate. *Sensors* **2017**, *17*, 1442. [CrossRef]

47. Kang, Y.J. Periodic and simultaneous quantification of blood viscosity and red blood cell aggregation using a microfluidic platform under in-vitro closed-loop circulation. *Biomicrofluidics* **2018**, *12*, 024116. [CrossRef]

48. Shin, S.; Nam, J.-H.; Hou, J.-X.; Suh, J.-S. A transient microfluidic approach to the investigation of erythrocyte aggregation: The threshold shear-stress for erythrocyte disaggregation. *Clin. Hemorheol. Microcirc.* **2009**, *42*, 117–125. [CrossRef]

49. Baskurt, O.K.; Uyuklu, M.; Meiselman, H.J. Time Course of Electrical Impedance during Red Blood Cell Aggregation in a Glass Tube: Comparison with Light Transmittance. *IEEE Trans. Biomed. Eng.* **2010**, *57*, 969–978. [CrossRef]

50. Yeom, E.; Lee, S.-J. Microfluidic-based speckle analysis for sensitive measurement of erythrocyte aggregation: A comparison of four methods for detection of elevated erythrocyte aggregation in diabetic rat blood. *Biomicrofluidics* **2015**, *9*, 024110. [CrossRef]

51. Kang, Y.J.; Kim, B.J. Multiple and periodic measurement of RBC aggregation and ESR in parallel microfluidic channels under on-off blood flow control. *Micromachines* **2018**, *9*, 318. [CrossRef] [PubMed]

10

Blood Cells Separation and Sorting Techniques of Passive Microfluidic Devices: From Fabrication to Applications

Susana O. Catarino [1,†], Raquel O. Rodrigues [1,†], Diana Pinho [2,3,†,‡], João M. Miranda [3], Graça Minas [1] and Rui Lima [3,4,*]

[1] Center for MicroElectromechanical Systems (CMEMS-UMinho), University of Minho, Campus de Azurém, 4800-058 Guimarães, Portugal
[2] Research Centre in Digitalization and Intelligent Robotics (CeDRI), Instituto Politécnico de Bragança, Campus de Santa Apolónia, 5300-253 Bragança, Portugal
[3] CEFT, Faculdade de Engenharia da Universidade do Porto (FEUP), Rua Roberto Frias, 4200-465 Porto, Portugal
[4] MEtRICs, Mechanical Engineering Department, University of Minho, Campus de Azurém, 4800-058 Guimarães, Portugal
*   Correspondence: rl@dem.uminho.pt
†   These authors contributed equally to this work.
‡   Current affiliation: INL – International Iberian Nanotechnology Laboratory, Av. Mestre José Veiga, 4715-330 Braga, Portugal.

Abstract: Since the first microfluidic device was developed more than three decades ago, microfluidics is seen as a technology that exhibits unique features to provide a significant change in the way that modern biology is performed. Blood and blood cells are recognized as important biomarkers of many diseases. Taken advantage of microfluidics assets, changes on blood cell physicochemical properties can be used for fast and accurate clinical diagnosis. In this review, an overview of the microfabrication techniques is given, especially for biomedical applications, as well as a synopsis of some design considerations regarding microfluidic devices. The blood cells separation and sorting techniques were also reviewed, highlighting the main achievements and breakthroughs in the last decades.

Keywords: microfluidics; red blood cells (RBCs); microfabrication; polymers; separation and sorting techniques

1. Introduction

Since the development of the first microfluidic device, microfluidics heralded the promise to change life science and industry [1]. Despite the enormous scientific achievements that microfluidics have had in the last decades in the field of biomedical applications, this technology is still considered in its "adolescence" [2]. Among the pullbacks, are the difficulty to achieve a cost-effective large-scale production that allows its commercialization for clinical application, the so-called lab-on-a-chip, and the complete understanding of the physics of fluids at the microscale level over the biological species, such as blood and blood cells.

Blood and blood cells are important for scientific and clinical purposes because they can be used as indicators of many pathological conditions, including arterial hypertension, ischemia, inflammation, and diabetes [3,4]. Based on the fact that abnormal blood cells typically have distinctive biological and physicochemical properties (e.g., size, deformability and chemical composition), with different hydrodynamic properties when compared to healthy ones, these features can be used for rapid, low-cost cell separation and diagnosis.

In parallel, recent developments in microfabrication with polymers and elastomers made possible to fabricate low-cost transparent micrometre-sized channels and, as a result, several studies have been proposed using microfluidics to measure the motion and dynamic behaviour of cells flowing through microfluidic devices [5–12]. Taken into consideration that since its origins, microfluidics has flourished and paved its path in parallel with the development of new fabrication technologies, the present review aims to give an overview perspective of this technology for blood cells separation and sorting from the fabrication to application, and thus, revising the main achievements and breakthroughs in the last decades.

This review is organized as follows: Section 2 presents a description of different techniques for the fabrication of microfluidic devices, as well as a comparison between them; Section 3 approaches design considerations regarding microfluidic devices for biomedical applications; Section 4 describes and compares the main passive methods for cells sorting and separation; and Section 5 briefly discusses future challenges and perspectives regarding microfluidic devices and their applications.

2. Fabrication of Polymeric Microfluidic Devices

The beginning of microfluidics and its early systems, in the late 1970s (Figure 1), were derived from microelectronics and microelectromechanical systems (MEMS) technology and techniques, such as photolithography and etching, which were highly developed at the time [2,13].

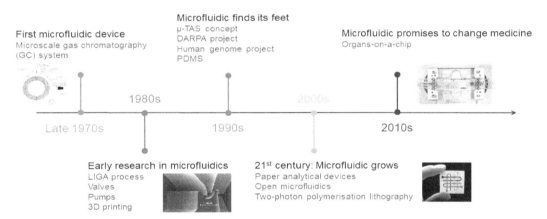

Figure 1. Timeline of the main microfluidics achievements from the first microfluidic device until the present.

Initially, silicon and glass were the select material to produce those microfluidic devices. Although, silicon had a big impact in microelectronics, initiating the Silicon Valley revolution, the material has some disadvantages for microfluidics, such as its opacity in the Ultra-Violet/Visible (UV/Vis) region of the electromagnetic spectrum and relative high cost [13,14]. Glass, on the other hand, is transparent, but due to its amorphous structure is difficult to etch compared with pure SiO_2. For the pattern of small size structures, sandblast and wet etching are the most used techniques. Nevertheless, sandblast is typically limited for patterns below 100 m and leads to rough surfaces, while wet etching allows smooth sidewalls but has low aspect ratio [15]. Therefore, among the glass micromachining limitations are the low etching aspect ratio and rate, limited mask selectivity and surface roughness [15]. Other disadvantages are that both materials required that each device is made in cleanroom facilities and its sealing made with high voltages and temperatures, which makes the microfabrication laborious and expensive [13]. In contrast to glass and silicon, polymers and elastomers, are less expensive and the channels can be obtained by molding or embossing that makes the fabrication faster and less expensive [14]. Among the most popular polymers used to fabricate microfluidic devices are poly(methyl methacrylate) (PMMA), cyclic olefin copolymer (COC), poly(styrene) (PS), poly(carbonate) (PC), poly(ethyleneterephthalate glycol) (PETG) and poly(dimethylsiloxane) (PDMS) [14]. Derived from this effort to find alternative materials, PDMS, a transparent elastomeric polymer pioneered by George Whitesides and his group at Harvard in the 1990s, quickly become the most popular material used in microfluidic devices [2]. The use of this new material made possible the massification of soft-lithography technique, with rapid prototyping and replica molding (Figure 2).

Figure 2 shows the main steps involved in the design and fabrication of microfluidic devices using the soft-lithography technique. The detailed description of these steps is well described elsewhere [13].

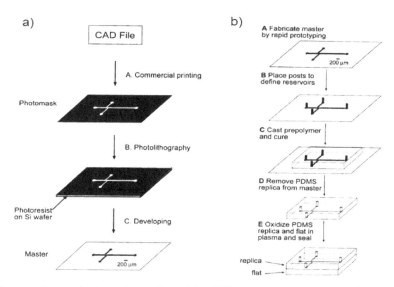

Figure 2. Soft lithography technique introduced by Whitesides and co-workers in 1998. (**a**) Rapid prototyping using photolithography and (**b**) replica molding with poly(dimethylsiloxane) (PDMS). Reproduced with permission from [13].

This innovation allowed the growth of microfluidics field due to the many advantages of this material: (i) high fidelity to replicate by molding features at the micro-scale level; (ii) its optically transparent down to 280 nm; (iii) low temperature and time to cure; (iv) biocompatibility and nontoxicity to cells; (v) possibility to change surface chemistry accordingly to the application needs; (vi) gas permeability, allowing culture of cells; (vii) reversal and self-bonding, among others [13,16,17].

In general, soft-lithography follows four major steps: (i) pattern design, drawn in computer-aided design (CAD) software programs for the fabrication of photomasks on transparency films (Figure 2a); (ii) fabrication of the mask and master, photomasks on transparency films are designed in high-resolution printers followed by photolithography technique (Figure 2a); (iii) fabrication of the PDMS stamp, fabricated by casting PDMS (pre-polymer mixed with cure agent) against a master whose surface has been patterned (Figure 2b) and (iv) fabrication of micro- and nanostructures with the stamp by printing, molding and embossing [18].

Although the several advantages of the soft-lithography method with PDMS, the standard prototyping method (i.e., photolithography) requires the access to cleanroom facilities and high-trained people. Additionally, the replica molding with PDMS is achieved by casting the masters one by one, which make the large-scale production slow. Nevertheless, this process is an ideal and fast solution to test prototypes. Another important aspect is that despite the common statement that BioMEMS is straightforward and inexpensive, the fabrication of microfluidic devices is, in general, complex and costly. For instance, it is estimated that the user fee in the United States for a fully staffed cleanroom, in a major research university, is in the order of $100/h per student [19]. This must include the typical time for training that can take several weeks for the basic operation of equipment and familiarization of techniques, such as spin coater, masker aligner and developing station [19]. An alternative is the contract of manufacturers that can provide custom master molds for a relatively low fee. However, this process can take several weeks from manufacturing to shipping [20]. To suppress the high cost and constrains of photolithography, alternatives have been developed in the last decade for the low-cost of microstructures without the need of cleanroom facilities. An example of this effort was published by Pinto et al., 2014 [21], describing the fabrication and optimization of microstructures in SU-8 (commonly used as epoxy-based negative photoresist), without the need of cleanroom facilities. The proposed fabrication technique uses an alternative photomask printed in transparent photographic sheet using standard tools and equipment employed in the printed circuit board (PCB) industry. Even though the outstanding achievement of the proposed technique, the SU-8 shows a resolution limitation of 10 m and the need to control the room temperature and humidity to optimize the fabrication procedure.

In parallel, alternative non-lithographic techniques have also emerged from these requirements of specific facilities and equipment that has inhibited many scientific groups to pursue new microfluidic innovations, namely print and peel techniques, e.g., xurography, micromilling or direct laser plotting (Figure 3), which are well reviewed elsewhere [22].

Briefly, xurography allows the generation of master molds (or masks) using a cutting plotter machine and adhesive vinyl film. Recently, Pinto et al. (2014) [23] have shown that xurography can be used as a rapid technique with good resolution to produce microfluidic structures down to 500 m. By using this technique Bento et al. [24] were able to successfully produce microchannels contractions with dimensions down to 350 m and as a result they have investigated how Taylor bubbles disturb the blood flow at the scale of blood cells.

Micromilling, is another low-cost fabrication technique that creates microscale structures by removing bulk material with cutting tools [25]. This technique was shown by Lopes and co-workers to have the ability to produce reusable microfluidic devices with widths down to 30 m [26].

Direct laser plotting is a microfabrication technique similar to micromilling that uses laser beams to create microchannels. This technique can typically generate microchannels widths up to 100 m. Although it has been shown the possibility to down to 20 m by using short laser pulses [22].

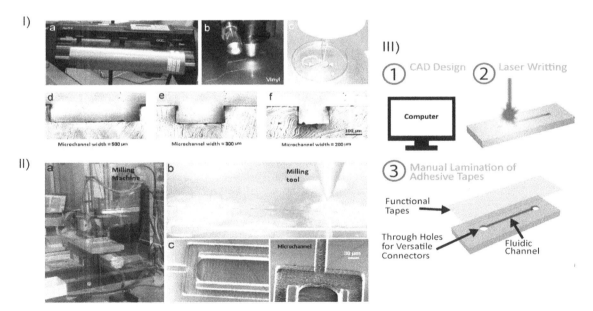

Figure 3. Low-cost print-and-peel microfabrication techniques. (**I**) Xurography: (**a**) cutting plotter machine; (**b**) features being cut by the cutting plotter; (**c**) PDMS being added to a petri dish containing the vinyl mask; (**d**), (**e**) and (**f**) Cross sections of microchannels with 500, 300 and 200 m of width, respectively. (**II**) Micromilling; (**a**) milling machine; (**b**) operating milling tool and (**c**) microchannels. Reproduced with permission from [22]. (**III**) Direct laser plotting main steps. Reproduced with permission from [27].

3D-printing fabrication techniques have also gained a growing interest to fabricate microfluidic devices, offering the possibility to generate devices with complex architectures from a broader range of materials and avoiding multi-step processing [28]. The main 3D-printing techniques are stereolithography (SLA), fused deposition modelling (FDM), selective laser sintering (SLS) and direct ink writing (inkjet) [28–30], allowing a broad range of applications. Among the advantages, the simplicity, fast and efficient prototyping with no need of photomask and cleanroom facilities, are some of the most important.

FDM, is the most simple and low-cost 3D-printing method, working by extruding a thermoplastic polymer through a hot nozzle to print layers of the object. The technique can be used to produce directly the microfluidic devices or the 3D mask that combined with PDMS replication molding allows the fabrication of 3D-biomodels, such as macro and micro-scale vascular system models [30,31].

An overview of the main advantages and disadvantages of the most representative fabrication techniques used to develop microfluidic devices in polymer substrates is given in Table 1.

Table 1. Main advantages, disadvantages, resolution range and aspect ratio of microfabrication techniques used to develop microfluidic devices using polymer substrates. Adapted from [14].

Fabrication Technique	Advantages	Disadvantages	Resolution Range and Aspect Ratio
Hot embossing	Precise and rapid in the replication of microstructures. Mass production.	Restricted to thermoplastics. Time-consuming. Complex 3D structures are difficult to be fabricated.	Resolution between sub-100 nm and millimetre. Moderate aspect ratio (5:1) [32,33]
Injection molding	Mass production. Fine features. Low cycle time. Highly automated.	Restricted to thermoplastics. High cost mold. Nano-size precision is limited.	Resolution between sub-100 nm and millimetre. High aspect ratio (20:1) [34]
Laser photoablation	Rapid. Large format production.	Limited materials. Multiple treatment session. Difficulties for mass production. Micro-size precision is limited.	Resolution between micrometre and millimetre. High aspect ratio (30:1) [35,36]
X-ray lithography	High-resolution. Straight and smooth walls.	Complex and difficult master fabrication. Time consuming and high cost process.	Resolution between few nanometres and micrometres. Ultra-high aspect ratio (350:1) [37]
Soft-lithography	High-resolution and 3D geometries. Cost-effective. Excellent micro-size precision.	Pattern deformation and vulnerability to defects. Difficult to fabricate circular 3D geometries.	Resolution between 30 nm and 500 m. High aspect ratio (20:1) [18]
Xurography	Low-cost and rapid technique.	Complex 3D structures are difficult to be fabricated. Micro-size precision is limited.	Resolution between 150 m and millimetre. Moderate aspect ratio (8:1) [21,23,38,39]
Direct laser plotting	Low-cost and rapid technique. Free-mask technique. Good micro-size precision.	Complex 3D structures are difficult to be fabricated. Micro-size precision is limited. Reproducibility of the microdevices.	Resolution between 10–500 m. Moderate aspect ratio (7:1) [40,41]

Table 1. *Cont.*

Fabrication Technique	Advantages	Disadvantages	Resolution Range and Aspect Ratio
Micromilling	Low-cost and rapid technique. Free-mask technique.	Complex 3D structures are difficult to be fabricated. Micro-size precision is limited. Reproducibility of the microdevices. Roughness.	Resolution between 30 m and millimetre. Moderate aspect ratio (8:1) [26,42]
Desktop fused deposition modeling (FDM), 3D-printing	Low-cost and rapid technique to fabricate prototypes.	Micro-size precision is limited. High roughness and complex to perform flow visualizations. Not suitable for mass production.	Resolution between 100 m and millimetre. Moderate aspect ratio (10:1) [43–45]
Nanofabrication	High-resolution of 2D and 3D geometries. Excellent nano-size precision. Highly repeatable, periodical structures.	High cost. Multiple process steps. Limited for microfluidic applications.	Resolution between 1–800 nm. Ultra-high aspect ratio (100:1) [17,46]

With the recent development of nanotechnology for several applications and fields, nanofabrication techniques for microfluidic devices have also been developed. In general, these new techniques are based in advanced nanoscale photolithographic methods, such as extreme ultraviolet, electron beam and nanoimprint lithography, or non-lithographic methods, such as anodic aluminium oxidation. All these new nanofabrication approaches are well described elsewhere [17]. With the ability to generate features with just a few nanometres, the main application of these nanofabrication techniques are lab-on-a-chip microdevices, with high potentiality to medicine, biology and chemical applications [47–49].

3. Design of Microfluidic Devices for Biomedical Applications

Biomedical science found a fruitful field in microfluidics to replace routine analysis and diagnosis tests, as well as to conduct fundamental biological studies in cells and diseases. Among the biomedical applications, microfluidics research has allowed the emerging of a wide range of promising applications from microscale genomic and proteomic analysis kits, biosensors, point-of-care diagnostic devices, drug screening and delivery platforms, implantable devices, novel biomaterials to tissue engineering and single cell studies [50].

Depending on the final application of the microfluidic device, different micro- or nanofabrication techniques are available and can be used. In general, most of the research groups try to pursue a time-cost effectiveness to fabricate their own microdevices. Based on this standpoint, Figure 4 gives an overview of the fabrication techniques listed in Table 1, from a time and cost perspective.

The material selection also has an important role in the application. For biomedical applications the selection of the material must consider important parameters, namely biocompatibility, bio-culture, permeability and porosity, protein crystallization, reusability and disposable device use. Some of these characteristics are listed in Table 2, for the most common materials used for biomedical applications.

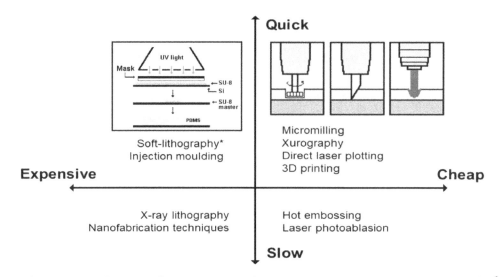

Figure 4. Fabrication techniques from a time and cost perspective. Adapted from [14]. * Despite standard soft-lithography technique is considered expensive, new alternatives without the need of cleanroom facilities significantly drop the cost, being considered as low-cost, as the work published by Pinto et al., 2014 [21].

Table 2. Significant characteristics of the most common materials used for biomedical applications. Adapted from [51].

Characteristics	Silicon	Glass	Thermoplastics	Elastomers (PDMS)
Protein crystallization	Poor	Poor	Good	Moderate
Droplet formation	Excellent	Excellent	Good	Moderate
Porosity	Poor	Poor	Moderate	Moderate
Permeability	Poor	Poor	Moderate	Good
Bio-culture	Moderate	Moderate	Moderate	Good
Reusability	Yes	Yes	Yes	No
Disposable device use	Expensive	Expensive	Good	Good

Another important aspect for the fabrication of microfluidic devices is the interfacing and/or integration of modules for the applications that the device is being designed. Among them, integration of microheaters, valves, sensors, electroosmotic fluid pumps, readout electronics, among others, can be accomplished to complete microfluidic devices with remarkable capabilities [52].

4. Microfluidic Cell Separation and Sorting Techniques

Despite all the research and development of microfluidic systems, several challenges remain related to the miniaturization of the lab-on-a-chip devices. At the microscale level, the mixture, pumping, separation and control of fluids are limited, on the one hand, by the minimum sample volumes and flow rates required by the biological analysis and, on the other hand, by the microscale dimensions of the systems. The dominant physical and chemical effects at the microscale level are different from the ones at the macroscale, leading to an increased complexity of the flow and mass transport phenomena. In order to overcome those limitations, significant research efforts have been performed for improving the design of micropumps, valves, mixers and separation devices that can be incorporated on lab-on-a-chip devices [53–55], while addressing the non-Newtonian behaviour of the majority of physiological fluids [56,57].

Microfluidic systems can integrate different kinds of sorting methods based on the physical parameters of cells, providing a perfect interface for the manipulation of single cells and access forces in a variety of ways and allowing a fully autonomous measurement of physical parameters [58].

Particularly, cell separation techniques have been developed for cell concentration purposes (removal of plasma and increase of the cell concentration, mainly haematocrit increase); plasma enrichment (removal of cells from plasma and cells dilution); blood fractioning (separation of blood into different components); cell sorting (separation of cells by type); and cell removal (specific cell sorting that removes only some specific cells), that can work as cell isolation or removal of pathogenics [59].

The manipulating of forces for the separation techniques can be active, passive or both (label-free cell sorting mechanism), as shown in Figure 5. Apart from these, there are other methods such as paper-based [60,61] and CD based [62,63] methods to separate mainly the plasma from blood [64]. Active technologies, based on microelectromechanical systems, improve the control of fluids using mobile parts or external mechanical forces, and can be based on dielectrophoresis, magnetophoresis, acoustophoresis and optical tweezers mechanisms [58,64]. Passive technologies for controlling fluids do not include external forces or mobile parts, and their control is promoted by diffusion as a function of the channel geometry [64–70], or intrinsic hydrodynamic forces, such as punch flow fraction, deterministic lateral displacement, inertial forces and intrinsic physical property of the cells [69–74], including sieving, which uses the size of micropores, microweirs, membranes and the gap between micropillars arrays for the separation of cells [26,69–78]. The passive microfluidic technologies bring more interest in the lab-on-a-chip and microfluidics research field due to its precise manipulation, low cost fabrication, simple structure, simple integration and lower maintenance in lab-on-a-chip devices and high throughput [79–82].

Therefore, this paper presents, in addition to an overview over the microfabrication techniques using polymers as substrates, a review and discussion of different passive techniques and microfluidic devices for separation of cells, categorized according to the separation phenomena: hydrodynamic phenomena (as punch flow, inertial forces or deterministic lateral displacement); hemodynamic phenomena (based on the intrinsic physical properties of the cells); and filters and physical filtration (based on micropores, microweirs, membranes and the gap between micropillars), as shown in Figure 5.

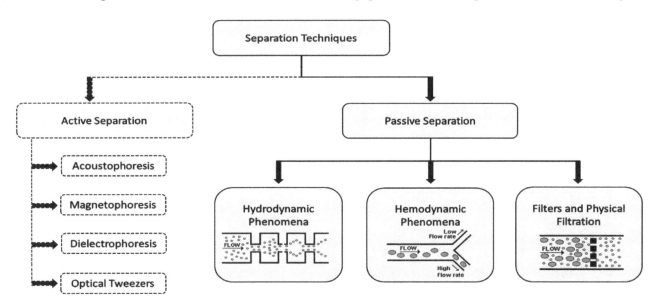

Figure 5. Classification of the main active and passive separation techniques used in microfluidic systems.

4.1. Hydrodynamic Separation and Sorting Techniques

The hydrodynamic separation techniques are adequate for low Reynolds number flows (Re < 1) in the microfluidic devices. In a purely hydrodynamic flow separation technique, the laminar flow conditions exist, i.e., viscous forces are strong enough to have any disturbances in the pumped flow through the microchannel. In this process, the aligned cells are separated through multiple side branching outlets (Figure 6b), so that particles of different sizes will follow different paths, achieving size-based separation [83]. The hydrodynamic focusing is able to achieve narrow streams through sheath flows unlike the inertial focusing that occurs in a single flow stream.

Particles or cells exposed to a shear flow experience a lift force perpendicular to the flow direction and a force from the wall. The equilibrium of these two forces is responsible for the cells or particles migration and depends on several factors, such as channel geometry, flow rate, rheological properties of the carrier fluid and mechanical properties of the elements, as in Figure 6a. By manipulating the flow, for example, controlling the flow rate through one or more inlets, it is possible to achieve size-based cell separation and sorting [84].

The inertial separation methods generate the deflection of larger particles away from the flow, while smaller ones are carried on or near the original flow streamline. These mechanisms occur in curved and focused flow segments, and result from the combination of asymmetrical sheath flows and specific channel geometries, which are able to create a soft inertial force on the fluid. By using channels with curvature (as in Figure 6e), an additional drag force arising from secondary flows (called Dean vortices) enhances the speed of particle migration to more stable equilibrium positions, achieving a faster focusing of cells and particles than in straight channels, with high-throughput and continuous blood separation [64,70]. The inertial migration phenomenon has been widely recognised by the counteraction of two inertial effects, i.e., the shear gradient lift and the wall lift forces [85]. Many of the microfluidic devices have combined this separation inertial focusing strategy with other microfluidic methodologies to enhance blood cells separation, as different examples are presented in Figure 6.

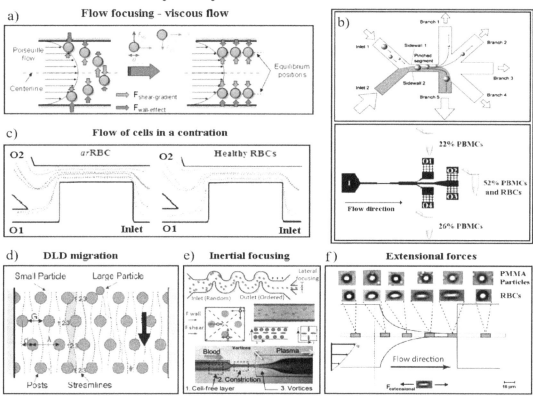

Figure 6. Hydrodynamic methods of separation: (**a**) the implied forces in a Poiseuille flow for cell separation. Reproduced with permission from [86] (**b**) the principle of hydrodynamic filtration in a microchannel with many outlets. Reproduced with permission from [81,84]. (**c**) trajectories analysis of rigid and deformable cells through a contraction for cell separation in two outlets. Reproduced with permission from [87]. (**d**) principle of deterministic lateral displacement. Reproduced with permission from [86]. (**e**) separation using inertial flow forces and at high flow rates creating vortices downstream a contraction. Reproduced with permission from [64,88]. (**f**) extensional forces for cell separation and mechanical analysis. Reproduced with permission from [89].

Wang et al. [90], reported an inertial microfluidic device for continuous extraction of large particles or cells with high size-selectivity (under 2 μm) and high efficiency (above 90%). The authors developed a simple geometry with four key parts: a main microchannel, with a high-aspect-ratio geometry, to assure the inertial particle flow; two chambers for the formation of microvortexes, symmetrically positioned; two side outlets, positioned at the chambers' corners, for the creation of sheath flow and removal of large particles; and, finally, an outlet for the small particles.

One of the hydrodynamic separation methods is based on the principle known as deterministic lateral displacement (DLD). This method employs arrays of pillars placed within a microchannel (array of obstacles). The laminar flow together with interactions in the array, forces the particles or cells to flow with specific trajectories through the device. The distance among the pillars is tailored according to the size of the cells or the particles to be sorted. The array pattern determines the displacement of cells or particles [84], i.e., the gap between posts and their offset determines the critical particle size for the fractionation. If the particles and/or cells are smaller than the critical size, they tend to flow through the array gaps without net displacement from the original central streamline. If the particles are bigger than the critical size, they will displace laterally, traveling at an angle predetermined by the posts offset distance (as shown in Figure 6d) [84]. Liu et al. [91] developed a rapid and label-free microfluidic structure for isolation of cancer cells from peripheral whole blood, using deterministic lateral displacement arrays (based on the size-dependent hydrodynamic forces), and achieved cells separation efficiency between 80% and 99% with a 2 mL/min throughput [91]. A high-throughput cytometry microsystem was reported by Rosenbluth et al. [92], to distinguish and quantify blood cell properties and help to prevent different hematologic problems (as sepsis, occlusion or leukastasis). The proposed microsystem presents a trifurcation into two bypass channels, and a network of bifurcations that split into 64 parallel capillary-like microchannels.

4.2. Hemodynamic Phenomena on Cell Separation Techniques

Microfluidic biomimetic cell separation techniques are based on mimicking the hemodynamic phenomena and the intrinsic properties of plasma and blood cells when flowing in microvessels. Different hemodynamic phenomena have been observed in vivo and replicated in microfluidic systems, including: plasma layer; Fåharaeus–Lindqvist effect (decrease of the apparent viscosity of blood in small vessels), which causes the tendency of the RBCs to migrate toward the centre of the microchannel, creating the cell-free layer (CFL) [11,93] (Figure 7b); leukocyte margination (migration of leukocytes, that are less deformable than RBCs, to the wall of the microchannel due to collisions between leucocytes and erythrocytes) [86]; plasma skimming (uneven distribution of red blood cells and plasma between the small side branch and the main channel); and the Zweifach–Fung bifurcation effect (in asymmetric bifurcations in which the vessel with the smaller flow rate gets a higher concentration of plasma), as represented in Figure 7c [64,93]. A number of microdevices have been developed to take advantage of these effects. For instance, in blood vessels with luminal diameter less than 300 μm, RBCs tend to migrate radially to the axial centre line of the vessel (Fåharaeus–Lindqvist effect), as shown in Figure 7a. Figure 7 summarizes the main hemodynamic phenomena of cell separation in microdevices. In microcirculation, the Zweifach–Fung bifurcation law is a relevant effect describing the cells tendency to travel to the daughter channel with a higher flow rate [86,88,94].

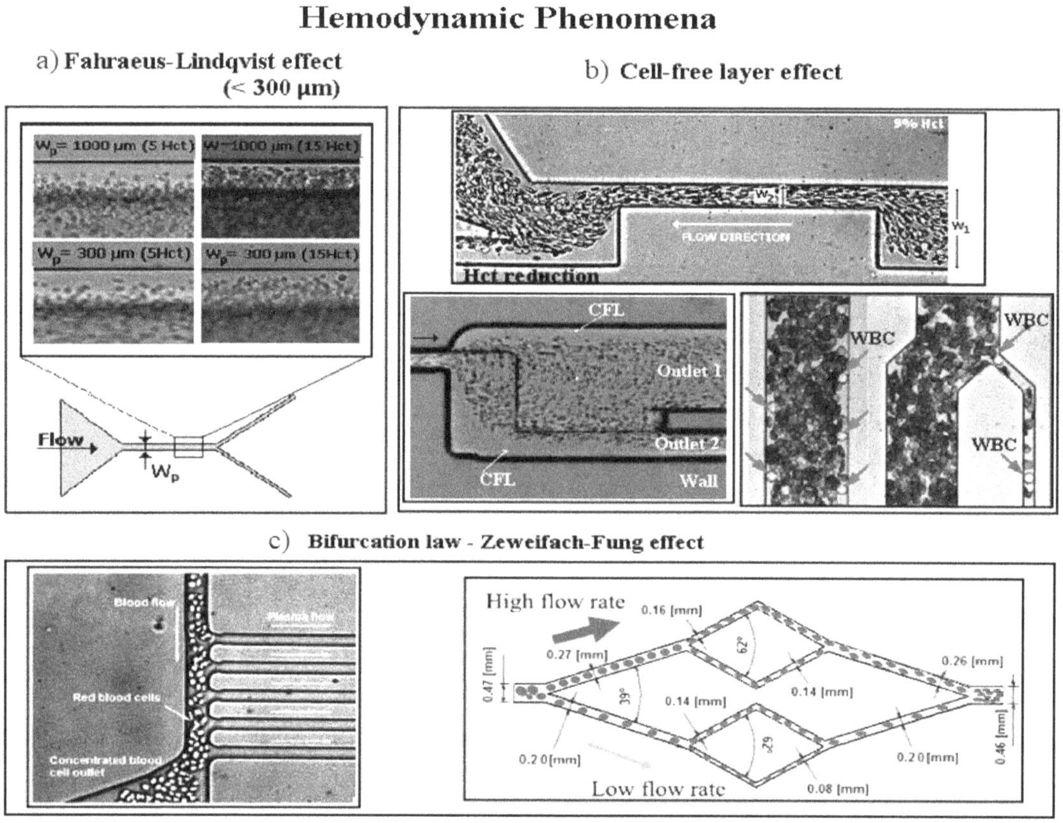

Hemodynamic Phenomena

a) Fahraeus-Lindqvist effect
(< 300 μm)

b) Cell-free layer effect

c) Bifurcation law - Zeweifach-Fung effect

Figure 7. Blood separation microdevices based on hemodynamic flow separation techniques: (a) the Fåharaeus–Lindqvist effect in a microchannels with dimensions < 300 μm. Reproduced with permission from [23]. (b) cell-free layer as an advantage for cell and plasma separation and plasma skimming effect, WBCs margination. Adapted from [86,95,96]. (c) the Bifurcation law manipulated to remove cell-free plasma from blood and to mimic the microvasculature networks. Reproduced with permission from [86,97].

Jaggi et al. [94] developed a poly(methyl methacrylate) (PMMA) microdevice for blood plasma separation at high flow rates, based on the bifurcation law. The authors obtained, for Hct 4.5% and whole blood Hct of 45%, at a 5 mL/min^{-1} flow rate, separation efficiencies of 92% and 30%, respectively. The plasma yield obtained was 4% for the 45% Hct. The authors reported shear stress values much lower than the shear stress at which hemolysis occurs [94]. Lopes et al. [26] developed a microfluidic device able to perform separation of RBCs from plasma due to the cell-free layer (CFL) created upstream a contraction in a microchannel. The authors produced the device using a micromilling technique, and concluded that the geometric contraction produced by that technique was able to enhance the CFL, resulting in a low cost and efficient way to separate blood cells from plasma [26]. Faivre et al. [98] developed a microchannel with a constriction-expansion region for studying the Fahraeus effect, showing the increase of the cell-free region downstream of the constriction region. The authors collected almost pure plasma with Hct 16% at a flow rate of 200 μL·h^{-1}, with a 24% yield (the separation efficiency was not mentioned explicitly). Lima et al. [99] successfully studied the behavior of RBCs in a 75 μm circular polydimethylsiloxane (PDMS) microchannel. The authors tracked individual RBCs (for 3% and 23% hematocrit) and observed that the trajectories of the solutions with higher RBC concentrations exhibit higher fluctuations in the direction normal to the flow. Additionally, the authors concluded that the RBCs flowing in a higher concentration environment tend to undergo multi-body collisions, increasing the amplitude of the RBCs' lateral motion. Yang et al. [13] described a PDMS microfluidic device based on the Zweifach–Fung bifurcation law. The separation efficiency was defined in terms of hematocrit and quantified using an image processing program. The authors obtained, with the microdevice continuously running during 30 min without clogging, a separation efficiency of

100% for an inlet Hct of 45%, using defibrinated sheep blood, at a 10 μL·h^{-1} flow rate, with a yield or plasma volume percentage obtained of 15–25% [65]. During the last decade, Ishikawa et al., [67], Leble et al., [9] and Pinto et al., [23] have performed in vitro blood flow studies in simple microchannels with symmetric bifurcations and confluences and more recently Bento et al. [100,101] have performed similar studies in more complex geometries such as in microchannel networks. In those works, it was observed a clear cell-depleted layer at the region of the confluence apex that can be used to perform blood plasma separation.

4.3. Microfluidic Filters-Physical Filtration Techniques

Combined with the mentioned separation techniques, microfluidic filters are usually introduced to increment the efficiency of the microfluidic devices [82,102]. Microscale filters, such as micropillar arrays, microweir structures or microporous membranes, are able to separate cells and particles based on their size and/or deformability. Although these filters allow the precise adjustment of the filter pore size to the required needs, they need to overcome different challenges, such as clogging of the microchannels, fouling and heterogeneity of the cell sizes [84]. Additionally, the design of the filters and barriers needs to take into consideration the different physical properties of the cells, including density, shape and deformability. Physical filtration microstructures, besides being a simple and non-destructive separation method, also allow the integration with other separation strategies. A major problem of the latter separation methodology is the high tendency to have clogging, jamming and possible blockage of the microdevice [103]. One way to minimize such a problem is by using cross-flow filters [83,104–106], since in cross-flow filtration, the fluid flows tangentially rather than through the filter as it does in membrane filtration (see Figure 8). This technique allows the particles to stay in a suspended state, avoiding their deposition, and can be used for separation of particles and cells. Crowley et al., [107] fabricated a passive crossflow filtration microdevice, operating entirely on capillary action, for the isolation of plasma from whole blood. Another method is by using micro-pillars that are suitably placed within the microchannel in a way that cells larger than the critical diameter follow a deterministic path while smaller cells maintain an average downward flow direction around the pillars, leading to the formation of multiple streams based size [86]. Chen et al., [105] developed a set of microfluidic chips based on the crossflow filtration principle, in which parallel micropillar-array and parallel microweirs were used to separate cells via their different sizes. Under the optimal conditions, more than 95% of the RBCs in a sample can be removed from the initial whole blood, while 27.4% of the white blood cells (WBCs) can be obtained. Plasma, WBCs and RBCs can be simultaneously separated and collected at different outlet ports with multilevel filtration barriers [105]. This principle is presented in Figure 8.

Zhang et al., [108] combined the use of hydrodynamic forces with passive filters comprised of artificial microbarriers of varying dimensions (that range in size from 15 to 7 μm, following the direction of fluid flow) in a chip to promote the flow and the separation of cells. By combining hydrodynamic forces with passive filters, the authors reported the separation of cancer cells based on their deformability. Additionally, by arranging the microbarriers in a rectangular, matrix-like structure, and by placing wide channels between post arrays, the authors ensured that the most flexible cells were able to seek alternate routes in the event of a blockage, as well as to regulate and equalize hydrodynamic pressure throughout the chip. The microscale geometry of the flow channels and post arrays ensured that the fluid flow is laminar, resulting in continuous cell movement and deformation in the device [108].

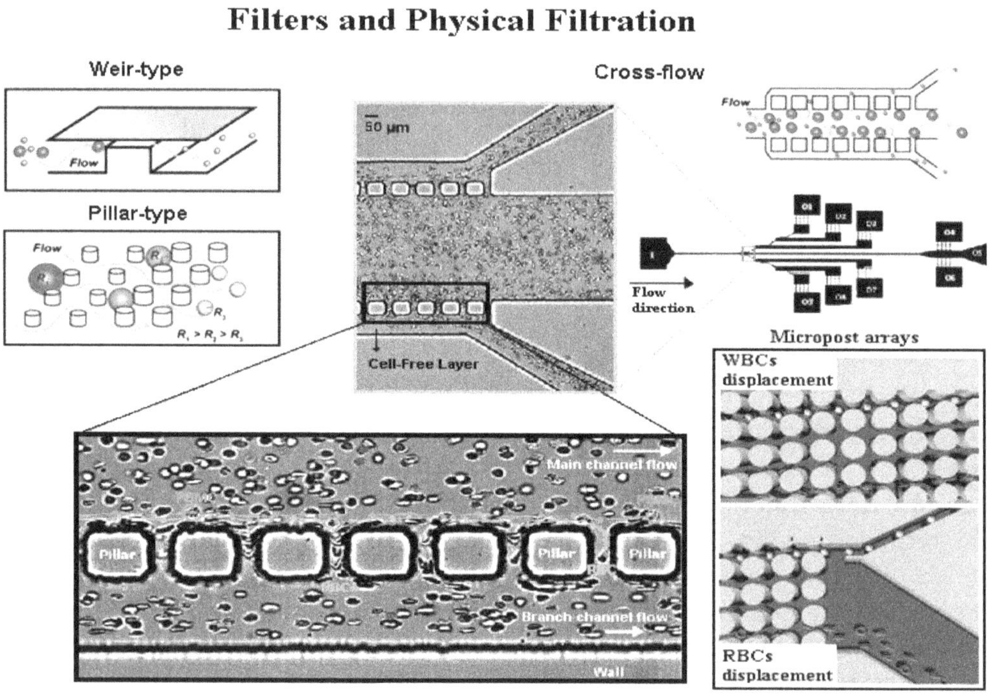

Filters and Physical Filtration

Figure 8. Schematic illustration for weir, pillar and cross-flow microfluidic filters. Images adapted from [81,84,109].

4.4. Comparison between the Separation Methods

Table 3 presents a comparison between the different categories of microfluidic cell separation, in terms of separation criteria, efficiency and throughput.

Table 3. Comparison between the passive separation phenomena.

Method	Hydrodynamic Separation	Hemodynamic Separation	Physical Filtration
Separation criteria	Size	Size, deformability, cells concentration (hematocrit), cell aggregation [102]	Size, shape, deformability
Target sample	Cells, microparticles	RBCs, WBCs, plasma	Cells, particles
Separation Efficiency	Above 90% [90,110]; 80–99% [91]; 62.2% [111]	100% separation efficiency with 15–25% plasma separation volume [65]; 92% separation efficiency with diluted blood (Hct 4.5%) and 37% with whole blood (Hct 45%) [94]	More than 95% of the RBCs and 27% of the WBCs removed from whole blood [105]; 65–100% [102]; 98%, 8% (plasma from whole blood) [112,113]
Throughput	2 mL/min [91]; 10^6 cells/min [110]; 1.2 mL/h (10^{10} cells/min) [111]	3–4 µL/min [112]; 5 mL/min [94]	2×10^3 cells/s [112,113]
Potential effects on cells	Shear stress	Shear stress	Clogging, fouling, shear stress
Required instrumentation	Fluidic pumps	Fluidic pumps	Fluidic pumps
Processing layout	Continuous flow	Continuous flow	Batch; Continuous flow

The referred passive separation methods are able to separate cells in a simple and non-destructive way and, furthermore, they allow easy integration of other processes in a single microdevice [114]. Ideally, a lab-on-a-chip platform should be small, simple and portable, by combining simple fluid driving mechanisms, reaction chambers and integrated detection systems for easy readout, making it able to be used by an end user or as a research tool, as a support for other laboratory technology [115].

Several authors have been approaching attempts for integration of passive separation of target cells and analysis, particularly of RBCs deformability assessment in a single microfluidic chip, which is still a challenge. Shevkoplyas et al. [116] developed a passive microfluidic device with a microvascular network perfusion system for cells separation and for measuring of the RBCs deformability. Faustino et al. [117] developed a microfluidic device in PDMS, with pillars and geometric variations, for the passive separation of RBCs, as well as to deform the cells and assess their deformability, by analyzing the acquired images. However, the proposed device is not fully integrated yet, since it still requires an external microscope for images evaluation and an external pumping system [117]. The described examples open new opportunities for research and show that lab-on-a-chip devices have high potential for integration of separation and detection tools in a single microfluidic platform.

There are still a lot of challenges to overcome regarding the integration of passive separation techniques in autonomous, functional and portable microdevices. Particularly, clogging, hematocrit, the amount of the sample and preparation time, mechanical stress (under relatively high pressure in microfluidic structures, several biological entities are at risk of rupturing, such as RBCs, or starting an adverse activation, such as platelets), contamination and biocompatibility are still challenging for the design and implementation of blood separation devices [64]. However, they also open new avenues for the miniaturization of analysis systems, requiring multidisciplinary synergies to assure the integration of microfluidics, actuation, detection, and readout systems in a single chip.

5. Perspectives

The research in the lab-on-a-chip area opens new possibilities for the miniaturization of analysis systems, requiring multidisciplinary synergies to assure the integration of microfluidics, actuation, detection, and readout systems in a single chip. All the developed efforts in this field are focused on the development of low-cost, portable, autonomous, multifunctional and commercial devices, with high sensitivity.

This paper presented an overview of the techniques used for separation of RBCs and the respective micro- and nanofabrication techniques, as well as examples of lab-on-a-chip devices with high potential for the integration of separation and detection tools in a single microfluidic platform. However, the use of these methods for separation of RBCs and detection of their properties has still a lot of challenges to overcome. Particularly, most separation methods, despite being able to separate particles, still need further development to be able to separate large cells, as RBCs, in microdevices, and require additional external equipment, which limits the methods' portability.

As the lab-on-a-chip devices become multifunctional tools for separation and analysis of cells, without altering their state, efforts are converging into new analytical chemistry, diagnostic and treatment applications [118,119]. Further advances include lab-on-a-cell platforms [120,121] for isolation and individual characterization of cells and organ-on-a-chip devices for, among other applications, oxygenation studies [122,123], improvement of the clinical translation of nanomaterials for cancer theranostics, drug screening and personalized medicine [124,125].

Author Contributions: Conceptualization, S.O.C., R.O.R., D.P. and R.L.; Writing-Original Draft Preparation, S.O.C., R.O.R. and D.P.; Writing-Review & Editing, J.M.M., G.M. and R.L.; Supervision, G.M. and R.L.; Funding Acquisition, S.O.C, G.M. and R.L.

References

1.   Whitesides, G.M. The origins and the future of microfluidics. *Nature* **2006**, *442*, 368–373. [CrossRef] [PubMed]
2.   Convery, N.; Gadegaard, N. 30 years of microfluidics. *Micro Nano Eng.* **2019**, *2*, 76–91. [CrossRef]
3.   Mchedlishvili, G.; Maeda, N. Blood flow structure related to red cell flow: A determinant of blood fluidity in narrow microvessels. *Jpn. J. Physiol.* **2001**, *51*, 19–30. [CrossRef] [PubMed]
4.   Bukowska, D.M.; Derzsi, L.; Tamborski, S.; Szkulmowski, M.; Garstecki, P.; Wojtkowski, M. Assessment

of the flow velocity of blood cells in a microfluidic device using joint spectral and time domain optical coherence tomography. *Opt. Express* **2013**, *21*, 24025–24038. [CrossRef] [PubMed]

5.   Abkarian, M.; Faivre, M.; Stone, H.A. High-speed microfluidic differential manometer for cellular-scale hydrodynamics. *Proc. Natl. Acad. Sci. USA* **2006**, *103*, 538–542. [CrossRef] [PubMed]

6.   Bhattacharya, S.; DasGupta, S.; Chakraborty, S. Collective dynamics of red blood cells on an in vitro microfluidic platform. *Lab Chip* **2018**, *18*, 3939–3948.

7.   Zhao, R.; Antaki, J.F.; Naik, T.; Bachman, T.N.; Kameneva, M.V.; Wu, Z.J. Microscopic investigation of erythrocyte deformation dynamics. *Biorheology* **2006**, *43*, 747–765. [PubMed]

8.   Fujiwara, H.; Ishikawa, T.; Lima, R.; Matsuki, N.; Imai, Y.; Kaji, H.; Nishizawa, M.; Yamaguchi, T. Red blood cell motions in high-hematocrit blood flowing through a stenosed microchannel. *J. Biomech.* **2009**, *42*, 838–843. [CrossRef]

9.   Leble, V.; Lima, R.; Dias, R.; Fernandes, C.; Ishikawa, T.; Imai, Y.; Yamaguchi, T. Asymmetry of red blood cell motions in a microchannel with a diverging and converging bifurcation. *Biomicrofluidics* **2011**, *5*, 044120. [CrossRef]

10. Manouk, A.; Magalie, F.; Renita, H.; Kristian, S.; Catherine, A.B.-P.; Howard, A.S. Cellular-scale hydrodynamics. *Biomed. Mater.* **2008**, *3*, 034011.

11. Lima, R.; Ishikawa, T.; Imai, Y.; Yamaguchi, T. Blood Flow Behavior in Microchannels: Past, Current and Future Trends. In *Single and Two-Phase Flows on Chemical and Biomedical Engineering*; Dias, R., Martins, A.A., Lima, R., Mata, T.M., Eds.; Bentham Science: Sharjah, UAE, 2012; pp. 513–547.

12. Tomaiuolo, G.; Barra, M.; Preziosi, V.; Cassinese, A.; Rotoli, B.; Guido, S. Microfluidics analysis of red blood cell membrane viscoelasticity. *Lab Chip* **2011**, *11*, 449–454. [CrossRef] [PubMed]

13. McDonald, J.C.; Duffy, D.C.; Anderson, J.R.; Chiu, D.T.; Wu, H.; Schueller, O.J.; Whitesides, G.M. Fabrication of microfluidic systems in poly(dimethylsiloxane). *Electrophoresis* **2000**, *21*, 27–40. [CrossRef]

14. Rodrigues, R.O.; Lima, R.; Gomes, H.T.; Silva, A.M.T. Polymer microfluidic devices: An overview of fabrication methods. *U. Porto J. Eng.* **2015**, *1*, 67–79. [CrossRef]

15. Van Toan, N.; Toda, M.; Ono, T. An Investigation of Processes for Glass Micromachining. *Micromachines* **2016**, *7*, 51. [CrossRef] [PubMed]

16. Halldorsson, S.; Lucumi, E.; Gómez-Sjöberg, R.; Fleming, R.M.T. Advantages and challenges of microfluidic cell culture in polydimethylsiloxane devices. *Biosens. Bioelectron.* **2015**, *63*, 218–231. [CrossRef] [PubMed]

17. Gale, B.; Jafek, A.; Lambert, C.; Goenner, B.; Moghimifam, H.; Nze, U.; Kamarapu, S. A Review of current methods in microfluidic device fabrication and future commercialization prospects. *Inventions* **2018**, *3*, 60. [CrossRef]

18. Qin, D.; Xia, Y.; Whitesides, G.M. Soft lithography for micro- and nanoscale patterning. *Nat. Protoc.* **2010**, *5*, 491. [CrossRef] [PubMed]

19. Folch, A. *Introduction to BioMEMS*; CRC Press: Boca Raton, FL, USA, 2013; p. 528.

20. Walsh, D.I.; Kong, D.S.; Murthy, S.K.; Carr, P.A. Enabling microfluidics: From clean rooms to makerspaces. *Trends Biotechnol.* **2017**, *35*, 383–392. [CrossRef]

21. Pinto, V.C.; Sousa, P.J.; Cardoso, V.F.; Minas, G. Optimized SU-8 processing for low-cost microstructures fabrication without cleanroom facilities. *Micromachines* **2014**, *5*, 738–755. [CrossRef]

22. Faustino, V.; Catarino, S.O.; Lima, R.; Minas, G. Biomedical microfluidic devices by using low-cost fabrication techniques: A review. *J. Biomech.* **2016**, *49*, 2280–2292. [CrossRef] [PubMed]

23. Pinto, E.; Faustino, V.; Rodrigues, R.; Pinho, D.; Garcia, V.; Miranda, J.; Lima, R. A rapid and low-cost nonlithographic method to fabricate biomedical microdevices for blood flow analysis. *Micromachines* **2015**, *6*, 121–135. [CrossRef]

24. Bento, D.; Sousa, L.; Yaginuma, T.; Garcia, V.; Lima, R.; Miranda, J.M. Microbubble moving in blood flow in microchannels: Effect on the cell-free layer and cell local concentration. *Biomed. Microdevices* **2017**, *19*, 6. [CrossRef] [PubMed]

25. Guckenberger, D.J.; de Groot, T.E.; Wan, A.M.D.; Beebe, D.J.; Young, E.W.K. Micromilling: A method for ultra-rapid prototyping of plastic microfluidic devices. *Lab Chip* **2015**, *15*, 2364–2378. [CrossRef] [PubMed]

26. Lopes, R.; Rodrigues, R.O.; Pinho, D.; Garcia, V.; Schütte, H.; Lima, R.; Gassmann, S. Low cost microfluidic device for partial cell separation: Micromilling approach. In Proceedings of the 2015 IEEE International Conference on Industrial Technology (ICIT), Seville, Spain, 17–19 March 2015; pp. 3347–3350.

27. Ren, Y.; Ray, S.; Liu, Y. Reconfigurable Acrylic-tape Hybrid Microfluidics. *Sci. Rep.* **2019**, *9*, 4824. [CrossRef] [PubMed]

28. Gaal, G.; Mendes, M.; de Almeida, T.P.; Piazzetta, M.H.; Gobbi, Â.L.; Riul, A., Jr.; Rodrigues, V. Simplified fabrication of integrated microfluidic devices using fused deposition modeling 3D printing. *Sens. Actuators B Chem.* **2017**, *242*, 35–40. [CrossRef]

29. Li, Z.A.; Yang, J.; Li, K.; Zhu, L.; Tang, W. Fabrication of PDMS microfluidic devices with 3D wax jetting. *RSC Adv.* **2017**, *7*, 3313–3320. [CrossRef]

30. Faria, C.L.; Pinho, D.; Santos, J.; Gonçalves, L.M.; Lima, R. Low cost 3D printed biomodels for biofluid mechanics applications. *J. Mech. Eng. Biomech.* **2018**, *3*, 1–7. [CrossRef]

31. Rodrigues, R.O.; Pinho, D.; Bento, D.; Lima, R.; Ribeiro, J. Wall expansion assessment of an intracranial aneurysm model by a 3D Digital Image Correlation System. *Measurement* **2016**, *88*, 262–270. [CrossRef]

32. Miller, R.; Glinsner, T.; Kreindl, G.; Lindner, P.; Wimplinger, M. *Industrial Applications Demanding Low and High Resolution Features Realized by Soft UV-NIL and Hot Embossing*; SPIE: Bellingham, WA, USA, 2009; 72712J.

33. He, Y.; Fu, J.-Z.; Chen, Z.-C. Research on optimization of the hot embossing process. *J. Micromech. Microeng.* **2007**, *17*, 2420–2425. [CrossRef]

34. Stormonth-Darling, J.M.; Pedersen, R.H.; How, C.; Gadegaard, N. Injection molding of ultra high aspect ratio nanostructures using coated polymer tooling. *J. Micromech. Microeng.* **2014**, *24*, 075019. [CrossRef]

35. Sarig-Nadir, O.; Livnat, N.; Zajdman, R.; Shoham, S.; Seliktar, D. laser photoablation of guidance microchannels into hydrogels directs cell growth in three dimensions. *Biophys. J.* **2009**, *96*, 4743–4752. [CrossRef] [PubMed]

36. Yang, C.-R.; Hsieh, Y.-S.; Hwang, G.-Y.; Lee, Y.-D. Photoablation characteristics of novel polyimides synthesized for high-aspect-ratio excimer laser LIGA process. *J. Micromech. Microeng.* **2004**, *14*, 480–489. [CrossRef]

37. Hartley, F.T.; Malek, C.G.K. Nanometer X-ray Lithography. In Proceedings of the Asia Pacific Symposium on Microelectronics and MEMS, Gold Coast, Australia, 8 October 1999.

38. Hizawa, T.; Takano, A.; Parthiban, P.; Doyle, P.S.; Iwase, E.; Hashimoto, M. Rapid prototyping of fluoropolymer microchannels by xurography for improved solvent resistance. *Biomicrofluidics* **2018**, *12*, 064105. [CrossRef] [PubMed]

39. Bartholomeusz, D.A.; Boutte, R.W.; Andrade, J.D. Xurography: Rapid prototyping of microstructures using a cutting plotter. *J. Microelectromech. Syst.* **2005**, *14*, 1364–1374. [CrossRef]

40. Lamont, A.C.; Alsharhan, A.T.; Sochol, R.D. Geometric Determinants of In-Situ Direct Laser Writing. *Sci. Rep.* **2019**, *9*, 394. [CrossRef] [PubMed]

41. Do, M.T.; Li, Q.; Nguyen, T.T.N.; Benisty, H.; Ledoux-Rak, I.; Lai, N.D. High aspect ratio submicrometer two-dimensional structures fabricated by one-photon absorption direct laser writing. *Microsyst. Technol.* **2014**, *20*, 2097–2102. [CrossRef]

42. Friedrich, C.R.; Vasile, M.J. The micromilling process for high aspect ratio microstructures. *Microsyst. Technol.* **1996**, *2*, 144–148. [CrossRef]

43. Kitson, P.J.; Rosnes, M.H.; Sans, V.; Dragone, V.; Cronin, L. Configurable 3D-Printed millifluidic and microfluidic 'lab on a chip' reactionware devices. *Lab Chip* **2012**, *12*, 3267–3271. [CrossRef]

44. Au, A.K.; Huynh, W.; Horowitz, L.F.; Folch, A.V. 3D-Printed microfluidics. *Angew. Chem. Int. Ed.* **2016**, *55*, 3862–3881. [CrossRef]

45. Waheed, S.; Cabot, J.M.; Macdonald, N.P.; Lewis, T.; Guijt, R.M.; Paull, B.; Breadmore, M.C. 3D printed microfluidic devices: Enablers and barriers. *Lab Chip* **2016**, *16*, 1993–2013. [CrossRef]

46. Chang, C.; Sakdinawat, A. Ultra-high aspect ratio high-resolution nanofabrication for hard X-ray diffractive optics. *Nat. Commun.* **2014**, *5*, 4243. [CrossRef] [PubMed]

47. Isobe, G.; Kanno, I.; Kotera, H.; Yokokawa, R. Perfusable multi-scale channels fabricated by integration of nanoimprint lighography (NIL) and UV lithography (UVL). *Microelectron. Eng.* **2012**, *98*, 58–63. [CrossRef]

48. Kim, J.; Gale, B.K. Quantitative and qualitative analysis of a microfluidic DNA extraction system using a nanoporous AlOx membrane. *Lab Chip* **2008**, *8*, 1516–1523. [CrossRef] [PubMed]

49. Zhang, R.; Larsen, N.B. Stereolithographic hydrogel printing of 3D culture chips with biofunctionalized complex 3D perfusion networks. *Lab Chip* **2017**, *17*, 4273–4282. [CrossRef] [PubMed]

50. Yeo, L.Y.; Chang, H.C.; Chan, P.P.; Friend, J.R. Microfluidic devices for bioapplications. *Small* **2011**, *7*, 12–48. [CrossRef] [PubMed]

51. Ren, K.; Zhou, J.; Wu, H. Materials for Microfluidic Chip Fabrication. *Acc. Chem. Res.* **2013**, *46*, 2396–2406. [CrossRef] [PubMed]

52. Friend, J.; Yeo, L. Fabrication of microfluidic devices using polydimethylsiloxane. *Biomicrofluidics* **2010**, *4*, 026502. [CrossRef] [PubMed]

53. Cardoso, V.F.; Minas, G. Micro Total Analysis Systems. In *Microfluidics and Nanofluid. Handbook: Fabrication, Implementation and Applications*; CPTF Group, Ed.; LLC Publishers: Boca Raton, FL, USA, 2011; Volume 5, pp. 319–366.

54. Haeberle, S.; Zengerle, R. Microfluidic platforms for lab-on-a-chip applications. *Lab Chip* **2007**, *7*, 1094–1110. [CrossRef]

55. Rife, J.C.; Bell, M.I.; Horwitz, J.S.; Kabler, M.N.; Auyeung, R.C.Y.; Kim, W.J. Miniature valveless ultrasonic pumps and mixers. *Sens. Actuators A Phys.* **2000**, *86*, 135–140. [CrossRef]

56. Fung, Y.C. *Biomechanics-Circulation*; Springer: New York, NY, USA, 1997.

57. Roselli, R.J.; Diller, K.R. *Biotransport: Principles and Applications*; Springer: New York, NY, USA, 2011.

58. Mohamed, M. Use of Microfluidic Technology for Cell Separation. In *Blood Cell-An Overview of Studies in Hematology*; InTech: London, UK, 2012.

59. Shields, C.W., 4th; Reyes, C.D.; Lopez, G.P. Microfluidic cell sorting: A review of the advances in the separation of cells from debulking to rare cell isolation. *Lab Chip* **2015**, *15*, 1230–1249. [CrossRef]

60. Songjaroen, T.; Dungchai, W.; Chailapakul, O.; Henry, C.S.; Laiwattanapaisal, W. Blood separation on microfluidic paper-based analytical devices. *Lab Chip* **2012**, *12*, 3392–3398. [CrossRef] [PubMed]

61. Kim, J.-H.; Woenker, T.; Adamec, J.; Regnier, F.E. Simple, Miniaturized blood plasma extraction method. *Anal. Chem.* **2013**, *85*, 11501–11508. [CrossRef] [PubMed]

62. Haeberle, S.; Brenner, T.; Zengerle, R.; Ducrée, J. Centrifugal extraction of plasma from whole blood on a rotating disk. *Lab Chip* **2006**, *6*, 776–781. [CrossRef] [PubMed]

63. Amasia, M.; Madou, M. Large-volume centrifugal microfluidic device for blood plasma separation. *Bioanalysis* **2010**, *2*, 1701–1710. [CrossRef] [PubMed]

64. Kersaudy-Kerhoas, M.; Sollier, E. Micro-scale blood plasma separation: From acoustophoresis to egg-beaters. *Lab Chip* **2013**, *13*, 3323–3346. [CrossRef] [PubMed]

65. Yang, S.; Undar, A.; Zahn, J.D. A microfluidic device for continuous, real time blood plasma separation. *Lab Chip* **2006**, *6*, 871–880. [CrossRef]

66. Shevkoplyas, S.S.; Yoshida, T.; Munn, L.L.; Bitensky, M.W. Biomimetic autoseparation of leukocytes from whole blood in a microfluidic device. *Anal. Chem.* **2005**, *77*, 933–937. [CrossRef]

67. Ishikawa, T.; Fujiwara, H.; Matsuki, N.; Yoshimoto, T.; Imai, Y.; Ueno, H.; Yamaguchi, T. Asymmetry of blood flow and cancer cell adhesion in a microchannel with symmetric bifurcation and confluence. *Biomed. Microdevices* **2011**, *13*, 159–167. [CrossRef]

68. Karimi, A.; Yazdi, S.; Ardekani, A.M. Hydrodynamic mechanisms of cell and particle trapping in microfluidics. *Biomicrofluidics* **2013**, *7*, 21501. [CrossRef]

69. Martel, J.M.; Toner, M. Inertial focusing in microfluidics. *Annu. Rev. Biomed. Eng.* **2014**, *16*, 371–396. [CrossRef]

70. Zhang, J.; Yan, S.; Yuan, D.; Alici, G.; Nguyen, N.T.; Warkiani, M.E.; Li, W. Fundamentals and applications of inertial microfluidics: A review. *Lab Chip* **2016**, *16*, 10–34. [CrossRef] [PubMed]

71. Lee, C.-Y.; Chang, C.-L.; Wang, Y.-N.; Fu, L.-M. Microfluidic mixing: A review. *Int. J. Mol. Sci.* **2011**, *12*, 3263–3287. [CrossRef] [PubMed]

72. Suh, Y.K.; Kang, S. A Review on mixing in microfluidics. *Micromachines* **2010**, *1*, 82–111. [CrossRef]

73. Pamme, N.; Manz, A. On-chip free-flow magnetophoresis: Continuous flow separation of magnetic particles and agglomerates. *Anal. Chem.* **2004**, *76*, 7250–7256. [CrossRef] [PubMed]

74. Pamme, N. Continuous flow separations in microfluidic devices. *Lab Chip* **2007**, *7*, 1644–1659. [CrossRef] [PubMed]

75. Lee, G.-H.; Kim, S.-H.; Ahn, K.; Lee, S.-H.; Park, J.Y. Separation and sorting of cells in microsystems using physical principles. *J. Micromech. Microeng.* **2015**, *26*, 013003. [CrossRef]

76. Kang, T.G.; Yoon, Y.-J.; Ji, H.; Lim, P.Y.; Chen, Y. A continuous flow micro filtration device for plasma/blood separation using submicron vertical pillar gap structures. *J. Micromech. Microeng.* **2014**, *24*, 087001. [CrossRef]

77. Pinho, D.; Rodrigues, R.O.; Faustino, V.; Yaginuma, T.; Exposto, J.; Lima, R. Red blood cells radial dispersion in blood flowing through microchannels: The role of temperature. *J. Biomech.* **2016**, *49*, 2293–2298. [CrossRef]

78. Hou, H.W.; Bhagat, A.A.; Chong, A.G.; Mao, P.; Tan, K.S.; Han, J.; Lim, C.T. Deformability based cell margination–a simple microfluidic design for malaria-infected erythrocyte separation. *Lab Chip* **2010**, *10*, 2605–2613. [CrossRef]

79. Chung, Y.C.; Hsu, Y.L.; Jen, C.P.; Lu, M.C.; Lin, Y.C. Design of passive mixers utilizing microfluidic self-circulation in the mixing chamber. *Lab Chip* **2004**, *4*, 70–77. [CrossRef]

80. Khosravi Parsa, M.; Hormozi, F.; Jafari, D. Mixing enhancement in a passive micromixer with convergent–divergent sinusoidal microchannels and different ratio of amplitude to wave length. *Comput. Fluids* **2014**, *105*, 82–90. [CrossRef]

81. Rodrigues, R.O.; Pinho, D.; Faustino, V.; Lima, R. A simple microfluidic device for the deformability assessment of blood cells in a continuous flow. *Biomed. Microdevices* **2015**, *17*, 108. [CrossRef] [PubMed]

82. Squires, T.M.; Quake, S.R. Microfluidics: Fluid physics at the nanoliter scale. *Rev. Mod. Phys.* **2005**, *77*, 977–1026. [CrossRef]

83. Tsutsui, H.; Ho, C.-M. Cell separation by non-inertial force fields in microfluidic systems. *Mech. Res. Commun.* **2009**, *36*, 92–103. [CrossRef] [PubMed]

84. Gossett, D.R.; Weaver, W.M.; Mach, A.J.; Hur, S.C.; Tse, H.T.; Lee, W.; Amini, H.; Di Carlo, D. Label-free cell separation and sorting in microfluidic systems. *Anal. Bioanal. Chem.* **2010**, *397*, 3249–3267. [CrossRef] [PubMed]

85. Di Carlo, D. Inertial microfluidics. *Lab Chip* **2009**, *9*, 3038–3046. [CrossRef] [PubMed]

86. Bhagat, A.A.; Bow, H.; Hou, H.W.; Tan, S.J.; Han, J.; Lim, C.T. Microfluidics for cell separation. *Med. Biol. Eng. Comput.* **2010**, *48*, 999–1014. [CrossRef] [PubMed]

87. Pinho, D.; Rodrigues, R.O.; Yaginuma, T.; Faustino, V.; Bento, D.; Fernandes, C.S.; Garcia, V.; Pereira, A.I.; Lima, R. Motion of rigid particles flowing in a microfluidic device with a pronounced stenosis: Trajectories and deformation index. In Proceedings of the 1th World Congress on Computational Mechanics, Barcelona, Spain, 20–25 July 2014.

88. Yu, Z.T.F.; Aw Yong, K.M.; Fu, J. Microfluidic blood cell sorting: Now and beyond. *Small* **2014**, *10*, 1687–1703. [CrossRef] [PubMed]

89. Calejo, J.; Pinho, D.; Galindo-Rosales, F.J.; Lima, R.; Campo-Deaño, L. Particulate blood analogues reproducing the erythrocytes cell-free layer in a microfluidic device containing a hyperbolic contraction. *Micromachines* **2015**, *7*, 4. [CrossRef] [PubMed]

90. Wang, X.; Zhou, J.; Papautsky, I. Vortex-aided inertial microfluidic device for continuous particle separation with high size-selectivity, efficiency, and purity. *Biomicrofluidics* **2013**, *7*, 44119. [CrossRef] [PubMed]

91. Liu, Z.; Huang, F.; Du, J.; Shu, W.; Feng, H.; Xu, X.; Chen, Y. Rapid isolation of cancer cells using microfluidic deterministic lateral displacement structure. *Biomicrofluidics* **2013**, *7*, 11801. [CrossRef] [PubMed]

92. Rosenbluth, M.J.; Lam, W.A.; Fletcher, D.A. Analyzing cell mechanics in hematologic diseases with microfluidic biophysical flow cytometry. *Lab Chip* **2008**, *8*, 1062–1070. [CrossRef]

93. Pinho, D.; Campo-Deaño, L.; Lima, R.; Pinho, F.T. In vitro particulate analogue fluids for experimental studies of rheological and hemorheological behavior of glucose-rich RBC suspensions. *Biomicrofluidics* **2017**, *11*, 054105. [CrossRef]

94. Jäggi, R.D.; Sandoz, R.; Effenhauser, C.S. Microfluidic depletion of red blood cells from whole blood in high-aspect-ratio microchannels. *Microfluid. Nanofluid.* **2007**, *3*, 47–53. [CrossRef]

95. Singhal, J.; Pinho, D.; Lopes, R.; C Sousa, P.; Garcia, V.; Schütte, H.; Lima, R.; Gassmann, S. Blood Flow Visualization and Measurements in Microfluidic Devices Fabricated by a Micromilling Technique. *Micro Nanosyst.* **2015**, *7*, 148–153. [CrossRef]

96. Pinho, D.; Yaginuma, T.; Lima, R. A microfluidic device for partial cell separation and deformability assessment. *Biochip J.* **2013**, *7*, 367–374. [CrossRef]

97. Cidre, D.; Rodrigues, R.O.; Faustino, V.; Pinto, E.; Pinho, D.; Bento, D.; Correia, T.; Fernandes, C.S.; Dias, R.P.; Lima, R. Flow of red blood cells in microchannel networks: In vitro studies. In *Perspectives in Fundamental and Applied Rheology*; Rubio-Hernández, F.J., Gómez-Merino, A.I., Pino, C., Parras, L., Campo-Deaño, L., Galindo-Rosales, F.J., Velázquez-Navarro, J.F., Eds.; In Iberian Meeting on Rheology: Málaga, Spain, 2013; pp. 271–275.

98. Faivre, M.; Abkarian, M.; Bickraj, K.; Stone, H.A. Geometrical focusing of cells in a microfluidic device: An approach to separate blood plasma. *Biorheology* **2006**, *43*, 147–159. [PubMed]

99. Lima, R.; Oliveira, M.S.; Ishikawa, T.; Kaji, H.; Tanaka, S.; Nishizawa, M.; Yamaguchi, T. Axisymmetric polydimethysiloxane microchannels for in vitro hemodynamic studies. *Biofabrication* **2009**, *1*, 035005. [CrossRef]

100. Bento, D.; Pereira, A.I.; Lima, J.; Miranda, J.M.; Lima, R. Cell-free layer measurements of in vitro blood flow in a microfluidic network: An automatic and manual approach. *Comput. Methods Biomech. Biomed. Eng. Imaging Vis.* **2018**, *6*, 629–637. [CrossRef]

101. Bento, D.; Fernandes, C.S.; Miranda, J.M.; Lima, R. In vitro blood flow visualizations and cell-free layer (CFL) measurements in a microchannel network. *Exp. Therm. Fluid Sci.* **2019**, *109*, 109847. [CrossRef]

102. Tripathi, S.; Varun Kumar, Y.V.B.; Prabhakar, A.; Joshi, S.S.; Agrawal, A. Passive blood plasma separation at the microscale: A review of design principles and microdevices. *J. Micromech. Microeng.* **2015**, *25*, 083001. [CrossRef]

103. Bacchin, P.; Meireles, M.; Aimar, P. Modelling of filtration: From the polarised layer to deposit formation and compaction. *Desalination* **2002**, *145*, 139–146. [CrossRef]

104. Keskinler, B.; Yildiz, E.; Erhan, E.; Dogru, M.; Bayhan, Y.K.; Akay, G. Crossflow microfiltration of low concentration-nonliving yeast suspensions. *J. Membr. Sci.* **2004**, *233*, 59–69. [CrossRef]

105. Chen, X.; Cui, D.F.; Liu, C.C.; Li, H. Microfluidic chip for blood cell separation and collection based on crossflow filtration. *Sens. Actuators B Chem.* **2008**, *130*, 216–221. [CrossRef]

106. Lee, Y.; Clark, M.M. Modeling of flux decline during crossflow ultrafiltration of colloidal suspensions. *J. Membr. Sci.* **1998**, *149*, 181–202. [CrossRef]

107. Crowley, T.A.; Pizziconi, V. Isolation of plasma from whole blood using planar microfilters for lab-on-a-chip applications. *Lab Chip* **2005**, *5*, 922–929. [CrossRef] [PubMed]

108. Zhang, W.; Kai, K.; Choi, D.S.; Iwamoto, T.; Nguyen, Y.H.; Wong, H.; Landis, M.D.; Ueno, N.T.; Chang, J.; Qin, L. Microfluidics separation reveals the stem-cell-like deformability of tumor-initiating cells. *Proc. Natl. Acad. Sci. USA* **2012**, *109*, 18707–18712. [CrossRef] [PubMed]

109. Choi, J.; Hyun, J.-C.; Yang, S. On-chip Extraction of Intracellular Molecules in White Blood Cells from Whole Blood. *Sci. Rep.* **2015**, *5*, 15167. [CrossRef] [PubMed]

110. Kuntaegowdanahalli, S.S.; Bhagat, A.A.; Kumar, G.; Papautsky, I. Inertial microfluidics for continuous particle separation in spiral microchannels. *Lab Chip* **2009**, *9*, 2973–2980. [CrossRef] [PubMed]

111. Lee, M.G.; Choi, S.; Kim, H.J.; Lim, H.K.; Kim, J.H.; Huh, N.; Park, J.K. Inertial blood plasma separation in a contraction–expansion array microchannel. *Appl. Phys. Lett.* **2011**, *98*, 253702. [CrossRef]

112. Van Delinder, V.; Groisman, A. Perfusion in microfluidic cross-flow: Separation of white blood cells from whole blood and exchange of medium in a continuous flow. *Anal. Chem.* **2007**, *79*, 2023–2030. [CrossRef] [PubMed]

113. Van Delinder, V.; Groisman, A. Separation of plasma from whole human blood in a continuous cross-flow in a molded microfluidic device. *Anal. Chem.* **2006**, *78*, 3765–3771. [CrossRef] [PubMed]

114. Yang, X.; Yang, J.M.; Tai, Y.-C.; Ho, C.-M. Micromachined membrane particle filters. *Sens. Actuators A Phys.* **1999**, *73*, 184–191. [CrossRef]

115. Streets, A.M.; Huang, Y. Chip in a lab: Microfluidics for next generation life science research. *Biomicrofluidics* **2013**, *7*, 11302. [CrossRef] [PubMed]

116. Shevkoplyas, S.S.; Yoshida, T.; Gifford, S.C.; Bitensky, M.W. Direct measurement of the impact of impaired erythrocyte deformability on microvascular network perfusion in a microfluidic device. *Lab Chip* **2006**, *6*, 914–920. [CrossRef] [PubMed]

117. Faustino, V.; Catarino, S.O.; Pinho, D.; Lima, R.A.; Minas, G. A passive microfluidic device based on crossflow filtration for cell separation measurements: A spectrophotometric characterization. *Biosensors* **2018**, *8*, 125. [CrossRef] [PubMed]

118. Catarino, S.O.; Lima, R.; Minas, G. Smart devices: Lab-on-a-chip. In *Bioinspired Materials for Drug Delivery and Analysis*; Rodrigues, L., Mota, M., Eds.; Woodhead Publishing: Cambridge, UK, 2017; pp. 331–369.

119. Minas, G.; Catarino, S.O. Lab-on-a-chip devices for chemical analysis. In *Encyclopedia of Microfluidics and Nanofluidics*; Li, D., Ed.; Springer: New York NY, USA, 2015; pp. 1511–1531.

120. Clausell-Tormos, J.; Lieber, D.; Baret, J.C.; El-Harrak, A.; Miller, O.J.; Frenz, L.; Blouwolff, J.; Humphry, K.J.; Köster, S.; Duan, H.; et al. Droplet-based microfluidic platforms for the encapsulation and screening of mammalian cells and multicellular organisms. *Chem. Biol.* **2008**, *15*, 427–437. [CrossRef] [PubMed]

121. Wang, M.; Orwar, O.; Olofsson, J.; Weber, S.G. Single-cell electroporation. *Anal. Bioanal. Chem.* **2010**, *397*, 3235–3248. [CrossRef] [PubMed]

122. Wood, D.K.; Soriano, A.; Mahadevan, L.; Higgins, J.M.; Bhatia, S.N. A biophysical indicator of vaso-occlusive risk in sickle cell disease. *Sci. Transl. Med.* **2012**, *4*, 123ra26. [CrossRef]

123. Di Caprio, G.; Stokes, C.; Higgins, J.M.; Schonbrun, E. Single-cell measurement of red blood cell oxygen affinity. *Proc. Natl. Acad. Sci. USA* **2015**, *112*, 9984–9989. [CrossRef]

124. Bhise, N.S.; Ribas, J.; Manoharan, V.; Zhang, Y.S.; Polini, A.; Massa, S.; Dokmeci, M.E.R.; Khademhosseini, A. Organ-on-a-chip platforms for studying drug delivery systems. *J. Control. Release* **2014**, *190*, 82–93. [CrossRef] [PubMed]

125. Zhang, B.; Radisic, M. Organ-on-a-chip devices advance to market. *Lab Chip* **2017**, *17*, 2395. [CrossRef] [PubMed]

11

Deformation of a Red Blood Cell in a Narrow Rectangular Microchannel

Naoki Takeishi [1,*], Hiroaki Ito [2,3], Makoto Kaneko [2] and Shigeo Wada [1]

[1]   Graduate School of Engineering Science, Osaka University, 1-3 Machikaneyama, Toyonaka, Osaka 560-8531, Japan; shigeo@me.es.osaka-u.ac.jp

[2]   Department of Mechanical Engineering, Osaka University, Suita, Osaka 565-0871, Japan; ito@hh.mech.eng.osaka-u.ac.jp (H.I.); mk@mech.eng.osaka-u.ac.jp (M.K.)

[3]   Department of Physics, Graduate School of Science, Chiba University, Chiba 263-8522, Japan

*   Correspondence: ntakeishi@me.es.osaka-u.ac.jp

Abstract: The deformability of a red blood cell (RBC) is one of the most important biological parameters affecting blood flow, both in large arteries and in the microcirculation, and hence it can be used to quantify the cell state. Despite numerous studies on the mechanical properties of RBCs, including cell rigidity, much is still unknown about the relationship between deformability and the configuration of flowing cells, especially in a confined rectangular channel. Recent computer simulation techniques have successfully been used to investigate the detailed behavior of RBCs in a channel, but the dynamics of a translating RBC in a narrow rectangular microchannel have not yet been fully understood. In this study, we numerically investigated the behavior of RBCs flowing at different velocities in a narrow rectangular microchannel that mimicked a microfluidic device. The problem is characterized by the capillary number Ca, which is the ratio between the fluid viscous force and the membrane elastic force. We found that confined RBCs in a narrow rectangular microchannel maintained a nearly unchanged biconcave shape at low Ca, then assumed an asymmetrical slipper shape at moderate Ca, and finally attained a symmetrical parachute shape at high Ca. Once a RBC deformed into one of these shapes, it was maintained as the final stable configurations. Since the slipper shape was only found at moderate Ca, measuring configurations of flowing cells will be helpful to quantify the cell state.

Keywords: red blood cells; Lattice–Boltzmann method; finite element method; immersed boundary method; narrow rectangular microchannel; computational biomechanics

1. Introduction

It is well known that many blood-related diseases are associated with alterations in the geometry and membrane properties of red blood cells (RBCs) that result in reduced functionality [1]. For instance, RBCs in patients with diabetes mellitus exhibit impaired cell deformability [2], as do those in patients with sepsis [3]. As another example, malaria-infected RBCs demonstrate membrane stiffening as well as shape distortion [4–6]. Hence, cell deformability may be an important indicator of cell state, and might be used to diagnoses relevant blood diseases. To date, various experimental techniques have been proposed to evaluate RBC deformability, e.g., optical tweezers and atomic force microscopy, but they usually suffer from low throughput. Recently, several microfluidic techniques that are capable of high-throughput measurement have been developed [7–11]. For instance, Ito et al. (2017) successfully developed a novel high-throughput assay to quantify the mechanical response of RBCs after spatial constriction, and found a characteristic mechanical response to long-term deformation that may have been related to chemical energy content [9].

Along with these experimental studies, recent computer simulation techniques have successfully been used to investigate aspects of cell dynamics such as stresses, velocities, and deformations, and have been shown to reproduce single-cell dynamics [12–14]. Mokbel et al. (2017) quantitatively related cell deformation to mechanical parameters in an experiment involving microfluidic flow through a square channel [13]. To elucidate patient-specific blood rheology, RBCs in diabetes mellitus and sickle-cell anemia were modeled in terms of cell rigidity and membrane viscosity, and their hydrodynamic interactions were quantified [15,16]. Since such numerical models allow us to investigate cell behavior in large parameter spaces, the coupling of experimental and numerical approaches may constitute a usefull bioengineering strategy to quantify the cell state.

Despite the studies referred to above, much is still unknown about the behavior of flowing RBCs, especially in a confined microchannel or between two closely spaced parallel plates (i.e., Hele-Shaw cell). Since the deformation of a RBC in a narrow rectangular microchannel is limited to an almost two-dimensional space, it is relatively easy to quantify the deformed configuration [17,18]. Although a number of studies using microfluidic devices have reported cellular-scale dynamics [19–24] as well as numerical studies [20,25–28], the dynamics of a translating RBC in a narrow rectangular microchannel have not yet been fully investigated. Recent our developed on-chip feedback manipulation system allowed us to investigate the two-dimensionally projected shape profile of RBCs, and showed RBC heterogeneity in a narrow rectangular microchannel [17,18]. However, a precise deformation especially in thickness direction of RBCs cannot be captured by means of the experimental observation.

One of the pioneering theoretical works about the behavior of the cell membrane in a confined channel was reported by Secomb & Skalak (1982) [29]. More recently, Tahiri et al. (2013) systematically investigated the shape transition of confined RBCs modeled as vesicles, and showed a phase diagram of the mode of RBCs [28]. Since these works were limited to the two-dimensional behavior of RBCs, it is unknown whether their insights are applicable to estimating the three-dimensional deformation of a RBC in a narrow rectangular microchannel. Fedosov et al. (2014) systematically investigated the behavior of a single RBC in cylindrical microchannels for a wide range of channel confinements ($2a/D$, being the radius of the RBC a and the channel diameter D) using a three-dimensional dissipative particle dynamics model [30]. However, their microchannels ($2a/D < 0.8$) had relatively large cross-sectional area comparing to a narrow rectangular microchannel represented in [17,18,31]. Zhu et al. (2016) numerically investigated the behavior of a droplet in a Hele-Shaw cell, and identified characteristic flow structures that were induced by the translating droplet [31]. Since forces acting on an interface depend on the constitutive law, it is expected that the hydrodynamic interaction between the fluid and cell membrane will differ from that observed in the droplet model.

The objective in this study, therefore, is to clarify the detailed behavior of translating RBCs in a narrow rectangular microchannel. The RBCs was modeled as a biconcave capsules, whose membranes followed the Skalak constitutive law [32]. We quantified the stable configuration of deformed RBCs in a narrow rectangular microchannel, mimicking a microfluidic device [17], for different values of the capillary number Ca, which is the ratio between the fluid viscous force and the membrane elastic force. We also investigated the effect on this configuration of altering parameters such as bending rigidity and viscosity ratio. To accelerate numerical simulations, we resorted to computing with a graphics processing unit (GPU), using the Lattice–Boltzmann method (LBM) for the inner and outer fluids and the finite element method to follow the deformation of the RBC membrane. These models were previously successfully applied to the analysis of cellular hydrodynamic interactions in channel flows [12,33–35].

2. Materials and Methods

2.1. Flow and RBC Model

We considered a cellular flow consisting of an external/internal fluid and a RBC membrane with radius a in a rectangular box representing a microfluidic device with 10 μm × 3.5 μm along the wall-normal and span-wise directions (Figure A1a). Representative images of a flowing RBC in a microfluidic device (Figure A1b,c) are shown in Figure A1d. The stream-wise distance for the computational domain was set to be 50 μm (Figure 1). Each RBC was modeled as a biconcave capsule, or a Newtonian fluid enclosed by a thin elastic membrane, with a major diameter 8 μm (=2a) and maximum thickness 2 μm (= $a/2 = t^R$). The flow was driven by a pressure gradient. Periodic boundary conditions were imposed on the inlet and outlet. To reproduce in vivo human RBC condition experimentally, the cytoplasmic viscosity was taken to be $\mu_1 = 6.0 \times 10^{-3}$ Pa·s, which is five times higher than the external fluid viscosity, $\mu_0 = 1.2 \times 10^{-3}$ Pa·s. Hence, the viscosity ratio λ (=μ_1/μ_0) was set to be 5. The computational domain and the initial state or steady deformed state of the RBC are shown in Figure 1. The problem was characterized by the capillary number (Ca),

$$Ca = \frac{\mu_0 \dot{\gamma} a}{G_s},$$ (1)

where G_s is the surface shear elastic modulus, and $\dot{\gamma}$ (=U_m^∞/H) is the shear rate defined by the mean velocity of the external fluid without cell U_m^∞ and channel height H (=10 μm). Since the inertial effect can be negligible in the microfluidic device, we set Re as small enough to assume the Stokes flow. To reduce the computational costs, we set $Re = \rho U^\infty H/\mu_0 = 0.2$, where ρ is the external fluid density and U^∞ is the maximum velocity of the external fluid with no cell. This value accurately represents the capsule dynamics solved by the boundary integral method in Stokes flow [12,33].

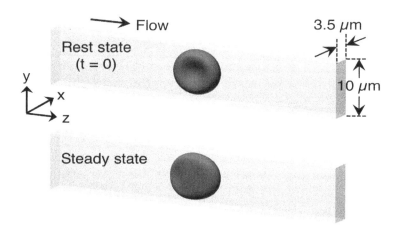

Figure 1. Computational domain to reproduce a translating red blood cell (RBC) in the narrow rectangular microchannel. The domain mimicked a microfluidic device as shown in Figure A1. The domain cross-section was 10 μm × 3.5 μm along the wall-normal and span-wise directions, respectively, and the stream-wise distance was set to be 50 μm. Flow direction is from left to right.

The membrane was modeled as an isotropic and hyperelastic material that followed the Skalak constitutive (SK) law [32]. The strain energy w and principal tensions in the membrane T_1 and T_2 ($T_1 \geq T_2$) of the SK law are given by

$$w = \frac{G_s}{4}\left(I_1^2 + 2I_1 - 2I_2 + CI_2^2\right),$$ (2)

and

$$T_1 = \frac{G_s \lambda_1}{\lambda_2}\left[\lambda_1^2 - 1 + C\lambda_2^2\left(\lambda_1^2\lambda_2^2 - 1\right)\right], \quad \text{(likewise for } T_2\text{)},$$ (3)

where C is a coefficient representing the area incompressibility, $I_1 (=\lambda_1^2 + \lambda_2^2 - 2)$ and I_2 (= $\lambda_1^2\lambda_2^2 - 1 = J_s^2 - 1$) are the first and second invariants of the strain tensor, λ_1, λ_2 are the two principal in-plane stretch ratios, and $J_s = \lambda_1\lambda_2$ is the Jacobian, which expresses the ratio of the deformed to reference surface areas. If I_2 equals zero (i.e., $J_s = 1$), the membrane satisfies perfect incompressibility. In this study, the surface shear elastic modulus and area incompressibility coefficient of RBCs were determined to be G_s = 4.0 μN/m and $C = 10^2$, respectively [6,33]. The bending resistance k_b was also considered [36], with a bending modulus $k_b = 1.2 \times 10^{-19}$ J, according to the order of the value of k_b [37].

2.2. Numerical Simulation

We used the LBM [38] coupled with the finite element method (FEM) [39]. The membrane mechanics were solved by the FEM, and are given by

$$\int_S \hat{\boldsymbol{u}} \cdot \boldsymbol{q} dS = \int_S \hat{\boldsymbol{\epsilon}} : \boldsymbol{T} dS, \tag{4}$$

where $\boldsymbol{T}$ is the Cauchy stress tensor, $\boldsymbol{q}$ is the load on the membrane, $\hat{\boldsymbol{u}}$ is the virtual displacement, and $\hat{\boldsymbol{\epsilon}} = (\nabla_s \hat{\boldsymbol{u}} + \nabla_s \hat{\boldsymbol{u}}^T)/2$ is the virtual strain tensor. The fluid mechanics were solved by the LBM [38] as,

$$f_i(\boldsymbol{x} + \boldsymbol{c}_i \Delta t, t + \Delta t) - f_i(\boldsymbol{x}, t) = -\frac{1}{\tau}[f_i(\boldsymbol{x}, t) - f_i^{eq}(\boldsymbol{x}, t)] + F_i \Delta t, \tag{5}$$

where f_i is the particle distribution function for ideal particles with velocity $\boldsymbol{c}_i$ at position $\boldsymbol{x}$, Δt is the time step size, f_i^{eq} is the equilibrium distribution, τ is the nondimensional relaxation time, and F_i is the external force term. Subscript i represents the distribution direction of an ideal particle (i = 0–18). The D3Q19 LBM was used. FEM and LBM were coupled by the immersed boundary method [40]. All procedures were fully implemented on a GPU to accelerate the numerical simulation [41]. Our coupling method has been successfully applied to numerical analyses of cellular flow [33–35] and cell adhesion [12]. The solid and fluid mesh sizes were set to be 125 nm (an unstructured mesh with 20,480 elements was used for the RBC membrane). This resolution has been shown to successfully represent single-cell dynamics in a channel [12]. The results of cell deformation did not change with twice the fluid-mesh resolution (Figure 2b).

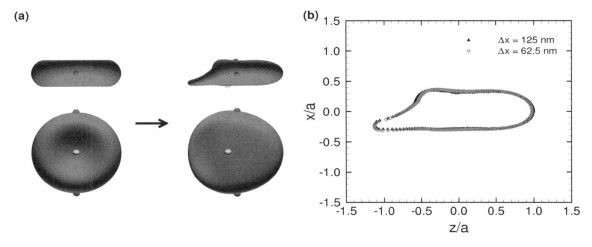

Figure 2. (a) Typical snapshots of a deformed RBC subjected to Ca = 0.15 at the initial state (left) and steady state (right). Two views, from the span-wise and stream-wise directions, are shown above and below, respectively. The markers represent node points. (b) Superposition of the fully deformed RBC projected on the x-z plane at Ca = 0.15 . The two lines obtained with Δx = 125 nm (black) and 62.5 nm (red), respectively. The membrane position is normalized by the reference radius a.

3. Results

3.1. Deformation of a Translating RBC in a Narrow Rectangular Microchannel

We performed numerical simulations to reproduce a translating RBC in a narrow rectangular microchannel, as shown in Figure A1d, and found that the RBC demonstrated an asymmetrical shape, the so-called slipper shape [42], which was also observed in the experiment as shown in Figure A2 (see also Videos S1 and S2). A typical asymmetrical shape of a deformed RBC subjected to $Ca = 0.15$ is shown in Figure 2a, where the markers represent membrane node points. The result clearly shows that the membrane does not rotate; in other words, the RBC stably translates without a tank-treading motion. The outlines of the deformed RBC at different fluid mesh resolutions are shown in Figure 2b, projected on the z-x plane. The result remains the same with twice the fluid mesh resolution ($\Delta x = 62.5$ nm). Therefore, the present resolution ($\Delta x = 125$ nm) successfully reproduces the fluid dynamics between the membrane and wall, and will be used in this study.

Figure 3a shows snapshots of a stable RBC configuration for different Ca at fully developed flow. The RBC demonstrated an almost unchanged (symmetrical) biconcave shape at small $Ca = 10^{-3}$, then shifted to an asymmetrical slipper shape as Ca increased (see also Video S3 for $Ca = 0.1$), and finally attained a symmetrical parachute shape at $Ca \geq 0.35$ (see also Video S4 for $Ca = 0.5$). To quantify the symmetry of the stable configuration of the deformed RBC, we propose a symmetry index ID_{sym}, which is defined by the volume ratio of two volumes that are divided by a plane parallel to the flow direction at the midline of the channel, as shown in Figure 3b. Using volume 1 (Vol_1) and volume 2 (Vol_2), ID_{sym} is given as

$$ID_{sym} = \frac{\text{MIN}\left(Vol_1, Vol_2\right)}{\text{MAX}\left(Vol_1, Vol_2\right)}. \tag{6}$$

A complete symmetrical shape is expressed as $ID_{sym} = 1$. We show the results of ID_{sym} as a function of Ca in Figure 3c. An asymmetrical parachute shape abruptly appeared for $Ca \geq 0.01$, but it gradually recovered and finally reached $ID_{sym} = 1$ for $Ca \geq 0.35$. These results suggest that there exists the following specific range of Ca that allows a RBC to deform into an asymmetrical slipper shape: $5 \times 10^{-3} < Ca < 0.35$.

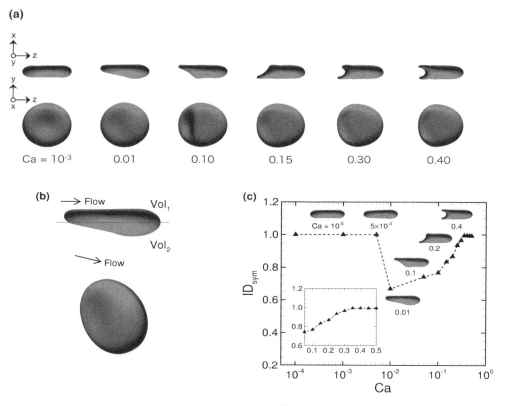

Figure 3. (**a**) Snapshots of a fully deformed RBC for different Ca. (**b**) Typical snapshots of a RBC at $Ca = 0.01$, where the blue plane denotes the center of the x-z-plane parallel to the flow direction, dividing the cell into the volume 1 (Vol_1) and volume 2 (Vol_2). (**c**) The symmetry index ID_{sym} as a function of Ca. The insets represent snapshots of deformed RBCs at specific Ca.

Figure 4a shows one example of the temporal history of the RBC centroid velocity V_c at $Ca = 0.01$, where V_c is normalized by the characteristic (maximum) fluid velocity without cell U^∞. The centroid velocity of RBC is calculated as a volume-averaged velocity, and is given by,

$$V_c = \frac{1}{\mathcal{V}} \int_{\mathcal{V}} v(x_m) d\mathcal{V} = \frac{1}{\mathcal{V}} \int_{\mathcal{V}} \nabla \cdot (v \otimes r) \, d\mathcal{V} = \frac{1}{\mathcal{V}} \int_{\mathcal{S}} n \cdot (v \otimes r) \, dS, \tag{7}$$

and

$$\mathcal{V} = \int_{\mathcal{V}} d\mathcal{V} = \frac{1}{3} \int_{\mathcal{V}} \nabla \cdot r d\mathcal{V} = \frac{1}{3} \int_{S} n \cdot r dS, \tag{8}$$

where $v(x_m)$ is the interfacial velocity of the membrane at the membrane node point x_m, r is the membrane position relative to the center of the RBC, n is the surface normal vector, $\mathcal{V}$ the volume of the RBC, and S is the surface area of the membrane. The velocity slightly ($\sim$3%) decreased when the RBC shape changed from a symmetrical to asymmetrical shapes at $Ca = 0.01$ (Figure 4a). Because the membrane of a slipper-shaped RBC is dragged by the fluid near the wall, V_c is slower than that of a symmetrically shaped RBC. Once the membrane deformed into an asymmetrical shape, that shape persisted. In this study, we defined the "steady state" as the condition wherein the centroid velocity reached a plateau (this time is hereafter referred to as $\dot{\gamma}t = 0$), and used data after $\dot{\gamma}t = 0$ to reduce the influence of the initial conditions. A time average was performed for the period $\dot{\gamma}t \geq 100$ after $\dot{\gamma}t = 0$. Figure 4b shows the time average of centroid velocity V_c and total fluid velocity V_{total} for different Ca, where those values are normalized by characteristic velocity U^∞. The tendency that V_c/U^∞ slightly decreases as Ca increases (Figure 4b) agrees with previous numerical results of a spherical capsule in a square channel [43] and constricted channel [44]. Note that the dimensional cell velocity basically increases as Ca increases, for instance, $V_c \sim 0.12$ μm/s for the lowest Ca ($=10^{-4}$) and $V_c \sim 1200$ μm/s for the highest Ca ($=0.5$).

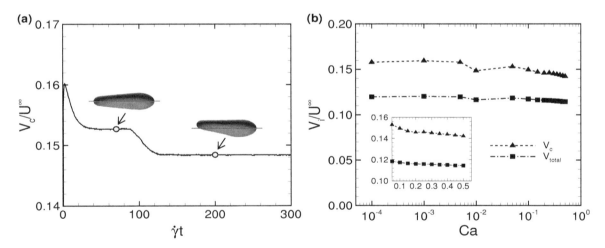

Figure 4. (a) Time history of the RBC centroid velocity (V_c) at $Ca = 0.01$, where $V_c = 24.7$ μm/s at $\dot{\gamma}t = 200$ corresponding to $t = 12$ s. The images represent snapshots of the deformed RBC at $\dot{\gamma}t = 70$ ($t = 4.2$ s) and 200 ($t = 12$ s), respectively. The blue line denotes the center axis of the channel. (b) Time average of the RBC centroid velocity V_c and total fluid velocity V_{total} as a function of Ca. The velocity V_i is normalized by the characteristic fluid velocity without cell U^∞, where V_i represents V_c and V_{total} by the index i = "c" or "total".

The deformation of each axis in a steady-state membrane is quantified by the deformation index L_i/L_i^{ref}, which is the ratio between each axis length of a deformed RBC L_i and each reference axis length L_i^{ref} (i.e., without flow), where subscript i represents the maximum, middle and minimum axes (i.e., i = "max", "mid", and "min"). The results of L_i/L_i^{ref} are shown in Figure 5a. We found that only the minimum axis (i.e., thickness) increases as Ca increases, while the maximum and middle axes decrease.

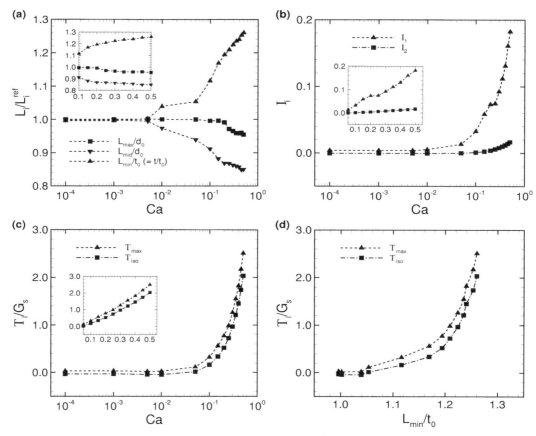

Figure 5. (a) Time average of the deformation index L_i/L_i^{ref} as a function of Ca, where the maximum, middle, and minimum axis lengths (L_{max}, L_{min}, and L_{mid}, respectively) are normalized by each reference length L_i^{ref} (i.e., no flow condition), where the reference major and minor axis lengths are d_0 and t_0 (thickness), respectively. (b) Averaged first and second invariants $\mathcal{I}_i$ ($i = 1$ and 2) as a function of Ca. (c) Averaged maximum and isotropic tensions; $\mathcal{T}_{max}$ and $\mathcal{T}_{iso}$, respectively. These values are normalized by the shear elastic modulus G_s. (d) The average of these tensions, $\mathcal{T}_i$, as a function of the deformation index L_{min}/t_0, which is the ratio between the minimum axis length of the deformed RBC (thickness) and the reference thickness.

To quantify the strain of an isotropic elastic membrane, the first and second invariants of the strain tensor I_i ($i = 1$ and 2) are calculated, and are given in Figure 5b. These are averaged by the total number of membrane meshes and the analysis duration, i.e.,

$$\mathcal{I}_i = \frac{1}{\mathscr{T}S} \int_t \int_S I_i(\boldsymbol{x}_g, t) dS dt \quad (i = 1 \text{ and } 2), \tag{9}$$

where $\mathscr{T}$ is the period of analysis duration, and $\boldsymbol{x}_g$ is the centroid of the triangle element of the membrane. According to Figure 5b, the second invariant $\mathcal{I}_2$ is almost zero for $Ca \leq 0.1$, and only slightly increases for $Ca > 0.1$. Therefore, the membrane incompressibility is well maintained even after the membrane demonstrates the slipper/parachute shape. The first invariant $\mathcal{I}_1$, on the other hand, starts to increase from $Ca \geq 0.01$ and grows rapidly compared to $\mathcal{I}_2$. Therefore, the symmetrical parachute-like deformation results from greater membrane extension than the asymmetrical slipper-like deformation.

We also investigated the maximum in-plane principal tension T_{max} ($T_1 \geq T_2$) and the isotropic tension $T_{iso}(=T_1 + T_2)/2$ in the deformed RBC, and show the results in Figure 5c. We calculated the average value of those tensions as $\mathcal{T}_{max}$ and $\mathcal{T}_{iso}$ by using Equation (9). As expected, both tensions start to increase simultaneously when $\mathcal{I}_1$ increases (i.e., $Ca = 0.01$). The isotropic tension $\mathcal{T}_{iso}$ is always lower than the maximum principal tension $\mathcal{T}_{max}$. To demonstrate the relationship between tension and deformation, T_i is described as a function of the deformation index L_{min}/t_0 in Figure 5d. The result clearly shows the strain-hardening behavior of the RBC due to the nonlinearity of the SK law.

3.2. Effects of Perturbations on Stable Membrane Configuration

To clarify the reproducibility of the stable configuration of a deformed RBC in the narrow rectangular microchannel, we investigated the effects of potential perturbations, e.g., the initial centroid position x_0, bending rigidity k_b, and viscosity ratio λ. Figure 6 shows the centroid velocity V_c of a RBC subjected to low Ca (= 5×10^{-3}) and maximum Ca (= 0.5) for different initial centroid positions along the span-wise direction of the channel. When the centroid of the RBC was initially placed two fluid meshes away from the midline of the channel (i.e., $x_0 = -2\Delta x$), the RBC started to flow with an asymmetrical slipper shape, but gradually migrated to the channel axis due to the lift forces induced by the wall and shear gradient, and finally attained a symmetrical shape for both Ca values with the same velocity as that obtained with $x_0 = 0$ (Figure 4; see also Videos S5 and S6). Therefore, the stable configuration of the deformed RBC is insensitive to the initial position. Note that although the RBC subjected to low Ca (= 5.0×10^{-3}) did not perfectly orient parallel to the flow direction (Figure 6a) and suffered from decreasing the cell velocity, the symmetry index ID_{sym} remained the same (Figure 7a).

We also tested different values for bending rigidity k_b, where the value of k_b was set to a quarter of the original bending resistance ($k_b = 3.0 \times 10^{-20}$), and twice the original bending resistance ($k_b = 2.4 \times 10^{-19}$). As shown in Figure 7a, the symmetry index ID_{sym} remained same regardless of the value of k_b. Therefore, bending rigidity does not affect the stable configuration of the translating RBC in the narrow rectangular microchannel, at least within the parameter space that we investigated, namely $3.0 \times 10^{-20} \leq k_b \leq 2.4 \times 10^{-19}$.

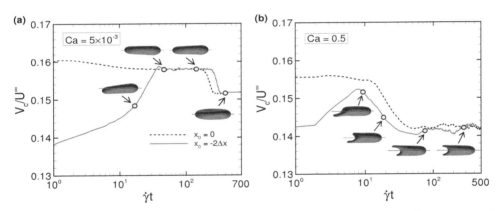

Figure 6. Time history of the RBC centroid velocity (V_c) at (**a**) low $Ca = 5 \times 10^{-3}$, and (**b**) high $Ca = 0.5$ for different initial positions along the span-wise direction x_0, where one RBC is initially placed at the midline of the channel ($x_0 = 0$, dashed line) and the other RBC is placed two fluid meshes away from the midline ($x_0 = -2\Delta x$, red line). The images represent snapshots of the RBC with $x_0 = -2\Delta x$ at the indicated times (see also Videos S5 and S6). Note that $V_c = 12.7$ μm/s for $Ca = 5 \times 10^{-3}$ at $\dot{\gamma}t = 500$ ($t = 60$ s), and $V_c = 1180$ μm/s for $Ca = 0.5$ at $\dot{\gamma}t = 500$ ($t = 0.6$ s).

However, DI_{sym} was affected by the viscosity ratio λ. When λ decreased to unity (i.e., $\lambda = 1$), the membrane tended to assume a symmetrical shape even at relatively low $Ca = 0.01$. The most asymmetrical shape was found at at $\lambda = 5$, and the minimum $DI_{sym}|_{\lambda=1}$ shifted to larger $Ca \approx 0.1$ (Figure 7a). The value of DI_{sym} at $\lambda = 1$ started to recover beginning at $Ca = 0.1$, and finally almost reached 1 at $Ca = 0.3$. To see the effect of λ, we compared the centroid velocity V_c and membrane tension T_i between different λ (= 1 and 5). V_c at $\lambda = 1$ tended to be larger, and was approximately 4% greater than that obtained with $\lambda = 5$ (Figure 7b). The results of T_i, on the other hand, tended to decrease as λ decreased (Figure 7c).

Figure 7d shows the membrane tensions as a function of the deformation index L_{min}/t_0. When L_{min}/t_0 was invariant, the tensions acting on the membrane T_i tended to be lower as λ decreased.

This tendency was inconsistent with the previous numerical results of the RBC in simple shear flow [45]. Compared with the previous results in [45], the similarities or discrepancies in the values of $\mathcal{T}_i$ (Figure 7c,d) for different λ would arise from different flow modes and confined geometries. Even though tensions acting on the membrane and deformation depend on λ, the RBC in the narrow rectangular microchannel underwent the same history of deformation as a function of Ca; the almost original biconcave shape at low Ca, and an asymmetrical slipper shape at low/moderate Ca, and finally a symmetrical parachute shape at high Ca. These results suggest that the stable configuration of the translating RBC in the narrow rectangular microchannel was reproducible independently of any perturbations that we investigated.

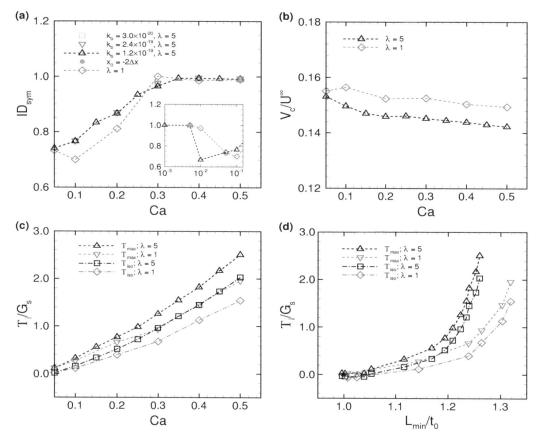

Figure 7. (a) The symmetry index ID_{sym} as a function of Ca for different values of bending modulus $k_b = 3.0 \times 10^{-20}$ J (square), 1.2×10^{-19} J (triangle), and 2.4×10^{-19} J (inverted triangle). The results obtained with a viscosity ratio of unity (i.e., $\lambda = 1$) are also displayed (diamond). The circular dot represents the result of $x_0 = -2\Delta x$ at low Ca ($= 5 \times 10^{-3}$) and high Ca ($= 0.5$) and $\lambda = 5$. These results were obtained with $k_b = 1.2 \times 10^{-19}$ J. (b) Time average of the RBC centroid velocity (V_c) as a function of Ca for different viscosity ratios ($\lambda = 1$ and 5). (c) Averaged maximum and isotropic tensions, $\mathcal{T}_{max}$ and $\mathcal{T}_{iso}$, respectively. (d) Averaged tension $\mathcal{T}_i$ as a function of the deformation index L_{min}/t_0.

4. Discussion

The asymmetric slipper shape of RBCs has been found in capillaries [42], and the motion has been systematically investigated both in experiments [19–23] and in numerical simulations [20,26,28,30]. An experiment using microfluidic devices showed that RBCs undergo a transition from a symmetrical parachute shape to an asymmetrical slipper shape as cell velocity increased [23]. Other experimental results showed that viscous shear stresses controlled this transition, and confinement was not necessary for the slipper shape [19]. The results reported in [19] are consistent with the numerical results obtained using a two-dimensional (2D) droplet model [26]. The numerical studies reported in [26] clearly showed that the shape transition in an unbounded Piseuille flow occurred when a dimensionless vesicle deflation number, representing shape stability, fell below a certain value. Other numerical results reported in [28] demonstrated that 2D droplets also assumed the slipper shape, not only in an unbounded Piseuille flow but also in a confined channel. These numerical studies also clarified the effect of the viscosity ratio λ on stable configuration, showing specifically that a droplet with $\lambda = 1$ transitioned from a parachute shape to a slipper shape as the flow strength decreased [26], while a droplet with $\lambda \approx 5$ made this same transition as the flow strength increased [28]; these findings were consistent with the experimental results reported in [23]. Since the above numerical analyses were performed using a 2D droplet model, it is uncertain whether their results are applicable to the dynamics of a translating three-dimensional (3D) RBC in a confined rectangular channel when taking membrane elasticity into account. Fedosov et al. (2014) systematically investigated the behavior of single RBC in cylindrical microchannels for a wide range of channel confinements ($2a/D$, being a channel diameter D) using a 3D dissipative particle dynamics model [30], but the cross-sectional area of the microchannels were relatively large ($2a/D < 0.8$) comparing to a narrow rectangular microchannel represented in [17], where the channel confinement is characterized as $2a/H = 0.8$ and $2a/W \sim 2.29$ using the wall-normal length H and span-wise length W (Figure A1a–c). We thus numerically investigated the behavior of translating RBCs in a narrow rectangular microchannel that mimicked a microfluidic device (Figure A1) [17] with different Ca. Our numerical results demonstrated that the confined RBCs maintained a nearly unchanged, biconcave shape at low Ca, then shifted to an asymmetrical slipper shape at low/moderate Ca, and finally attained a symmetrical parachute shape at high Ca. Such asymmetrical slipper shape was also observed in the experiment (Figure A2). The finding that RBCs tended to show a symmetrical shape with increasing Ca contradicted previous experimental results [23] as well as numerical results obtained using a 2D-droplet model with $\lambda \approx 5$ [28]. This discrepancy may have been caused by the effects of three-dimensional flow structures in a confined channel and by the membrane constitutive law. Our numerical results of the transition from slipper to parachute shapes qualitatively agree with those obtained in cylindrical microchannels for $2a/D < 0.8$ [30]. To the best of our knowledge, such shape transition in a narrow rectangular microchannel that was presented here is the first of its kind. We also showed that the stable configuration of the translating RBC in the narrow rectangular microchannel was reproducible independently of any perturbations that we investigated such as the initial centroid position, bending rigidity, and viscosity ratio. If the fully deformed configuration or the transition mode is related to membrane shear elasticity, which is characterized by Ca, these insights will help us identify the cell state. Since different motions of individual RBCs may affect the bulk suspension rheology [46], identifying a stable mode of RBCs in a channel will be also helpful to evaluate the blood rheology.

In our experiment using microfluidic devices, we observed a slipper-shaped RBC whose velocity was almost 1.2 mm/s (Figure A2), while the numerical results showed that a velocity this high resulted in a RBC with a symmetrical parachute shape (Figure 3c). This discrepancy may have been due to the duration of the observation. Since experimental observation periods are limited to 0.1 s or less, the slipper-shaped RBC in the microfluidic device may have been in the transition. According to our numerical results shown in Figure 6, the transition from slipper shape to parachute shape takes at least $\dot{\gamma}t \sim 300$, corresponding to $\sim$0.3 s for $Ca = 0.5$ ($V_c \sim 1.2$ mm/s). Another possible reason may have been due to RBC heterogeneity as reported in our previous experiments [17,18]. The experimental observations of an asymmetrical slipper shape in a microfluidic device are required for precise statistical analysis, which will be addressed in future study.

We are not sure what perturbations are needed to destroy the stable symmetrical shape. Thermal energy is unlikely to be affecting the state: indeed, although the RBC membrane usually demonstrates Brownian motion in the free state, the Peclet number ($Pe = \dot{\gamma}a/D_p$, being a radius of the RBC a and a diffusion coefficient D_p) is estimated as approximately $O(Pe) = 10^1$, even at $Ca = 10^{-4}$, by using the Stokes–Einstein equation, and thus the Brownian diffusion (thermal fluctuations) should have little effect. Although the membrane bending rigidity did not affect the stable membrane configuration at least for 3×10^{-20} J $\leq Ca \leq 2.4 \times 10^{-19}$ J, further investigation will be required for larger parameter spaces. In this study, we defined the initial shape of RBCs as a biconcave disc. Since some recent numerical studies have debated the stress-free shape of RBCs [47–49], it will be interesting to study how the reference shape (biconcave, oblate spheroid, and sphere) affects the stable configuration of translating RBCs in a narrow rectangular microchannel.

5. Conclusions

We numerically investigated the dynamics of translating RBCs in a narrow rectangular microchannel for different capillary numbers (Ca). Our numerical results demonstrated that a confined RBC in a narrow rectangular microchannel maintained a nearly unchanged, biconcave shape at low Ca, then assumed an asymmetrical slipper shape at moderate Ca, and finally attained a symmetrical parachute shape at high Ca. Once the RBC deformed into either of the latter two shapes, they sustained that shape as their final stable configurations. The membrane deformation as a function of Ca remained the same even when the viscosity ratio λ decreased from physiological relevant value ($\lambda = 5$) to unity. The final stable configuration was insensitive to bending resistance and initial position. If these shapes are found in diseased RBCs translating at specific velocities, the shapes will be an important indicator of cell state.

Video S1: experimental result at the speed of the cell being 1200 μm/s, corresponding to $Ca \approx 0.5$; Video S2: numerical result at $Ca = 0.01$; Video S3: numerical result at $Ca = 0.1$; Video S4: numerical result at $Ca = 0.5$; Videos S5 and Video S6: numerical results of initial RBC centroid position two meshes away from the midline for $Ca = 5 \times 10^{-3}$ and $Ca = 0.5$, respectively. These numerical results were obtained with $\lambda = 5$ and $k_b = 1.2 \times 10^{-19}$ J.

Author Contributions: N.T., analyzed data; H.I. performed experiments; N.T., and H.I. interpreted results of simulations and experiments; N.T. and H.I. prepared figures; N.T. and H.I. drafted manuscript; N.T. and H.I. edited and revised manuscript; N.T., H.I., M.K., and S.W. approved final version of manuscript; N.T. contributed to research conception and design.

Acknowledgments: We thank M. Chimura, T. Ohtani, and Y. Sakata for providing blood samples. Last but not least, Naoki Takeishi thanks Yohsuke Imai and also Toshihiro Omori for helpful discussions.

Abbreviations

The following abbreviations are used in this manuscript:

RBC   Red blood cell
LBM   Lattice–Boltzmann method
FEM   Finite element method
IBM   Immersed boundary method
GPU   Graphics processing unit

Appendix A. Sample Preparation and Observation

Adult blood was drawn from healthy donors based on the informed consent. All the experiments and experimental protocols in microchannels were approved by the Ethical Committee of Osaka University and performed according to the appropriate guidelines and regulations. Immediately after the blood was drawn, it was maintained in an intact condition by dispersal at a concentration of 1% (v/v) in standard saline.

A microfluidic channel was constructed between a glass slide and poly (dimethylsiloxane) (PDMS) that was designed and printed from a master mold made of SU-8 photoresist using standard photolithography. The cross-section of the rectangular microchannel was 10 μm × 3.5 μm (Figure A1a,b). The experimental system was composed of a high-speed camera (IDP-Express R2000, Photron) and microscope (IX71, Olympus) equipped with an × 40 (N.A. = 0.6) or × 50 (N.A. = 0.42) objective lenses. Images were captured at 1000 frames/s with exposure time of 1 ms. The spatial resolutions of captured images were 0.24 μm/pixel (Figure A1d) and 0.26 μm/pixel (Figure A2) for × 40 and × 50 objective lenses, respectively. Flow of the solution inside the microchannel was basically driven by a constant pressure difference between the inlet and outlet of the channel, maintained by atmospheric pressure and gravitational force.

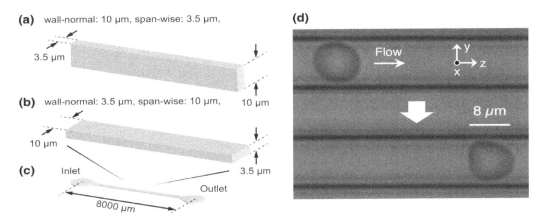

Figure A1. Detailed channel geometry. Magnified view of the channels with the cross-sections of (**a**) 10 μm × 3.5 μm and (**b**) 3.5 μm × 10 μm, which were used in Figure A2 and Figure A1, respectively. (**c**) Schematic view of the whole channel, whose stream-wise length was 8000 μm. (**d**) Representative images of a flowing RBC in a microfluidic device. Flow direction is from left to right.

Figure A2 shows representative snapshot images of a RBC flowing at a velocity of 1200 μm/s; imaging was performed at 1000 frames/s, perpendicular to the span-wise direction of the microchannel. The RBC deformed into an asymmetrical shape, the so-called slipper shape [42]. Interestingly, this configuration was also found in a numerical simulation with $Ca = 0.01$, where the RBC centroid velocity was $V_c \sim 25$ μm/s (Figure A2). Although we reported RBC heterogeneity in [17], the asymmetrical shape of RBCs by means of the experimental observations is required for a precise statistical analysis, which is however future study.

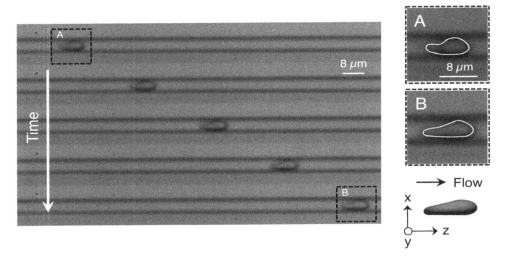

Figure A2. Representative images of the flowing RBC at frame numbers 0 (top), 20, 40 60, and 80 (bottom), respectively, where the speed of the cell is 1200 μm/s (see also Video S1). A representative numerical result of a stable slipper-shaped RBC subjected to $Ca = 0.01$ (calculated centroid velocity $V_c \sim 25$ μm/s) is also displayed (see also Video S2).

References

1.   Chen, S. Red cell deformability and its relevance to blood flow. *Annu. Rev. Physiol.* **1987**, *49*, 177–192. [CrossRef]

2.   Caimi, G.; Presti, R.L. Techniques to evaluate erythrocyte deformability in diabetes mellitus. *Acta Diabetol.* **2004**, *41*, 99–103. [CrossRef] [PubMed]

3.   Johannes, M.B.P.; Leray, C.; Ruef, P.; Cazenave, J.P.; Linderkamp, O. Endotoxin binding to erythrocyte membrane and erythrocyte deformability in human sepsis and in vitro. *Crit. Care Med.* **2003**, *31*, 924–928.

4.   Glenister, F.K.; Coppel, R.L.; Cowman, A.F.; Mohandas, N.; Cooke, B.M. Contribution of parasite proteins to altered mechanical properties of malaria-infected red blood cells. *Blood* **2002**, *99*, 1060–1063. [CrossRef]

5.   Park, Y.; Diez-Silva, M.; Popescu, G.; Lykotrafitis, G.; Choi, W.; Feld, M.S.; Suresh, S. Refractive index maps and membrane dynamics of human red blood cells parasitized by Plasmodium falciparum. *Proc. Natl. Acad. Sci. USA.* **2008**, *112*, 6068–6073. [CrossRef] [PubMed]

6.   Suresh, S.; Spatz, J.; Mills, J.P.; Micoulet, A.; Dao, M.; Lim, C.T.; Beil, M.; Seufferlein, T. Connections between single-cell biomechanics and human disease states: Gastrointestinal cancer and malaria. *Acta Biomater.* **2005**, *1*, 15–30. [CrossRef]

7.   Fregin, B.; Czerwinski, F.; Biedenweg, D.; Girardo, S.; Gross, S.; Aurich, K.; Otto, O. High-throughput single-cell rheology in complex samples by dynamic real-time deformability cytometry. *Nat. Commun.* **2019**, *10*, 415. [CrossRef] [PubMed]

8.   Gossett, D.R.; Tse, H.T.K.; Lee, S.A.; Ying, Y.; Lindgren, A.G.; Yang, O.O.; Rao, J.; Clark, A.T.; Carloa, D.D. Hydrodynamic stretching of single cells for large population mechanical phenotyping. *Proc. Natl. Acad. Sci. USA* **2012**, *109*, 7630–7635. [CrossRef]

9.   Ito, H.; Murakami, R.; Sakuma, S.; Tsai, C.-H.D.; Gutsmann, T.; Brandenburg, K.; Poöschl, J.M.B.; Arai, F.; Kaneko, M.; Tanaka, M. Mechanical diagnosis of human eryhrocytes by ultra-high speed manipulation unraveled critical time window for global cytoskeletal remodeling. *Sci. Rep.* **2017**, *7*, 43134. [CrossRef]

10. Otto, O.; Rosendahl, P.; Mietke, A.; Golfier, S.; Herold, C.; Klaue, D.; Girardo, S.; Pagliara, S.; Ekpenyong, A.; Jacobi, A.; et al. Real-time deformability cytometry: On-the-fly cell mechanical phenotyping. *Nat. Methods* **2015**, *12*, 199–202. [CrossRef]

11. Tsai, C.-H.D.; Tanaka, J.; Kaneko, M.; Horade, M.; Ito, H.; Taniguchi, T.; Ohtani, T.; Sakata, Y. An on-chip RBC deformability checker significantly improves velocity-deformation correlation. *Micromachines* **2016**, *7*, 176. [CrossRef]

12. Takeishi, N.; Imai, Y.; Ishida, S.; Omori, T.; Kamm, R.D.; Ishikawa, T. Cell adhesion during bullet motion in capillaries. *Am. J. Physiol. Heart Circ. Physiol.* **2016**, *311*, H395–H403. [CrossRef] [PubMed]

13. Mokbel, M.; Mokbel, D.; Mietke, A.; Traber, N.; Girardo, S.; Otto, O.; Guck, J.; Aland, S. Numerical simulation of real-time deformability cytometry to extract cell mechanical properties. *ACS Biomater. Sci. Eng.* **2017**, *3*, 2962–2973. [CrossRef]

14. Mauer, J.; Mendez, S.; Lanotte, L.; Nicoud, F.; Abkarian, M.; Gompper, G.; Fedosov, D.A. Flow-induced transitions of red blood cell shapes under shear. *Phys. Rev. Lett.* **2018**, *121*, 118103. [CrossRef] [PubMed]

15. Chang, H.-Y.; Yazdani, A.; Li, X.; Douglas, K.A.A.; Mantzoros, C.S.; Karniadakis, G.E. Quantifying platelet margination in diabetic blood flow. *Biophys. J.* **2018**, *115*, 1–12. [CrossRef]

16. Li, X.; Du, E.; Lei, H.; Tang, Y.-H.; Dao, M.; Suresh, S.; Karniadakis, G.E. Patient-specific blood rheology in sickle-cell anaemia. *Interf. Focus* **2016**, *6*, 20150065. [CrossRef] [PubMed]

17. Ito, H.; Takeishi, N.; Kirimoto, A.; Chimura, M.; Ohtani, T.; Sakata, Y.; Horade, M.; Takayama, T.; Wada, S.; Kaneko, M. How to measure cellular shear modulus inside a chip: Detailed correspondence to the fluid-structure coupling analysis. In Proceedings of the MEMS2019, Seoul, Korea, 27–31 January 2019; pp. 336–433.

18. Kirimoto, A.; Ito, H.; Tsai, C.D.; Kaneko, M. Measurement of both viscous and elasticc constants of a red blood cell in a microchannel. In Proceedings of the MEMS2018, Belfast, UK, 21–25 January 2018; doi:10.1109/MEMSYS.2018.8346569.

19. Abkarian, M; Faivre, M; Horton, R.; Smistrup, K.; Best-Popescu, C.A.; Stone, H.A. Cellular-scale hydrodynamics. *Biomed. Mater.* **2008**, *3*, 034011. [CrossRef] [PubMed]

20. Guckenberger, A.; Kihm, A.; John, T.; Wagner, C.; Gekle, S. Numerical-experimental observation of shape bistability of red blood cells flowing in a microchannel. *Soft Matter.* **2018**, *14*, 2032–2043. [CrossRef]

21. Prado, G.; Farutin, A.; Misbah, C.; Bureau, L. Viscoelastic transient of confined red blood cells. *Biophys. J.* **2015**, *108*, 2126–2136. [CrossRef]

22. Suzuki, Y.; Tateishi, N.; Soutani, M.; Maeda, N. Deformation of erythrocytes in microvessels and glass capillaries: Effects of erythrocyte deformability. *Microcirculation* **1996**, *3*, 49–57. [CrossRef]

23. Tomaiuolo, G.; Simeone, M.; Martinelli, V.; Rotolib, B.; Guido, S. Red blood cell deformation in microconfined flow. *Soft Matter* **2009**, *5*, 3736–3740. [CrossRef]

24. Tomaiuolo, G.; Lanotte, L.; D'Apolito, R.; Cassinese, A.; Guido, S. Microconfined flow behavior of red blood cells. *Med. Eng. Phys.* **2016**, *38*, 11–16. [CrossRef] [PubMed]

25. Brust, M.; Aouane, O.; Thiébaud, M.; Flormann, D.; Verdier, C.; Kaestner, L.; Laschke, M.W.; Selmi, H.; Benyoussef, A.; Podgorski, T.; et al. The plasma protein fibrinogen stabilizes clusters of red blood cells in microcapillary flows. *Sci. Rep.* **2014**, *4*, 4348. [CrossRef] [PubMed]

26. Kaoui, B.; Biros, G.; Misbah, C. Why do red blood cells have asymmetric shapes even in a symmetric flow? *Phys. Rev. Lett.* **2009**, *103*, 188101. [CrossRef] [PubMed]

27. Lázaro, G.R.; Hernández-Machadoa, A.; Pagonabarraga, I. Rheology of red blood cells under flow in highly confined microchannels. II. Effect of focusing and confinement. *Soft Matter* **2014**, *10*, 7207–7217. [CrossRef] [PubMed]

28. Tahiri, N.; Biben, T.; Ez-Zahraouy, H.; Benyoussef, A; Misbah, C. On the problem of slipper shapes of red blood cells in the microvasculature. *Microvasc. Res.* **2013**, *85*, 40–45. [CrossRef] [PubMed]

29. Secomb, T.W.; Skalak, R. A two-dimensional model for capillary flow of an asymmetric cell. *Microvasc. Res.* **1982**, *24*, 194–203. [CrossRef]

30. Fedosov, D.A.; Peltomäki, M.; Gompper, G. Deformation and dynamics of red blood cells in flow through cylindrical microchannels. *Soft Matter* **2014**, *10*, 4258–4267. [CrossRef]

31. Zhu, L.; Gallaire, F. A pancake droplet translating in a Hele-Shaw cell: Lubrication film and flow field. *J. Fluid Mech.* **2016**, *798*, 955–969. [CrossRef]

32. Skalak, R.; Tozeren, A.; Zarda, R.P.; Chien, S. Strain energy function of red blood cell membranes. *Biophys. J.* **1973**, *13*, 245–264. [CrossRef]

33. Takeishi, N.; Imai, Y.; Nakaaki, K.; Yamaguchi, T.; Ishikawa, T. Leukocyte margination at arteriole shear rate. *Physiol. Rep.* **2014**, *2*, e12037. [CrossRef] [PubMed]

34. Takeishi, N.; Imai, Y.; Yamaguchi, T.; Ishikawa, T. Flow of a circulating tumor cell and red blood cells in microvessels. *Phys. Rev. E* **2015**, *92*, 063011. [CrossRef]

35. Takeishi, N.; Imai, Y. Capture of microparticles by bolus of red blood cells in capillaries. *Sci. Rep.* **2017**, *7*, 5381. [CrossRef] [PubMed]

36. Li, J.; Dao, M.; Lim, C.T.; Suresh, S. Spectrin-level modeling of the cytoskeleton and optical tweezers stretching of the erythrocyte. *Phys. Fluid* **2005**, *88*, 3707–6719. [CrossRef] [PubMed]

37. Puig-de-Morales-Marinkovic, M.; Turner, K.T.; Butler, J.P.; Fredberg, J.J.; Suresh, S. Viscoelasticity of the human red blood cell. *Am. J. Physiol. Cell Physiol.* **2007**, *293*, C597–C605. [CrossRef] [PubMed]

38. Chen, S.; Doolen, G.D. Lattice boltzmann method for fluid flow. *Annu. Rev. Fluid. Mech.* **1998**, *30*, 329–364. [CrossRef]

39. Walter, J.; Salsac, A.V.; Barthès-Biesel, D.; Le Tallec, P. Coupling of finite element and boundary integral methods for a capsule in a stokes flow. *Int. J. Numer. Meth. Eng.* **2010**, *83*, 829–850. [CrossRef]

40. Peskin, C.S. The immersed boundary method. *Acta Numer.* **2002**, *11*, 479–517. [CrossRef]

41. Miki, T.; Wang, X.; Aoki, T.; Imai, Y.; Ishikawa, T.; Takase, K.; Yamaguchi, T. Patient-specific modeling of pulmonary air flow using GPU cluster for the application in medical particle. *Comput. Meth. Biomech. Biomed. Eng.* **2012**, *15*, 771–778. [CrossRef] [PubMed]

42. Skalak, R.; Branemark, P.I. Deformation of red blood cells in capillaries. *Science* **1969**, *164*, 717–719. [CrossRef] [PubMed]

43. Kuriakose, S.; Dimitrakopoulos, P. Motion of an elastic capsule in a square microfluidic channel. *Phys. Rev. E* **2011**, *84*, 011906. [CrossRef]

44. Rorai, C.; Touchard, A.; Zhu, L.; Brandt, L. Motion of an elastic capsule in a constricted microchannel. *Eur. Phys. J. E* **2015**, *38*, 49. [CrossRef]

45. Omori, T.; Ishikawa, T.; Barthès-Biesel, D.; Salsac, A.-V.; Imai, Y.; Yamaguchi, T. Tension of red blood cell membrane in simple shear flow. *Phys. Rev. E* **2012**, *86*, 056321. [CrossRef]

46. Lanotte, L.; Mauer, J.; Mendez, S.; Fedosov, D.A.; Fromental, J.-M.; Claveria, V.; Nicoul, F.; Gompper, G.; Abkarian, M. Red cells' dynamic morphologies govern blood shear thinning under microcirculatory flow conditions. *Proc. Natl. Acad. Sci. USA* **2016**, *113*, 13289–13294. [CrossRef]

47. Peng, Z.; Mashayekh, A.; Zhu, Q. Erythrocyte responses in low-shear-rate flows: Effects of non-biconcave stress-free state in the cytoskeleton. *J. Fluid. Mech.* **2014** *742*, 96–118. [CrossRef]

48. Sinha, K.; Graham, M.D. Dynamics of a single red blood cell in simple shear flow. *Phys. Rev. E* **2015**, *92*, 042710. [CrossRef]

49. Tsubota, K.; Wada, S.; Liu, H. Elastic behavior of a red blood cell with the membrane's nonuniform natural state: Equilibrium shape, motion transition under shear flow, and elongation during tank-treading motion. *Biomech. Model. Mechanobiol.* **2014**, *13*, 735–746. [CrossRef]

12

Multiple and Periodic Measurement of RBC Aggregation and ESR in Parallel Microfluidic Channels under On-Off Blood Flow Control

Yang Jun Kang [1,*] **and Byung Jun Kim** [2]

[1]   Department of Mechanical Engineering, Chosun University, 309 Pilmun-daero, Dong-gu, Gwangju 61452, Korea
[2]   Department of Biomedical Science and Engineering, Gwangju Institute of Science and Technology (GIST), Gwangju 61005, Korea; gene392@gist.ac.kr
*   Correspondence: yjkang2011@chosun.ac.kr

Abstract: Red blood cell (RBC) aggregation causes to alter hemodynamic behaviors at low flow-rate regions of post-capillary venules. Additionally, it is significantly elevated in inflammatory or pathophysiological conditions. In this study, multiple and periodic measurements of RBC aggregation and erythrocyte sedimentation rate (ESR) are suggested by sucking blood from a pipette tip into parallel microfluidic channels, and quantifying image intensity, especially through single experiment. Here, a microfluidic device was prepared from a master mold using the xurography technique rather than micro-electro-mechanical-system fabrication techniques. In order to consider variations of RBC aggregation in microfluidic channels due to continuous ESR in the conical pipette tip, two indices (aggregation index (AI) and erythrocyte-sedimentation-rate aggregation index (EAI)) are evaluated by using temporal variations of microscopic, image-based intensity. The proposed method is employed to evaluate the effect of hematocrit and dextran solution on RBC aggregation under continuous ESR in the conical pipette tip. As a result, EAI displays a significantly linear relationship with modified conventional ESR measurement obtained by quantifying time constants. In addition, EAI varies linearly within a specific concentration of dextran solution. In conclusion, the proposed method is able to measure RBC aggregation under continuous ESR in the conical pipette tip. Furthermore, the method provides multiple data of RBC aggregation and ESR through a single experiment. A future study will involve employing the proposed method to evaluate biophysical properties of blood samples collected from cardiovascular diseases.

Keywords: red blood cell (RBC) aggregation; multiple microfluidic channels; master molder using xurography technique; RBC aggregation index; modified conventional erythrocyte sedimentation rate (ESR) method; regression analysis

1. Introduction

Normal red blood cell (RBC) in autologous plasma suspension tends to aggregate and form rouleaux (i.e., stacks-of-coins) under extremely low shear-rate conditions [1,2]. This reversible process is strongly dependent on several factors such as surface properties (membrane deformability and negative surface charge), plasma proteins (fibrinogen and globulins), shear stress, and hematocrit [3]. Additionally, RBC aggregation is considered a key determinant of blood viscosity, because it contributes to increasing blood viscosity at low shear rates. Thus, it causes to alter hemodynamic behaviors at low flow-rate regions of post-capillary venules [4,5]. Furthermore, RBC aggregation is significantly elevated in inflammatory or pathophysiological conditions [6,7]. As an indicator of RBC aggregation, erythrocyte sedimentation rate (ESR) is quantified by measuring setting distance of RBCs in a vertical tube (inner diameter = 2.55 mm, length = 300 mm, and blood volume = 5 mL) for 1 h. In other words, ESR is measured as the height of an RBC-depleted region (or plasma region) of a blood sample in a vertical tube with a specific elapse of time (t) (t = 1 h). The ESR is widely used in clinical medicine, because it is a simple and inexpensive method [6–12]. However, the method involves several disadvantages such as large volume consumption (~2 mL) and long measurement time (~1 h). Conversely, after blood flow in a microfluidic channel is agitated with external sources such as pressure source [13], syringe pump [2,14], and pinch valve [3], RBC aggregation is immediately quantified by constructing variations of image intensity [3,13–15], laser back-scattering [16], ultrasound signal [17], or electrical impedance [18] with an elapse of time (i.e., syllectogram). Previously, our group suggests the simple measurement method of ESR in the microfluidic device [15]. In other words, after setting a disposable syringe into a syringe pump, the syringe pump is reversely aligned with respect to gravitational direction. Then, blood is supplied from the top position of the syringe into a microfluidic device. Hematocrit of blood supplied into a microfluidic channel decreases over time due to continuous ESR in the disposable syringe. This variation in hematocrit is used to measure ESR by quantifying image intensity of blood within a region-of-interest (ROI) of a microfluidic channel [15]. The method is devised to monitor RBC-depleted region in a disposable syringe. However, it does not provide sufficient information on RBC aggregation of blood in a microfluidic channel. According to a previous study [17], RBC aggregation with microscopic, image-based intensity gave comparable value to RBC aggregation, compared with the ultrasonic method and conventional ESR methods. Recently, a simple method is devised to measure RBC aggregation under continuous ESR in a conical pipette tip [19]. According to the previous study [20], blood storage time at 25 °C should be limited to four hours for RBCs aggregation. Above four hours, RBC aggregation was varied with an elapse of time. In other words, when RBCs aggregation was varied over time, the repetitive test increased the scattering of the aggregation index significantly. Thus, multiple measurements of RBC aggregation were required to avoid large scattering due to repetitive tests being conducted for a long period of time. Thus, it is effective to obtain several data points without repetitive tests. Specifically, RBC aggregation should be quantified as mean ± standard deviation in single experiment with respect to an elapse of time. Thus, it does not require repetitive tests, which cause rheological properties to vary continuously.

In this study, multiple measurements of RBC aggregation under continuous ESR are proposed by sucking blood from a pipette tip into parallel microfluidic channels and quantifying image intensity, especially throughout a single experiment. Furthermore, two indices (aggregation index (AI), and erythrocyte-sedimentation-rate aggregation index (EAI) [19]) are evaluated to consider variations in RBC aggregation due to continuous ESR in a conical pipette tip. The proposed method is demonstrated by using a microfluidic device that is composed of an inlet port, an outlet port, and identical-parallel-microfluidic channels. The microfluidic device is prepared from master mold using xurography technique rather than MEMS (micro-electro-mechanical-system) fabrication techniques. A pipette tip is fitted into the inlet port, and the outlet port is then connected to a disposable syringe with a polyethylene tube. A disposable syringe is installed into a syringe pump. The syringe pump is set to a constant flow rate and operates in the withdrawal mode. A pinch valve is installed between the outlet port and a disposable syringe to control blood delivery from the pipette tip to a microfluidic device. The blood flow stops or runs in parallel microfluidic channels when the pinch valve is periodically clamped or released. The image intensity of blood in each microfluidic channel is quantified to obtain several data points of RBC aggregation over an interval of time. Thus, the proposed method measures several data points of RBC aggregation under continuous ESR in a single experiment without requiring additional repetitive tests.

The feasibility of the proposed method is evaluated by conducting experimental tests with two RBC aggregation indices such as EAI and AI. The EAI is applied to quantify RBC aggregation under continuous ESR in conical pipette tip. Furthermore, AI as a conventional aggregation index is used to compare EAI. In order to evaluate the performance of the proposed method, AI and EAI are quantified for several blood samples (hematocrit = 20%, 30%, 40%, and 50%) that are prepared by adding normal

RBCs into autologous plasma. In order to elevate RBC aggregation, blood samples are prepared using normal RBCs with three different concentrations of dextran solution ($C_{dextran}$ = 5 mg/mL, 15 mg/mL, and 20 mg/mL). Subsequently, the proposed method is employed to quantify the effect of dextran solution on the RBC aggregation under continuous ESR in the pipette tip.

2. Materials and Methods

2.1. Blood Sample Preparation

Blood samples were prepared by adding human RBCs to autologous plasma to evaluate RBC aggregation and ESR. Concentrated RBCs and plasma were provided by the Gwangju-Chonnam Blood Bank (Gwangju, Korea). In blood bank, RBCs were collected by removing plasma from whole blood. Then, the RBCs were stored in anticoagulant citrate phosphate dextrose adenine solution (CPDA-1). After concentrated RBCs packed within blood bag (~320 mL) were provided by blood bank, they were immediately stored at 4 °C. To collect pure RBCs from the concentrated RBCs, blood sample was prepared by adding concentrated RBCs (~8 mL) into 1× phosphate-buffered saline (PBS) solution (~8 mL). By operating centrifugal separator, pure RBCs were collected by removing buffy layer and PBS from the blood sample. This washing procedure was repeated three times. When blood storage time at 25 °C was over four hours, RBC aggregation was varied with an elapse of time [20]. Thus, after blood samples were prepared, they were stored at 4 °C before blood test. All experiments were finished within four hours. According to the previous studies [21,22], blood biophysical properties including blood viscosity, and RBC aggregation remained constant for up to 7 days of storage time. In other words, when storage time of RBCs was over 7 days, the RBCs were removed. Hematocrits of normal blood (H_{ct} = 20%, 30%, 40%, and 50%) were adjusted by adding normal RBCs to autologous plasma. In order to elevate RBC aggregation in blood samples, three different concentrations of dextran solution ($C_{dextran}$) ($C_{dextran}$ = 5 mg/mL, 15 mg/mL, and 20 mg/mL) were prepared by adding dextran (Leuconostoc spp., MW = 450–650 kDa, Sigma-Aldrich, St. Louis, MO, USA) to a 1× PBS solution. Hematocrit of blood samples was adjusted to 30% by adding normal RBCs into a specific dextran solution. A control blood sample ($C_{dextran}$ = 0) was prepared by adding normal RBCs into a 1× PBS solution.

2.2. Fabrication of a Microfluidic Device and Experimental Procedure

As shown in Figure 1A, a master mold was fabricated using a cutting plotter (i.e., xurography technique) [23–26]. Here, an adhesive sheet with a thickness of 100 μm was employed for 100 μm depth. A master mold was designed by using a commercial software program (AutoCAD 2014, Autodesk, San Rafael, CA, USA) [Figure 1A-a]. A cutter blade (CE6000-40, Graphtec, Irvine, CA, USA) was used to cut a cover of the adhesive sheet [Figure 1A-b]. The cover was peeled off from a liner [Figure 1A-c]. The master mold was finally prepared by attaching the liner on a glass slide [Figure 1A-d]. PDMS (polydimethylsiloxane) was mixed at a ratio of 10:1 with a curing agent, and the mixture was poured on the master mold positioned in a Petri dish. The air bubbles dissolved in the PDMS were completely removed by operating a vacuum pump for 1 h. The PDMS was cured in a convection oven at temperature of 75 °C for 1.5 h, and the PDMS block was peeled off from the master mold. Two biopsy punches were used, and the inlet port and outlet port was displayed through holes with diameters of 1.5 mm and 0.75 mm, respectively. Following the simultaneous treatment of oxygen plasma (CUTE-MPR, Femto Science Co., Gyeonggi, Korea) on the PDMS block and on a glass substrate, the microfluidic device was prepared by bonding the PDMS block to the glass substrate.

A microfluidic device was mounted on an optical microscope (IX53, Olympus, Tokyo, Japan) equipped with a 4× objective lens (numerical aperture (NA) = 0.1). As shown in Figure 1B, a pipette tip that was tightly fitted into inlet port after a pipette tip (50–1000 μL, Eppendorf, Germany) was cut approximately 34 mm from the top surface. The outlet port was connected to a disposable syringe with a polyethylene tube. The flow rate was set to 2 mL/h (i.e., Q = 2 mL/h) at the withdrawal mode. Blood (0.2 mL) was dropped into the pipette tip with a pipette. In order to avoid non-specific binding of plasma protein, microfluidic channels and the pipette tip were filled with 1% bovine serum albumin (BSA) diluted with $1\times$ PBS solution (pH 7.4, GIBCO, Life Technologies, Gangnam-gu, Korea) for 20 min. The BSA solution was removed from the microfluidic device by releasing the pinch valve. Subsequently, 0.2 mL of blood was dropped into the pipette tip, and it was ready to measure RBC aggregation under continuous hematocrit variations. As shown in Figure 1C-d, a high-speed camera (FASTCAM MINI, Photron, San Jose, CA, USA) was employed to capture blood flows in the microfluidic channels. The spatial resolution of the camera corresponded to 1280×1000 pixels. Each pixel corresponds to 10 μm. A function generator (WF1944B, NF Corporation, Tokyo, Japan) triggered the high-speed camera at an interval of 1 s to sequentially capture two microscopic images at a frame rate of 1 kHz. All experiments were conducted at a room temperature of 25 °C.

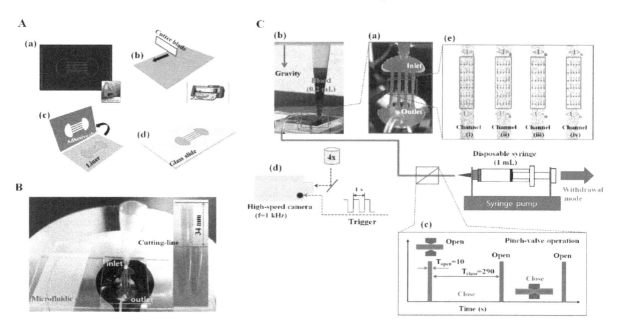

Figure 1. Details of a master mold using an adhesive sheet and a conical pipette tip, and schematic diagram of a proposed method for quantifying red blood cells (RBCs) aggregation and erythrocyte sedimentation rate (ESR) in a pipette tip. (**A**) Fabrication procedure for preparing an adhesive sheet for a master mold. (**A-a**) A pattern of master mold designed with commercial software. (**A-b**) A cutter blade to cut a cover of the adhesive sheet. (**A-c**) The cover was peeled off from a liner. (**A-d**) The master mold was finally prepared by attaching the liner on a glass slide. (**B**) A pipette tip tightly fitted into a microfluidic device. The pipette tip was prepared by cutting 34 mm from the top surface. (**C**) A schematic diagram of the proposed method including a pipette tip, a disposable microfluidic device, a pinch value, and a syringe pump. (**C-a**) A microfluidic device is composed of an inlet port, an outlet port, and parallel microfluidic channels ($N = 4$, width = 600 μm, depth = 100 μm, and length = 8 mm). (**C-b**) A pipette tip fitted into inlet port is filled with 0.2 mL blood. The outlet port is connected to a disposable syringe (1 mL) with a polyethylene tube (inner diameter = 250 μm, length = 600 mm). A disposable syringe is installed into the syringe pump. Flow rate is set to 2 mL/h (i.e., $Q = 2$ mL/h) at the withdrawal mode. (**C-c**) A pinch valve was installed in front of the disposable syringe to control blood flow in parallel microfluidic channels. A pinch valve was manually opened for 10 s ($T_{\text{open}} = 10$ s) and closed for 290 s ($T_{\text{close}} = 290$ s) during a single period ($T = 300$ s). (**C-d**) Image acquisition system including microscope, high-speed camera, and external trigger. (**C-e**) A specific region-of-interest (ROI) (80 pixel $\times$ 400 pixel) for each microfluidic channel was selected to determine average velocity ($<U>_{\text{i}}$, $<U>_{\text{ii}}$, $<U>_{\text{iii}}$ and $<U>_{\text{iv}}$) and average image intensity ($<I>_{\text{i}}$, $<I>_{\text{ii}}$, $<I>_{\text{iii}}$ and $<I>_{\text{iv}}$), which were calculated by conducting time-resolved micro-particle image velocimetry (PIV) technique and digital image processing, respectively.

2.3. The Proposed Method for Quantifying RBCs Aggregation and ESR over Time

A simple measurement technique of RBC aggregation under continuous ESR is proposed by sucking blood from a pipette tip into parallel microfluidic channels, and quantifying image intensity of blood over an interval of time. Several data of RBC aggregation are obtained throughout a single experiment at an interval of specific time duration.

Figure 1C shows a schematic diagram of the proposed method including a disposable microfluidic device, a pipette tip, a pinch valve, and a syringe pump. A microfluidic device is designed with an inlet port, an outlet port, and parallel microfluidic channels ($N = 4$, width = 600 μm, depth = 100 μm, and length = 8 mm) [Figure 1C-a]. A pipette tip (50–1000 μL, Eppendorf, Hamburg, Germany) is cut approximately 34 mm from the top surface [Figure 1B], and the pipette tip is tightly fitted into an inlet port (inner diameter = 1.5 mm). The outlet port is connected to a disposable syringe (1 mL) with a polyethylene tube (inner diameter = 250 μm and length = 600 mm). After the disposable syringe is installed into a syringe pump, the flow rate was set to 2 mL/h ($Q = 2$ mL/h) at the withdrawal mode. Subsequently, 0.2 mL blood is dropped into the pipette tip with a pipette [Figure 1C-b]. The RBC migrates towards the button position due to continuous ESR in the pipette tip, and thus the previous method quantifies ESR by measuring the height of the RBC-depleted region [15,17]. In contrast to previous ESR measurement, the proposed method is suggested to measure variations of RBC aggregation under continuous ESR by evaluating the microscopic image-based intensity of blood flow in microfluidic channels. Therefore, to evaluate variations in hematocrit due to continuous ESR in the pipette tip, blood is supplied from the conical pipette tip to the microfluidic channels over an interval of time. A pinch valve (Supa clip, Pankyo, Gyeonggi-do, Korea) was installed between the outlet port and the disposable syringe to periodically ensure blood delivery into the microfluidic device. A pinch valve is manually opened for 10 s ($T_{open} = 10$ s) and closed for 290 s ($T_{close} = 290$ s) during a single period ($T = 300$ s) [Figure 1C-c]. As shown in Figure 1C-e, a specific ROI (80 × 400 pixels) is selected for each microfluidic channel to determine an average value of blood velocity for each microfluidic channel ($<U>_i$, $<U>_{ii}$, $<U>_{iii}$ and $<U>_{iv}$) and an average value of image intensity for each microfluidic channel ($<I>_i$, $<I>_{ii}$, $<I>_{iii}$ and $<I>_{iv}$) that are calculated by conducting time-resolved micro-PIV technique and digital image processing, respectively.

As a preliminary study, blood with 30% hematocrit was prepared by adding normal RBCs into a specific dextran solution (i.e., $C_{dextran} = 15$ mg/mL). Figure 2A shows temporal variations of averaged image intensity ($<I>$) for individual microfluidic channel and averages blood velocity ($<U>$) through four microfluidic channels. Here, to monitor temporal variations of blood flow depending on the operation of the pinch value (i.e., open or close), velocity fields were obtained by conducting time-resolved micro-PIV technique. After guaranteeing the operation of the pinch valve sufficiently, we did not try to get velocity information. Sequential images for representing RBC-depleted regions in a pipette tip were captured with elapses of time (t) ([a] $t = 300$ s, [b] $t = 600$ s, [c] $t = 900$ s, and [d] $t = 1200$ s). With respect to an elapse of time, the RBC-depleted region tended to increase due to continuous ESR in conical tip. Additionally, image intensity ($<I>$) tended to decrease due to an increase in the hematocrit. As shown in Figure 2B, temporal variations of $<I>$ for each microfluidic channel are obtained for a single period ($T = 300$ s). Temporal variations of image intensity ($<I>$), which are called a syllectogram, are used to calculate three representative factors (S_A, S_B, and S_C) [19] as follows:

$$S_A = \int_{t=0}^{t=t_s} (<I> - <I>_{min})dt \qquad (1)$$

$$S_B = \int_{t=0}^{t=t_s} (<I>_{max} - <I>)dt \qquad (2)$$

$$S_C = \int_{t=0}^{t=t_s} <I>_{min} dt \qquad (3)$$

In Equations (1)–(3), $<I>_{min}$ and $<I>_{max}$ are denoted as $<I>_{min} = <I(t=0)>$ and $<I>_{max} = <I(t=t_s)>$, respectively. Furthermore, $<I>_{min}$ tended to decrease due to ESR in the pipette tip, and thus S_C was used to represent the dynamic behavior of ESR. According to most previous methods, a blood sample was directly dropped into an inlet port of the microfluidic device. Since hematocrit of the blood sample remained constant in a microfluidic channel, the previous methods did not require to consider the effect of continuous ESR in the reservoir on the RBCs aggregation. In other words, the previous method did not consider the effect of hematocrit variations on the syllectogram (i.e., $S_C = 0$). In other words, as shown in right panel of Figure 2B, RBC aggregation was quantified by calculating AI as $AI = S_A/(S_A + S_B)$. However, in this study, the proposed method involved simultaneously measuring RBC aggregation and ESR in conical pipette tip. The continuous ESR caused to increase hematocrit of blood supplied into a microfluidic channel. According to temporal variations of $<I>$, $<I>_{min}$ decreased due to increases in hematocrit. In order to quantify RBC aggregation due to ESR in the conical pipette tip, it was necessary to simultaneously consider variations in $<I>$ due to RBC aggregation (i.e., S_A) and $<I>_{min}$ due to ESR (i.e., S_C). Thus, EAI is evaluated as $EAI = S_A/S_C$. For convenience, t_s was fixed as $t_s = 250$ s. Sequential microscopic images for four microfluidic channels indicated that RBC tended to gradually aggregate with respect to an elapse of time (t) ([a] $t = 0$, [b] $t = 100$ s, [c] $t = 200$ s, and [d] $t = 300$ s). This preliminary result indicated that the proposed method measured variations of RBC aggregation under continuous ESR by quantifying image intensity of blood in each microfluidic channel.

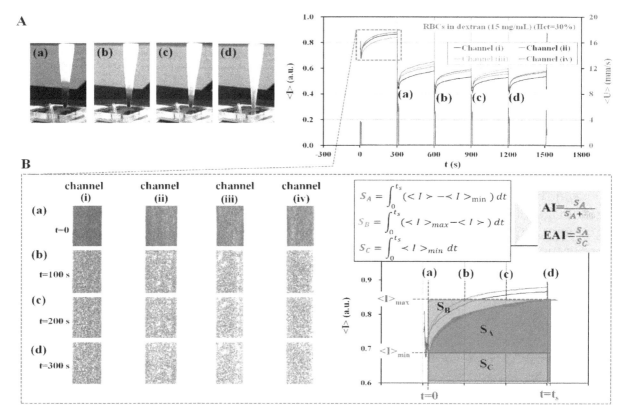

Figure 2. Quantification of two indices (AI and EAI) for quantifying RBCs aggregation and ESR in a conical pipette tip. (**A**) Temporal variations in $<I>$ for each microfluidic channel and average velocity ($<U>$) through four microfluidic channels. Sequential images for representing RBC-depleted regions in a pipette tip with an elapse of time (t) ([**A-a**] $t = 300$ s, [**A-b**] $t = 600$ s, [**A-c**] $t = 900$ s, and [**A-d**] $t = 1200$ s). (**B**) Temporal variations of $<I>$ for each microfluidic channel over a single period. Sequential microscopic images represent RBC aggregation for each microfluidic channel with an elapse of time (t) ([**B-a**] $t = 0$, [**B-b**] $t = 100$ s, [**B-c**] $t = 200$ s, and [**B-d**] $t = 300$ s). Two indices (AI and EAI) were defined as $AI = S_A/(S_A + S_B)$ and $EAI = S_A/S_C$ from a syllectogram obtained for 300 s.

2.4. Quantifications of Image Intensity (<I>) and Blood Velocity (<U>)

In order to evaluate variations in image intensity of blood with an elapse of time, a specific ROI (80 pixel × 400 pixel) was selected within each microfluidic channel as shown in Figure 1C-e. Average pixel values over the ROI ($<I>_i$, $<I>_{ii}$, $<I>_{iii}$, and $<I>_{iv}$) were estimated by performing digital image processing with a commercial software program (Matlab, Mathworks, Natick, MA, USA). To evaluate temporal variations of blood flow, velocity fields were obtained by conducting a time-resolved micro-PIV technique to evaluate temporal variations in blood flow. Specific ROIs (80 pixel × 400 pixel) were selected for each microfluidic channel to obtain velocity fields of blood flow. The size of the interrogation window corresponded to 16 × 16 pixels. The window overlap corresponded to 50%. The obtained velocity fields were validated with a median filter. The average velocities of blood flow for each microfluidic channel ($<U>_i$, $<U>_{ii}$, $<U>_{iii}$, and $<U>_{iv}$) were calculated as an arithmetic average over the ROI. Finally, average blood velocity in the parallel microfluidic channel (<U>) was calculated as $<U> = (<U>_i + <U>_{ii} + <U>_{iii} + <U>_{iv})/4$.

3. Results and Discussion

3.1. Variation of Width in Microfluidic Channel Fabricated by Using an Adhesive Sheet for Master Mold

In this study, the use of a liner cut from an adhesive sheet to form the master mold was employed to simplify the fabrication process, compared to MEMS fabrication. Variations of channel width were measured by analyzing microscopic images obtained from high-speed camera. After then, digital image processing was conducted to measure channel width of individual channel. Measurement for each channel was repeated ten times ($n = 10$). As shown in Figure 3A, the corresponding channel width (W) for each channel was measured as (a) $W = 615 \pm 12$ µm for (i) channel, (b) $W = 615 \pm 23$ µm for (ii) channel, (c) $W = 575 \pm 18$ µm for (iii) channel, and (d) $W = 571 \pm 33$ µm for (iv) channel. In other words, this simple technique could be employed to prepare microfluidic channel within 4% normal deviation in channel width of individual channel. Compared with MEMS fabrication, this simple technique was not feasible to fabricate a microfluidic channel with highly consistent dimensions. According to the previous studies, this xurography technique had poor resolution for dimensions smaller than 500 µm. However, it provides several advantages including inexpensive cost (material and equipment) and rapid fabrication without cleanroom [24,26]. Due to high advantages, it had been employed to fabricate biomedical device for blood flow analysis [25,27]. However, in this study, dynamic blood flow was required to disaggregate aggregated RBCs sufficiently. Since RBCs aggregation was quantified at stationary blood flows by clamping polyethylene tube with a pinch valve, blood flow in each channel does not have an influence on measurement of RBCs aggregation. Even though this technique has a little deviations in channel width, an adhesive sheet could be simply used as a master mold to prepare microfluidic device. On the other hand, to verify variations of each microfluidic device, channel width was measured with five microfluidic devices. Averaged channel width for each device was used to quantify device-to-device variation. Four channel widths of each device were arithmetically averaged as $W_{ave} = [W_{(i)} + W_{(ii)} + W_{(iii)} + W_{(iv)}]/4$. As shown in Figure 3B, averaged channel width (W_{ave}) remained consistent for five different devices. From these measurement results, the use of a liner cut from an adhesive sheet contributes to simplifying the fabrication process, and to preparing PDMS microfluidic channel reliably.

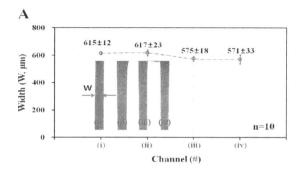
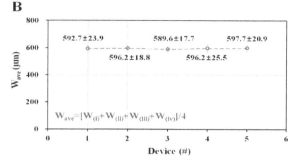

Figure 3. Quantitative measurement of width variations of four microfluidic channels fabricated by using an adhesive sheet for master mold. (**A**) Variations of channel width for four individual channels. (**B**) Variations of averaged channel width for five different devices.

3.2. Quantitative Evaluation of the Effects of Pinch-Valve Operation and Syringe Pump Flow-Rate

In order to analyze the dynamic effect of a microfluidic system (polyethylene tube and a microfluidic device) on the performance of the proposed method, image intensity ($<I>$) and blood velocity ($<U>$) of blood flow in parallel microfluidic channels were quantified with high resolution. Two sequential microscopic images were captured and recorded at an interval of 0.1 s. Hematocrit of blood was adjusted to 30% by adding normal RBCs into autologous plasma. A flow rate was set to 2 mL/h with a syringe pump. Figure 4A-a,A-b show temporal variations of image intensity ($<I>$) and average of blood velocity ($<U>$) obtained for specific durations of 120 s and 25 s. When a pinch valve clamps or releases the polyethylene tube, $<I>$ and $<U>$ showed transient behaviors with respect to time. The experimental results indicated that blood flow stopped shortly within 0.2 s. After clamping the tube, image intensity ($<I>$) tended to increase immediately. According to previous studies [17,28], blood flow decreased gradually based on the compliance effect of the microfluidic system when a syringe pump was used to control blood flow in a microfluidic channel in the delivery mode. In other words, when the syringe pump was set to zero value of the flow rate (i.e., $Q = 0$), RBC aggregation did not occur due to transient blood flow in the microfluidic channel. Thus, RBC aggregation was quantified by using temporal variations in image intensity after an elapse of 20 s [28] or 60 s [17]. For this reason, a glass capillary tube [2] or detour channel [14] was applied to minimize time delay due to the compliance effect of the microfluidic system. However, in the proposed method, a syringe pump sets to constant flow rate as withdrawal mode. The pinch valve clamped or released the polyethylene tube, and thus the blood flow stopped or ran within a very short time. The experimental results indicated that RBC aggregation was measured immediately after clamping the tube with a pinch valve (i.e., close mode). Additionally, the compliance effect of fluidic system on RBC aggregation and ESR was negligible.

To verify the effect of syringe pump flow-rate on RBC aggregation (i.e., AI) and ESR (i.e., EAI), temporal variations of image intensity ($<I>$) and velocity ($<U>$) were obtained by varying flow rate of the syringe pump (Q) ($Q = 0.5$ mL/h, 1 mL/h, and 2 mL/h). Figure 4B-a shows temporal variations of $<I>$ with respect to flow rate of syringe pump (Q). Here, $<I>$ denotes average values of image intensity in four microfluidic channels. With increasing syringe pump flow-rate, $<I>$ tends to decrease. For up to 600 s, minimum value of $<I>$ (i.e., $<I>_{min}$) tends to decrease gradually because of continuous ESR in the conical pipette tip. After 600 s, $<I>$ remained constant without respect to syringe pump flow-rate. In addition, amplitude of $<I>$ (i.e., ΔI) was decreased over time. Figure 4B-b shows temporal variations of $<U>$ with respect to syringe pump flow-rate (Q). Here, $<U>$ denotes averaged blood velocity through four microfluidic channels, especially for 10 s per each period. By increasing flow rate, blood velocity ($<U>$) tends to increase distinctively. In addition, at the higher syringe pump flow-rate of $Q = 1\sim2$ mL/h, blood velocity was decreased gradually from $t = 300$ s to $t = 900$ s. Then ($t > 900$ s), blood velocity remained constant over time. However, at the lower syringe pump flow-rate of $Q = 0.5$ mL/h, blood velocity remained constant over time. Using temporal variations of $<U>$ during a specific time duration of 1500 s, temporal variations of two indices (AI and EAI) were obtained by varying flow rates. As shown in

Figure 4B-c,B-d, AI as conventional RBC aggregation index remained constant without respect to flow rate but not with respect to the initial condition ($t = 0$). However, due to continuous ESR in the conical pipette tip, hematocrit of blood supplied from the conical tip into microfluidic channels was increased. Thus, EAI was decreased gradually over time. In addition, syringe pump flow-rate does not contribute to varying EAI. From these experimental demonstrations, it is found that syringe pump blood-flow rate does not have a significant influence on measurement of AI and EAI. In other words, the syringe pump flow-rate of $Q = 0.5$ mL/h is considered sufficient for removing and filling blood samples in each microfluidic channel for each period. In this study, for convenience, the higher syringe pump flow-rate of $Q = 2$ mL/h was selected to easily suck and remove blood samples from the bottom area of the pipette tip and change blood samples in each microfluidic channel.

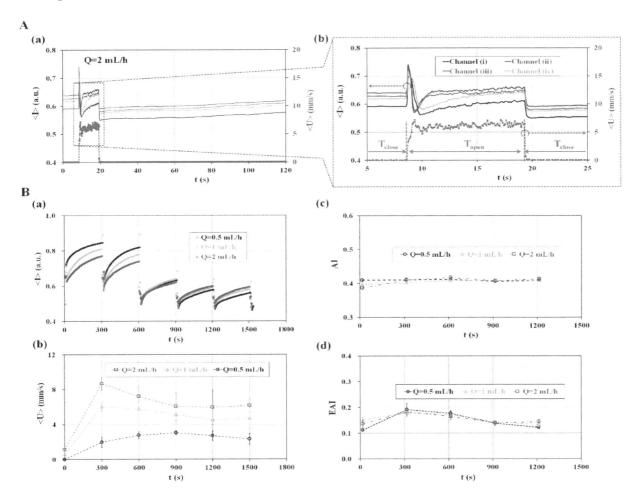

Figure 4. The quantitative evaluation of the effects of vital two factors including pinch-valve operation and syringe pump flow-rate on the measurement of RBC aggregation and ESR. (**A**) Dynamic characterization of image intensity (<I>) and blood velocity (<U>) based on operation of the pinch valve (open, close). To evaluate transient response with a high resolution, <I> and <U> were obtained at intervals of 0.1 s. Hematocrit of blood was adjusted to 30% by adding normal RBCs into the plasma solution. At the constant flow rate of 2 mL/h with syringe pump, temporal variations of <I> and <U> were obtained for specific duration of (**A-a**) 120 s and (**A-b**) 25 s. As a result, blood flow was stopped immediately within 0.2 s after clamping a tube with a pinch (i.e., close). (**B**) The effect of syringe pump flow-rate (Q) on the measurement of RBC aggregation (i.e., AI) and ESR (i.e., EAI). Temporal variations of <I> and <U> were obtained by varying flow rate of syringe pump (Q) ($Q = 0.5$, 1, and 2 mL/h). (**B-a**) Temporal variations of <I> with respect to blood flow rate. (**B-b**) Temporal variations of <U> with respect to syringe pump flow-rate. (**B-c**) Temporal variations of AI with respect to syringe pump flow-rate. (**B-d**) Temporal variations of EAI with respect to syringe pump flow-rate.

3.3. Quantitative Evaluation of the Channel Number for Evaluating Variations of AI and EAI

To find out the effect of the channel number on measurement of RBCs aggregation and ESR, the variations of RBC aggregation and ESR (i.e., AI and EAI) were evaluated with respect to number of channel (n) (n = 1,2, 3, and 4). Figure S1 (Supplementary Materials) showed microscopic images for microfluidic device with multiple numbers of channel (n) [(a) n = 1, (b) n = 2, (c) n = 3, and (d) n = 4]. Blood sample was prepared by adding normal RBCs into plasma. Hematocrit was fixed at 30%. As shown in Figure 5A, temporal variations of $<I>$ and $<U>$ were simultaneously measured with respect to channel number. As a result, $<I>$ and $<U>$ were decreased with increasing channel numbers. When removing pinch valve (i.e., open mode) for 10 s, blood velocity tended to decrease with increasing channel number. Furthermore, image intensity of stasis blood flow tended to decrease for rest time of each period (~290 s). In other words, blood velocity for short duration time (~10 s) contributed to changing image intensity of blood. Temporal variations of two indices (AI and EAI) were obtained by analyzing temporal variations of image intensity for each duration of period. As shown in Figure 5B-a, AI does not show significant difference with respect to channel number. To compare with scattering of AI, coefficient of variation (COV) (~standard deviation/mean) was estimated as less than 0.05 from two channels to four channels. However, since minimum value of image intensity ($<I>_{min}$) for each period was inserted to calculate EAI, higher number of channels contributed to decreasing EAI. As shown in Figure 5B-b, four channels showed lower values of EAI compared with the rest of channel numbers. In addition, COV of EAI remained within 0.1 from two channels to four channels.

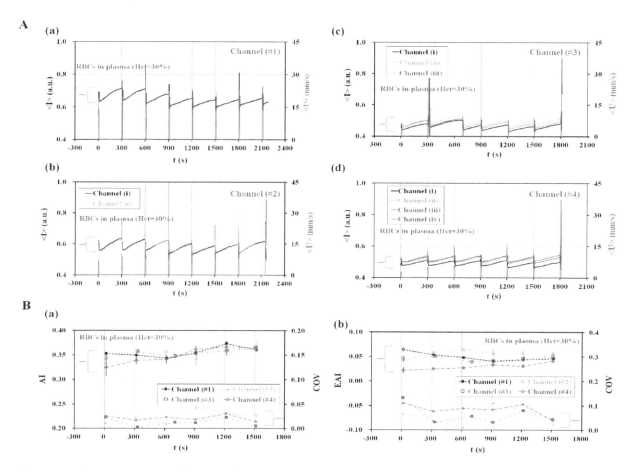

Figure 5. Quantitative evaluation of channel numbers for measuring scattering of two indices (AI and EAI). (**A**) Temporal variations of $<U>$ and $<I>$ with respect to channel number (n) ((**A-a**) n = 1, (**A-b**) n = 2, (**A-c**) n = 3, and (**A-d**) n = 4). (**B**) Temporal variations of AI and EAI with respect to channel number. (**B-a**) Temporal variation of AI and, coefficient of variation (COV) with respect to channel number. (**B-b**) Temporal variations of EAI and COV with respect to channel number.

3.4. Quantitative Evaluation of the Effect of Hematocrit Variations

In order to evaluate the effect of hematocrit on the RBC aggregation under continuous ESR, the four different hematocrits (H_{ct}) (H_{ct} = 20%, 30%, 40%, and 50%) were prepared by adding normal RBCs into autologous plasma. RBC aggregation and ESR were quantified using AI and EAI, respectively. Figure 6A shows temporal variations of <I> with respect to each microfluidic channel and hematocrit level (H_{ct}) ([a] H_{ct} = 20%, [b] H_{ct} = 30%, [c] H_{ct} = 40%, and [d] H_{ct} = 50%). Image intensity (<I>) varied over time with respect to each microfluidic channel and hematocrit. With respect to blood with 20% hematocrit, all RBCs were passed from a pipette tip to outlet port after 1200 s, and thus, variations in image intensity for four microfluidic channels were obtained up to 1200 s. With respect to blood with 30% hematocrit, variations of image intensity were obtained up to 1500 s. However, the other two blood types (H_{ct} = 40% and 50%) exhibited a lower value of ESR in a pipette tip, and thus, RBCs continued to exist in the microfluidic channels. Variations in image intensity were obtained up to 1800 s. Blood with lower hematocrit exhibited a higher value of S_A and S_C when compared with blood with higher hematocrit. This result indicated that blood sample with lower hematocrit exhibited higher values of ESR and RBC aggregation. Temporal variations of <I> were used for four microfluidic channels to obtain temporal variations of AI and EAI with respect to hematocrit. RBCs aggregation was quantified using temporal variations of image intensity from stasis blood flow (t = 0). The effect of shear rate on RBCs aggregation measurement was negligible (i.e., $\dot{\gamma}$ = 0). As shown in Figure 6A, since temporal variations of image intensity were obtained by analyzing microscopic images captured at stasis blood flows, RBCs aggregation only contributed to varying image intensity of blood sample in each microfluidic channel. As shown in Figure 6B-a, AI did not display significant differences with respect to hematocrit (H_{ct}) and measurement time (t). Additionally, blood with lower hematocrit exhibited a higher value of AI when compared with blood with higher hematocrit. Furthermore, AI remained constant over time. Conversely, temporal variations of EAI were obtained with respect to hematocrit to include the effect of ESR. As shown in Figure 6B-b, EAI shows a significant difference with respect to hematocrit when compared with AI. Therefore, blood with 20% hematocrit exhibited a higher value of EAI when compared with other blood. Moreover, blood with 40–50% hematocrit exhibited a similar value to EAI after 900 s. The result indicated that EAI was more effective at evaluating the effect of hematocrit on the RBC aggregation when compared with that of AI, because EAI included the effect of ESR in the pipette tip.

As quantitative comparison, the effect of hematocrit on ESR measurement was quantified by using a modified conventional method [15,17]. Here, hematocrit of blood (H_{ct}) were adjusted to H_{ct} = 20%, 30%, 40%, and 50% by adding normal RBCs into autologous plasma. After installing four disposable syringes vertically in base plate, blood with different hematocrit (~1 mL) was dropped into each syringe with a pipette as shown in Figure 6C-a. At intervals of 30 s, consecutive images were captured with a digital camera (D700, Nikon, Tokyo, Japan). The ESR was then quantified by measuring the height of RBCs-depleted layer (i.e., H) over time. As shown in Figure 6C-b, temporal variations of H were obtained by varying hematocrit. After then, to quantify relationship between proposed method (i.e., EAI) and conventional method (i.e., H), simple regression formula for each method was used as EAI = $a_1 + a_2 \exp(-t/\lambda_{EAI})$ and $H(t) = b_1 + b_2 \exp(-t/\lambda_H)$, respectively. Here, λ_{EAI} and λ_H denote corresponding time constants for proposed method and conventional method. By conducting nonlinear regression analysis with a commercial software (Matlab, Mathworks, Natick, MA, USA), variations of λ_{EAI} and λ_H were obtained with increasing hematocrit. As shown in Figure 6D-a, both time constants tend to increase gradually with respect to hematocrit. In other words, ESR is saturated within a short time for lower hematocrit, compared with higher hematocrit. In addition, EAI shows very similar trend with respect to hematocrit. To find out relationship between two time constants (λ_{EAI} and λ_H), linear regression analysis was conducted using EXCEL program (Microsoft^{TM}, Natick, MA, USA). As shown in Figure 6D-b, coefficient of R^2 shows sufficient high value of R^2 = 0.9521. From this result, both methods have significantly linear relation. Furthermore, it leads to conclusion that EAI as newly suggested index can be effectively employed to monitor variation of ESR through quantifying image intensity of blood flowing in microfluidic channels.

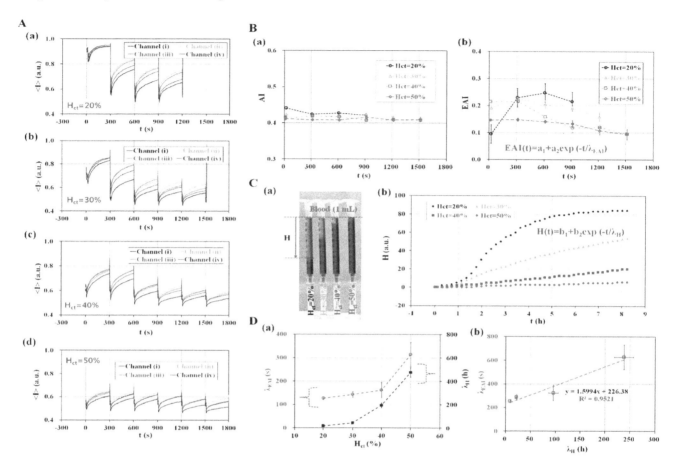

Figure 6. Quantitative evaluation of the effect of hematocrit on the performance of the proposed method. Specifically, RBC aggregation and ESR are quantified using two indices (AI and EAI). Hematocrit (H_{ct}) (H_{ct} = 20%, 30%, 40%, and 50%) was adjusted by adding normal RBCs into autologous plasma. (**A**) Temporal variations of <I> with respect to each microfluidic channel and hematocrit (H_{ct}) ([**A-a**] H_{ct} = 20%, [**A-b**] H_{ct} = 30%, [**A-c**] H_{ct} = 40%, and [**A-d**] H_{ct} = 50%). (**B**) Temporal variations of AI and EAI with respect to hematocrit. (**B-a**) Temporal variations of AI with respect to hematocrit. (**B-b**) Temporal variations of EAI with respect to hematocrit. (**C**) ESR measurement using a disposable syringe (~1 mL) as a conventional method. (**C-a**) Snapshot images for quantifying ESR method with respect to hematocrit. Here, H represents height in RBCs-depleted layer. (**C-b**) Temporal variations of H with respect to hematocrit. (**D**) Quantitative comparison between conventional method and proposed method. (**D-a**) Variations of λ_{EAI} and λ_{H} with respect to hematocrit (H_{ct}). (**D-b**) Linear relationship between λ_{EAI} and λ_{H}.

3.5. Quantitative Evaluation of RBC Aggregation under Continuous for Homogeneous Aggregated RBCs

A performance demonstration involved applying the proposed method to measure RBC aggregation under continuous ESR for homogeneous aggregated RBCs. In order to elevate RBC aggregation for normal RBCs, three different concentrations of dextran solution ($C_{dextran}$) ($C_{dextran}$ = 5 mg/mL, 15 mg/mL, and 20 mg/mL) were prepared by adding dextran into 1× PBS solution. Subsequently, hematocrit of the blood sample was adjusted to 30% by adding normal RBCs into three different concentrations of the dextran solution. Additionally, a control blood sample was prepared by adding normal RBCs into 1× PBS solution ($C_{dextran}$ = 0) to exclude the effect of RBC aggregation.

Figure 7A shows temporal variations of $<I>$ and $<U>$ for two different bloods prepared by adding normal RBCs into 20 mg/mL dextran solution and PBS solution, respectively. The tube opened shortly at an interval of 300 s, and thus, an average of blood velocity ($<U>$) was measured as a periodic pulse-like shape. Image intensity ($<I>$) tended to immediately increase over time when the pinch valve clamps the tube (i.e., in the close mode). A blood sample with a higher concentration of the dextran solution ($C_{dextran}$ = 20 mg/mL) exhibited larger variations in image intensity (i.e., S_A), when compared with that of the control blood sample ($C_{dextran}$ = 0). For two blood samples, a minimum value of $<I>$ ($<I>_{min}$) exhibited a significant decrease at t = 300 s. Following this, $<I>_{min}$ remained constant with an elapse of time. This result indicated that ESR occurs dominantly within 300 s. After 300 s, ESR remained constant with time elapses.

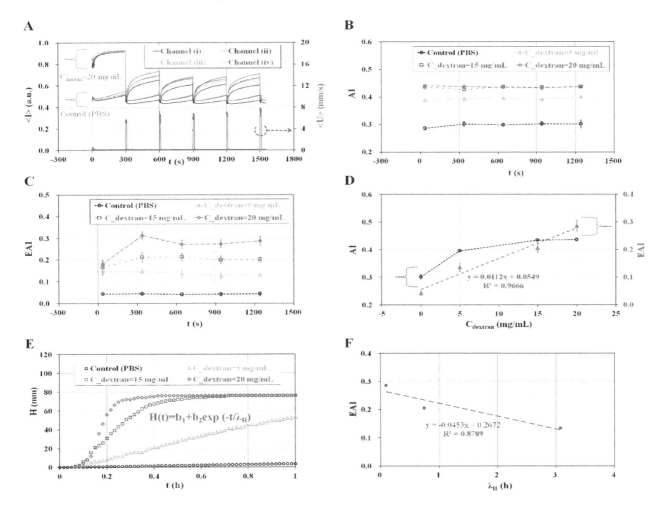

Figure 7. Quantitative evaluations of RBC aggregation (i.e., AI) and ESR (i.e., EAI) with the proposed method and the modified conventional ESR method. To elevate RBC aggregation and ESR, three concentrations of dextran solution ($C_{dextran}$) ($C_{dextran}$ = 5 mg/mL, 15 mg/mL, and 20 mg/mL) were prepared by adding dextran into a PBS solution. Hematocrit is adjusted to 30% by adding normal RBCs into three different concentrations of the dextran solution. (**A**) Temporal variations of $<I>$ and $<U>$ for two different blood samples ($C_{dextran}$ = 0, 20 mg/mL). (**B**) Temporal variations of AI with increasing concentrations of the dextran solution. (**C**) Temporal variations of EAI with increasing concentrations of the dextran solution. (**D**) Variations of AI and EAI with respect to the concentration of the dextran solution. (**E**) Temporal variations of H with respect to specific concentrations of dextran solution. Here, H denotes height of RBCs-depleted layer in a disposable syringe. (**F**) Linear relationship between proposed method (i.e., EAI) and the modified conventional ESR method (i.e., λ_H).

In order to quantify RBC aggregation under continuous ESR, two indices (AI and EAI) were calculated using temporal variations of <I> for each microfluidic channel. As shown in Figure 7B, the temporal variations of AI were obtained with respect to concentrations of the dextran solution. The control blood sample (i.e., normal RBC in PBS suspension) showed a lower value of AI = 0.30 ± 0.01 when compared with aggregated blood sample (i.e., normal RBCs in plasma), as shown in Figure 6B-a. Hence, the AI gives higher value of reference, since control blood sample was prepared to exclude RBC aggregation. Thus, it was estimated that lower hematocrit (H_{ct} = 30%) contributed to a higher value of AI as a reference value. Additionally, the blood sample exhibited a higher value of AI with increases in the concentration of the dextran solution. However, AI did not indicate significant differences for blood samples, with concentrations of the dextran solution ranging from $C_{dextran}$ = 15 mg/mL to $C_{dextran}$ = 20 mg/mL.

As shown in Figure 7C, temporal variation of EAI was calculated using temporal variations of image intensity (<I>) with respect to concentrations of the dextran solution. As a result, EAI remained constant after 2 cycles. Since each cycle is continued for five min., the proposed method requires at least 10 min. The proposed method does remove necessity of repetitive test as significant advantage. The control blood sample exhibited a significantly lower value of EAI (i.e., EAI = 0.04 ± 0.01) as a reference value when compared with that of the AI. Overall variations in EAI are significantly higher than those of AI within a specific dextran solution. Furthermore, EAI exhibited a significant difference at specific dextran concentrations ranging from $C_{dextran}$ = 15 mg/mL to $C_{dextran}$ = 20 mg/mL.

Finally, as shown in Figure 7D, variations of AI and EAI were displayed with respect to a specific dextran solution. The linear regression analysis indicated a high value of R^2 (i.e., R^2 = 0.9666), and thus, EAI linearly varied within a specific concentration of dextran solution. However, AI varied gradually below 15 mg/mL dextran solution. Furthermore, AI approached saturation above 15 mg/mL dextran solution. According to most previous methods, a blood sample was directly dropped into an inlet port of the microfluidic device. Since hematocrit of the blood sample remained constant in a microfluidic channel, the previous methods did not require to consider the effect of continuous ESR in the reservoir on the RBCs aggregation. In other words, the previous method did not consider the effect of hematocrit variations on the syllectogram (i.e., S_C = 0). Based on previous methods [2,3], the RBC aggregation was quantified by calculating AI as AI = $S_A/(S_A + S_B)$. However, in this study, the proposed method involved simultaneously measuring RBC aggregation and ESR in conical pipette tip. The continuous ESR caused to increase hematocrit of blood supplied into a microfluidic channel. According to temporal variations of <I>, minimum value of <I> (i.e., <I>$_{min}$) decreased due to increases in hematocrit. In order to quantify RBC aggregation due to ESR in the conical pipette tip, it was necessary to simultaneously consider variations in <I> due to RBC aggregation (i.e., S_A) and <I>$_{min}$ due to ESR (i.e., S_C). Thus, EAI is evaluated as EAI = S_A/S_C.

3.6. Quantitative Comparison between the Proposed Method and the Modified Conventional ESR Method

To compare with the experimental results obtained by the proposed method, blood was prepared by adding normal RBCs into a specific concentration of dextran solution ($C_{dextran}$) ($C_{dextran}$ = 0, 5 mg/mL, 15 mg/mL, and 20 mg/mL). Here, $C_{dextran}$ = 0 denotes 1× PBS solution. Thereafter, 1 mL blood was dropped into a disposable syringe (1 mL, BD Science, Singapore) as a modified conventional method [15,17]. Figure 7E shows temporal variations of H by varying various concentrations of dextran solution. As a result, dextran solution contributes to increasing H significantly, compared with control blood. To quantify variations of ESR, simple regression expression was suggested as $H(t) = b_1 + b_2 \exp(-t/\lambda_H)$. Then, time constant (i.e., λ_H) was obtained by conducting nonlinear regression analysis with commercial software. Figure 7F represents the quantitative comparison between proposed method (i.e., EAI) and the conventional method (i.e., λ_H). To verify the relationship between the proposed method and conventional method, a linear regression analysis was conducted with EXCEL program (Microsoft^{TM}, Natick, MA, USA). Since the coefficient of R^2 has higher value of R^2 = 0.8789, the EAI obtained by the proposed method can give comparable value of ESR, compared with the conventional method. As shown in Figure 6B-b, EAI of normal blood (H_{ct} = 30%) was varied from 0.16 to 0.22. According to Figure 7D, EAI was increased linearly with increasing concentration of dextran solution. Blood with lower concentration of dextran solution ($C_{dextran}$ = 5 mg/mL) had EAI = 0.134 $\pm$ 0.014. In other words, 5 mg/mL dextran solution played a similar ESR behavior, compared with plasma solution. Blood prepared with higher concentration of dextran solution ($C_{dextran}$ = 20 mg/mL) had EAI = 0.286 $\pm$ 0.019. From this result, maximum concentration of dextran solution (20 mg/mL) contributed to increasing EAI twice, compared with normal blood. According to previous study [22], using streptozotocin-induced rats, variations of ESR were measured by varying duration of diabetes ($D_{Diabetes}$). Compared with control, ESR was increased over twice. From this results, EAI obtained by the proposed method can be effectively used to detect variations of ESR or RBCs aggregation.

From this experimental demonstration, it is found that the suggested method is able to quantify variations of RBC aggregation under continuous ESR. In other words, EAI is more effective when compared with AI. Furthermore, the method provides multiple data of RBC aggregation and ESR through a single experiment. The rheological property varied continuously, and thus it is very effective at obtaining several data points without repetitive tests. Compared with the previous methods, this proposed method had some merits including fabrication, multiple channels, and quantitative comparison of ESR value. First, the use of a liner cut from an adhesive sheet to form the master mold was newly suggested to simplify the fabrication process, compared to MEMS fabrication. Since RBC aggregation is quantified under stasis blood flows or lower shear rates, it is not imperative that each microfluidic channel should have uniform sizes for consistent blood flows. Thus, this method can remove MEMS fabrications, which require high cost and technical expertise. Second, when RBC aggregation varied over time, the repetitive test caused to increase scattering of aggregation index largely. Thus, multiple measurement of RBC aggregation was required to avoid large scattering due to repetitive test conducted for long time. At last, ESR relationship between modified conventional method and proposed method was obtained by conducting regression analysis technique. As a result, the EAI obtained by the proposed method gave comparable value of ESR, compared with the modified conventional ESR method.

4. Conclusions

In this study, a simple measurement technique of RBC aggregation under continuous ESR was demonstrated by sucking blood from a conical pipette tip into parallel microfluidic channels and quantifying image intensity, especially throughout single experiment. Two indices (AI and EAI) were suggested to quantify variations of RBC aggregation due to ESR in the conical pipette tip. First, when clamping the fluidic tube with the pinch valve, blood flow in each microfluidic channel was stopped shortly within 0.2 s. RBCs aggregation was measured immediately after clamping the tube with a pinch valve (i.e., close mode). Additionally, the compliance effect of the fluidic system had a negligible effect on transient blood flows. In addition, AI and EAI remained constant without respect to flow rate (Q) (Q = 0.5 mL/h, 1 mL/h, and 2 mL/h). From this result, RBC aggregation and ESR were measured immediately by clamping the tube with a pinch valve, at the constant flow rate of 2 mL/h. Second, the proposed method was applied to measure the effect of hematocrit on the RBC aggregation under continuous ESR. AI remained over time with respect to hematocrit. However, EAI showed a significant difference with respect to hematocrit and measurement time. Compared with AI, EAI was more effective for evaluating continuous ESR in the conical pipette. After that, to quantify the relationship between the proposed method (i.e., EAI) and the modified conventional ESR method (i.e., H) with respect to hematocrit level, time constants (λ_{EAI}, λ_H) were obtained by conducting regression analysis with simple regression formula [i.e., EAI = a_1 + a_2 exp ($-t/\lambda_{EAI}$), H = b_1 + b_2 exp ($-t/\lambda_H$)]. For two time constants (λ_{EAI}, λ_H) with respect to hematocrit, linear regression analysis indicated that the coefficient of R^2 showed a sufficient high value of R^2 = 0.9521. Thus, EAI can be effectively employed to measure ESR in the reservoir, compared with a modified conventional ESR method. The proposed method was finally applied to evaluate RBC aggregation (AI) and ESR (EAI) for homogeneous aggregated RBCs. As a result, EAI and AI were gradually increased by varying concentration of dextran solution ranging from $C_{dextran}$ = 5 mg/mL to $C_{dextran}$ = 20 mg/mL. To evaluate the relationship between the proposed method and a modified conventional ESR method, EAI and λ_H were obtained at specific concentrations of dextran solution. Since regression analysis showed higher value of R^2 = 0.8789, the EAI obtained by the proposed method gave comparable value of ESR, compared with the modified conventional ESR method. These experimental demonstrations indicated that the proposed method simultaneously measures RBC aggregation and ESR by using two indices (AI and EAI). Moreover, the method provides multiple data of RBC aggregation and ESR through a single experiment. Future tests will involve employing the proposed method to evaluate biophysical properties of bloods collected from cardiovascular diseases.

Figure S1: Microscopic images for showing a microfluidic device with parallel microfluidic channel (n) [(a) n = 1, (b) n = 2, (c) n = 3, and (d) n = 4].

Author Contributions: Y.J.K. proposed this proposed method. Y.J.K and B.J.K. prepared the master mold with adhesive sheet. Y.J.K. devised all the experimental procedures including the microfluidic device and carried out experiments. Y.J.K. wrote the manuscript.

References

1. Lanotte, L.; Mauer, J.; Mendez, S.; Fedosov, D.A.; Fromental, J.-M.; Claveria, V.; Nicoud, F.; Gompper, G.; Abkarian, M. Red cells' dynamic morphologies govern blood shear thinning under microcirculatory flow conditions. *Proc. Natl. Acad. Sci. USA* **2016**, *113*, 13289–13294. [CrossRef] [PubMed]

2. Baskurt, O.K.; Meiselman, H.J. Time course of electrical impedance during red blood cell aggregation in a glass tube: Comparison with light transmittance. *IEEE Trans. Biomed. Eng.* **2010**, *57*, 969–978. [CrossRef] [PubMed]

3. Isiksacan, Z.; Erel, O.; Elbuken, C. A portable microfluidic system for rapid measurement of the erythrocyte sedimentation rate. *Lab Chip* **2016**, *16*, 4682–4690. [CrossRef] [PubMed]

4. Popel, A.S.; Johnson, P.C. Microcirculation and hemorheology. *Annu. Rev. Fluid Mech.* **2005**, *37*, 43–69. [CrossRef] [PubMed]

5. Bishop, J.J.; Popel, A.S.; Intaglietta, M.; Johnson, P.C. Rheological effects of red blood cell aggregation in the venous network: A review of recent studies. *Biorheology* **2001**, *38*, 263–274. [PubMed]

6. Yayan, J. Erythrocyte sedimentation rate as a marker for coronary heart disease. *Vasc. Health Risk Manag.* **2012**, *8*, 219–223. [CrossRef] [PubMed]

7. Bochen, K.; Krasowska, A.; Milaniuk, S.; Kulczyńska, M.; Prystupa, A.; Dzida, G. Erythrocyte sedimentation rate-an old marker with new applications. *JPCCR* **2011**, *5*, 50–55.

8. Piva, E.; Pajola, R.; Temporin, V.; Plebani, M. A new turbidimetric standard to improve the quality assurance of the erythrocyte sedimentation rate measurement. *Clin. Biochem.* **2007**, *40*, 491–495. [CrossRef] [PubMed]

9. Larsson, A.; Hansson, L.-O. Inflammatory activity: Capillary electrophoresis provides more information than erythrocyte sedimentation rate. *Upsala J. Med. Sci.* **2005**, *110*, 151–158. [CrossRef] [PubMed]

10. Fabry, T.L. Mechanism of erythrocyte aggregation and sedimentation. *Blood* **1987**, *70*, 1572–1576. [PubMed]

11. Cha, C.-H.; Park, C.-J.; Cha, Y.J.; Kim, H.K.; Kim, D.H.; Bae, J.H.; Jung, J.-S.; Jang, S.; Chi, H.-S.; Lee, D.S.; et al. Erythrocyte sedimentation rate measurements by test 1 better reflect inflammation than do those by the Westergren method in patients with malignancy, autoimmune disease, or infection. *Am. J. Clin. Pathol.* **2009**, *131*, 189–194. [CrossRef] [PubMed]

12. Plebani, M.; Toni, S.D.; Sanzari, M.C.; Bernardi, D.; Stockreiter, E. A New method for mMeasuring the erythrocyte sedimentation rate. *Am. J. Clin. Pathol.* **1998**, *110*, 334–340. [CrossRef] [PubMed]

13. Kaliviotis, E.; Sherwood, M.; Balabani, S. Partitioning of red blood cell aggregates in bifurcating microscale flows. *Sci. Rep.* **2017**, *7*, 44563. [CrossRef] [PubMed]

14. Kang, Y.J. Continuous and simultaneous measurement of the biophysical properties of blood in a microfluidic environment. *Analyst* **2016**, *141*, 6583–6597. [CrossRef] [PubMed]

15. Kang, Y.J.; Ha, Y.-R.; Lee, S.-J. Microfluidic-based measurement of erythrocyte sedimentation rate for biophysical assessment of blood in an in vivo malaria-infected mouse. *Biomicrofluidics* **2014**, *8*, 044114. [CrossRef] [PubMed]

16. Shin, S.; Hou, J.X.; Suh, J.-S. Measurement of cell aggregation characteristics by analysis of laser-backscattering in a microfluidic rheometry. *Korea-Aust. Rheol. J.* **2007**, *19*, 61–66.

17. Yeom, E.; Lee, S.J. Microfluidic-based speckle analysis for sensitive measurement of erythrocyte aggregation: A comparison of four methods for detection of elevated erythrocyte aggregation in diabetic rat blood. *Biomicrofluidics* **2015**, *9*, 024110. [CrossRef] [PubMed]

18. Zhbanov, A.; Yang, S. Effects of aggregation on blood sedimentation and conductivity. *PLoS ONE* **2015**, *10*, e0129337. [CrossRef] [PubMed]

19. Kang, Y.J. Microfluidic-based measurement method of red blood cell aggregation under hematocrit variations. *Sensors* **2017**, *17*, 2037. [CrossRef] [PubMed]

20. Uyuklu, M.; Cengiz, M.; Ulker, P.; Hever, T.; Tripette, J.; Connes, P.; Nemeth, N.; Meiselman, H.J.; Baskurt, O.K. Effects of storage duration and temperature of human blood on red cell deformability and aggregation. *Clin. Hemorheol. Microcirc.* **2009**, *41*, 269–278. [PubMed]

21. Lim, H.-J.; Nam, J.-H.; Lee, B.-K.; Suh, J.-S.; Shin, S. Alteration of red blood cell aggregation during blood storage. *Korea-Aust. Rheol. J.* **2011**, *23*, 67–70. [CrossRef]

22. Berezina, T.L.; Zaets, S.B.; Morgan, C.; Spillert, C.R.; Kamiyama, M.; Spolarics, Z.; Deitch, E.A.; Machiedo, G.W. Influence of storage on red blood cell rheological properties. *J. Surg. Res.* **2002**, *102*, 6–12. [CrossRef] [PubMed]

23. Bartholomeusz, D.A.; Boutté, R.; Andrade, J.D. Xurography: Rapid prototyping of microstructures using a cutting plotter. *J. Microelectromech. Syst.* **2005**, *14*, 1364–1374. [CrossRef]

24. Faustino, V.; Catarino, S.O.; Lima, R.; Minas, G. Biomedical microfluidic devices by using low-cost fabrication techniques: A review. *J. Biomech.* **2016**, *49*, 2280–2292. [CrossRef] [PubMed]

25. Pinto, E.; Faustino, V.; Rodrigues, R.O.; Pinho, D.; Garcia, V.; Miranda, J.M.; Lima, R. A rapid and low-cost nonlithographic method to fabricate biomedical microdevices for blood flow analysis. *Micromachines* **2015**, *6*, 121–135. [CrossRef]

26. Islam, M.; Natu, R.; Martinez-Duarte, R. A study on the limits and advantages of using a desktop cutter plotter to fabricate microfluidic networks. *Microfluid. Nanofluid.* **2015**, *19*, 973–985. [CrossRef]

27. Bento, D.; Sousa, L.; Yaginuma, T.; Garcia, V.; Lima, R.; Miranda, J.M. Microbubble moving in blood flow in microchannels: Effect on the cell-free layer and cell local concentration. *Biomed. Microdevices* **2017**, *19*, 6. [CrossRef] [PubMed]

28. Yeom, E.; Kim, H.M.; Park, J.H.; Choi, W.; Doh, J.; Lee, S.J. Microfluidic system for monitoring temporal variations of hemorheological properties and platelet adhesion in LPS-injected rats. *Sci. Rep.* **2017**, *7*, 1801. [CrossRef] [PubMed]

13

Assessment of the Deformability and Velocity of Healthy and Artificially Impaired Red Blood Cells in Narrow Polydimethylsiloxane (PDMS) Microchannels

Liliana Vilas Boas [1,2], **Vera Faustino** [1,3], **Rui Lima** [3,4], **João Mário Miranda** [4], **Graça Minas** [1], **Carla Sofia Veiga Fernandes** [2] **and Susana Oliveira Catarino** [1,*]

[1]   Microelectromechanical Systems Research Unit (CMEMS-UMinho), University of Minho, 4800-058 Guimarães, Portugal; liliana.sv.boas@gmail.com (L.V.B.); id5778@alunos.uminho.pt (V.F.); gminas@dei.uminho.pt (G.M.)

[2]   Instituto Politécnico de Bragança, ESTiG, C. Sta. Apolónia, 5300-253 Bragança, Portugal; cveiga@ipb.pt

[3]   MEtRICs, DEM, University of Minho, 4800-058 Guimarães, Portugal; rl@dem.uminho.pt

[4]   CEFT, University of Porto, 4000-008 Porto, Portugal; jmiranda@fe.up.pt

*   Correspondence: scatarino@dei.uminho.pt

Abstract: Malaria is one of the leading causes of death in underdeveloped regions. Thus, the development of rapid, efficient, and competitive diagnostic techniques is essential. This work reports a study of the deformability and velocity assessment of healthy and artificially impaired red blood cells (RBCs), with the purpose of potentially mimicking malaria effects, in narrow polydimethylsiloxane microchannels. To obtain impaired RBCs, their properties were modified by adding, to the RBCs, different concentrations of glucose, glutaraldehyde, or diamide, in order to increase the cells' rigidity. The effects of the RBCs' artificial stiffening were evaluated by combining image analysis techniques with microchannels with a contraction width of 8 μm, making it possible to measure the cells' deformability and velocity of both healthy and modified RBCs. The results showed that healthy RBCs naturally deform when they cross the contractions and rapidly recover their original shape. In contrast, for the modified samples with high concentration of chemicals, the same did not occur. Additionally, for all the tested modification methods, the results have shown a decrease in the RBCs' deformability and velocity as the cells' rigidity increases, when compared to the behavior of healthy RBCs samples. These results show the ability of the image analysis tools combined with microchannel contractions to obtain crucial information on the pathological blood phenomena in microcirculation. Particularly, it was possible to measure the deformability of the RBCs and their velocity, resulting in a velocity/deformability relation in the microchannel. This correlation shows great potential to relate the RBCs' behavior with the various stages of malaria, helping to establish the development of new diagnostic systems towards point-of-care devices.

Keywords: biomicrofluidics; red blood cells; deformability; velocity

1. Introduction

Malaria is a parasitic disease with more than half the world population at risk and around 500 thousand deaths per year, with 80% of infections occurring in children under 5 years old [1]. This disease is mainly widespread in underdeveloped regions, with lack of proper infrastructure and living conditions, worsening the chances of infection for the population. The control, effective treatment, and elimination of malaria require an early and accurate diagnosis. Currently, the malaria diagnosis is based on blood smear microscopy or rapid diagnostic tests (RDTs) [2,3], which have limitations in the detection limit (only detect above 50 parasites/µL of blood). Additionally, microscopy has limitations in the required time to perform the assays and in the need for specialized technicians and/or laboratories, compromising the reduction of global incidence. To fulfill these needs, innovative diagnosis based on molecular assays have been developed, with detection limits below 2 parasites/µL, particularly using loop-mediated isothermal amplification [4] or more advanced portable devices such as QuantuMDx/Q-POC [5]. However, these techniques require disposable reagents, technicians, more than 30 min to get the test results, and imply aseptic conditions (hard to maintain in endemic regions). Therefore, there is a huge need for fast, reagent-free, and low-cost malaria diagnostic systems, without requiring special training and independent of the genetic variability of the parasite, and overall the final ideal device should comprise all these concerns.

The malaria parasite lifecycle passes from the mosquito vector to the human host by entering the liver cells where it matures, to further being released into the blood stream, invading the red blood cells (RBCs). At this stage, the infected RBCs (iRBCs) suffer biochemical, optical, and morphological changes [6,7], making these cells more rigid and thicker, resulting in a decrease of the cells velocity (when the cells are infected with *Plasmodium falciparum* parasite) [8]. Hemodynamic studies help to obtain information regarding the evolution of the disease. Particularly, the RBCs' deformability and the RBCs' velocity when crossing a geometric contraction can work as relevant markers for malaria diagnostics applications, since they are directly related to the changes that the parasite causes throughout the evolution of the disease [9]. The literature reports different methods for assessment of the RBCs' deformability, including filtration [10], ektacytometry [11,12], optical tweezers [13,14], micropipette aspiration [15], and microfluidic geometrical constrictions [16–22]. Some numerical and experimental studies in the literature already report the relation between RBCs' deformability and hemodynamics [23,24], or between deformability and the individual RBCs' velocities in specific geometrical conditions [9,25–28]. This work will be focused on a microfluidic system to measure the RBCs' deformability and velocity, as well as to establish a relation between these properties when the cells cross geometric microcontractions, with the expectation to, in the future, compare this correlation with the real malaria effects in RBCs. The microfluidic systems are a potential alternative to the current diagnostic methods, since they are able to mimic the hemodynamic phenomena that happens in blood vessels and have advantages in terms of sample preparation and analysis (low volume of samples, easy handling, low-cost, and fast processing), eliminating the need for specialized personnel [22]. Additionally, microfluidic devices enhance the possibility of creating a fully automated and portable diagnostic device for malaria, when assembled in a microfluidic platform that includes microfluidic handling, control and readout electronics, and data acquisition.

In order to develop and evaluate those microfluidic methods for the deformability and velocity assessment, it is essential to synthetically impair the RBCs for mimicking malaria behavior, for testing the method's efficiency and reproducibility, without the constant need for parasites or infected samples, improving laboratorial safety, when testing, and decreasing the costs. For that purpose, glutaraldehyde, diamide, and glucose will be used for increasing the rigidity of the RBCs and, their effect in narrow constrictions will be compared [29–32]. When exposed to these chemicals, the RBCs will be rigidified and their dynamic behavior in narrow constrictions, relative to deformability and velocity, will be compared to healthy RBCs. The evaluation of the RBCs' velocity and deformability will be performed in a set of microchannels with abrupt constrictions, followed by abrupt expansions [25]. This approach takes advantage of the potential of these sudden geometrical contractions to deform the cells due to shear and extensional flows. The cells' behavior will be captured by a setup comprising a high-speed camera and a microscope, and the obtained images will be processed in two software tools (ImageJ and PIVLab) for determining both the RBCs' deformability and the RBCs' velocities, as well as determining the relationship between those properties.

2. Materials and Methods

This section presents the materials and samples used to perform the experimental assays, as well as the description of the microchannel fabrication method, experimental setup, and image processing techniques. In brief, RBC samples with low concentration (low hematocrit) will be exposed to glutaraldehyde, diamide, or glucose and will be tested in polydimethylsiloxane (PDMS) microchannels that comprise 8 μm widths abrupt contractions. The ability of the RBCs to flow through the microchannels contractions will be assessed.

2.1. Microchannels Fabrication

A polydimethylsiloxane (PDMS) microfluidic device was microfabricated by soft lithography techniques, using SU-8 molds (SU-8 purchased from Microchem Corporation, Westborough, MA, USA) [33,34]. PDMS (Sylgard 184 Silicone Elastomer kit obtained from Dow Corning, Midland, MI, USA) was chosen due to its transparency that is required for microscope visualization, easy fabrication, and low-cost for prototypes. The PDMS microchannels have a 25 μm height in order to reduce the flow volume and the number of RBCs within the microchannels, also making it easier to observe the RBCs. Each microchannel is composed by a linear transition zone followed by an abrupt contraction (at a 90° angle) with 8 μm width and 780 μm length (seen in Figure 1), designed to force the RBCs to deform and gain velocity when crossing it. The width of the contractions mimics capillary vessels with the same average dimensions of the RBCs (around 8 μm).

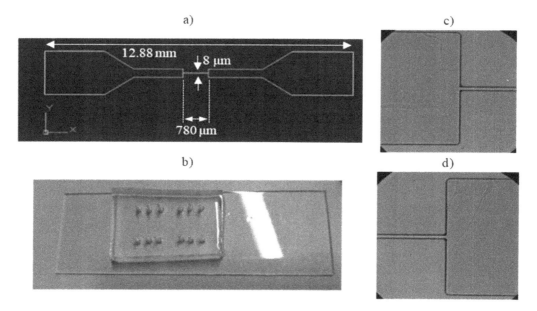

Figure 1. (a) 2D masks for microchannel fabrication. The narrow contractions in the central region of the microchannels have 8 μm width; **(b)** polydimethylsiloxane (PDMS) microchannels with a 12.8 mm total length; **(c)** Detail of the entrance of the 8 μm width contraction of the PDMS microchannel; **(d)** Detail of the outlet of the 8 μm width contraction of the PDMS microchannel. Magnification: 40×.

2.2. Samples

For the in vitro assays, samples containing human RBCs (hematocrit = 0.5%) in Dextran40 (Dx40) were used. Human RBCs have a biconcave shape and typical diameters in the 6–8 μm range, being highly deformable.

The healthy human whole blood samples were taken from a female volunteer and provided by Instituto Politécnico de Bragança (Bragança, Portugal). All procedures for the blood collection, transport, and in vitro experiments were carried out in compliance with the EU directives 2004/23/CE, 2006/17/CE, and 2006/86/CE and approved by the Unidade Local de Saúde do Nordeste (Bragança,

Portugal). In order to evaluate the RBCs' deformability and velocity in the microchannels, the RBCs were separated from the other blood constituents through centrifugation (15 min, 2000 rpm, at room temperature). After that, RBCs were re-suspended and washed twice in a physiological solution (PSS) (from B. Braun Medical, Melsungen, Germany) with a NaCl concentration of 0.9%. The Dx40 solution, where the RBCs were suspended, was used as a plasma-volume expander to prevent RBC sedimentation and maintain the ideal osmotic physiological conditions for the RBCs. This solution was synthetically produced by mixing 68 μL of $CaCl_2$ with 201 μL of KC, 7.35 mL of NaCl, and 5 g of Dx40 (for 1 M solution) (all reagents purchased from Sigma-Aldrich, St. Louis, MO, USA). The 0.5% hematocrit, representing a 0.5% volume of RBCs in 5 mL of Dx40, was considered in order to assure that the RBCs are isolated when crossing the microchannel contraction. Although the 0.5% hematocrit is significantly lower than the physiological one, it was decided to study diluted samples, to improve the visualizations and measurements of each individual RBC and, as a result, to avoid effects such as interactions and aggregation of RBCs. Preliminary tests performed with hematocrit values ranging from 0.5% up to 2% have shown that as the concentration of RBCs was increased, it was difficult to individually follow the RBCs and, consequently, to measure the RBCs' velocity and deformation index. Hence, the current study was performed with a hematocrit of 0.5%.

The RBC samples were then modified with glucose (COPAN Diagnostics Inc., Murrieta, CA, USA), glutaraldehyde (Sigma-Aldrich Corporation, St. Louis, MO, USA), and diamide (Sigma-Aldrich Corporation, St. Louis, MO, USA) solutions, in order to rigidify the cells at different levels. These chemicals were selected since they are commonly used to perform deformability studies, are accessible, and have simple preparation protocols, as well as they allow one to rigidify the cells at different levels, according to the added concentration. To modify the RBCs with glucose, four different concentrations of glucose were considered: 2%, 5%, 10%, and 20% (v/v). First, glucose (powder) was diluted in a phosphate buffered saline solution (PBS: pH 7.4). Then, the RBCs (already separated from the other blood constituents and suspended in Dx40) were incubated for 20 min, at room temperature, at each of the referred glucose concentrations. The cells were then washed in PSS to remove the excess of glucose from the samples and re-suspended in Dx40. To modify the cells with glutaraldehyde, at 0.00625%, 0.0125%, 0.025%, and 0.08% glutaraldehyde concentrations (v/v), the RBCs (already separated from the other blood constituents and suspended in Dx40) were incubated for 10 min at each of the referred concentrations, washed in PSS, re-suspended in Dx40, and used right away. The RBCs were also modified with diamide, at 0.00625%, 0.0125%, 0.025%, 0.08%, 0.32%, and 1% diamide concentrations (v/v), using the same protocol: Incubation for 10 min at each of the referred concentrations, washing in PSS, and re-suspension in Dx40.

2.3. Experimental Setup

The cells' deformability and velocity assays were performed with an experimental setup comprising the microfluidic device placed on the stage of an inverted microscope (IX71; Olympus Corporation, Tokyo, Japan). A flow rate of 5 μL/min was controlled using a syringe pump system (KD Scientific Inc., Holliston, MA, USA). For selecting the ideal flow rate, preliminarily studies were performed for four different flow rates (0.1, 1, 3, and 5 μL/min) and no significant differences were observed in the cells' deformability. Additionally, it was observed that the syringe pump system presented more stability for the highest tested flow rate, i.e., the 5 μL/min. The images of the RBCs were captured using a high-speed camera (Fastcam SA3, Photron, Motion Engineering Company, Westfield, IN, USA) at a 2000 frames/s rate and exported to a computer to be analyzed. Each assay was repeated 3 times.

2.4. Image Processing and Analysis Techniques

The images exported from the high-speed camera to the computer were analyzed using two software tools: ImageJ [35] and PIVLab [36,37]. For each assay, a sequence of 10,000 frames was considered. ImageJ was used to perform the pre-treatment of the acquired frames, in order to remove the noise and image artifacts, as well as convert them into binary images. Initially, the image sequence was imported and the crop function was executed to define the region of interest (ROI) as a rectangle with 308 µm × 332 µm dimension (Figure 2a). Then, by using the Z-Project function, the selected frames were stacked to determine an average of the frames. This averaged frame was subtracted from all the frames under analysis, eliminating all static objects, which resulted in frames comprising only the visible RBCs, without any additional information. Finally, by using a threshold function, the images were converted into binary images. The ImageJ software was also used to measure the cells size in order to calculate the RBCs' deformation index (DI). Using the ROI Manager and the Measure functions, it was possible to follow both the healthy and the impaired RBCs (example in Figure 2b) and calculate their DI along the microchannel, using the expression: $DI = (X - Y)/(X + Y)$, where X and Y represent the largest (X) and the smallest (Y) axis of the ellipse correspondent to the RBC under analysis. Typically, the RBCs' DI varies between 0 and 0.8, where 0 represents non-deformed cells and 0.8 represents cells at maximum elongation. For each assay, a group of RBCs was followed at the entrance and at the outlet of the contraction to measure their DI and determine an averaged value. Figure 2c presents the area at the entrance and at the outlet of the microchannel contraction (the areas inside the dashed lines in Figure 2c), where the deformability of the RBCs is measured. These areas were chosen after performing preliminary observations of the RBC flows. For the entrance of the contraction, a 121 µm × 237 µm region of interest was selected, since it is in this area that the RBCs experience the highest extensional flow and consequently start to deform to enter the narrowing. For the outlet, in the region immediately after exiting the contraction, the RBCs are at maximum deformation, and outside that region, the cells start to recover their original shape. Then, for assuring a standard area at the outlet for all assays, an 86 µm × 142 µm region of interest was selected. It should be noted that the evaluation area at the outlet of the contraction is significantly smaller than at the entrance. This difference is explained by the authors' intention, in future devices and prototypes, of integrating micro-sensors in the outlet of the contraction (occupying the smallest area possible) and, therefore, in this work it was expected to obtain relevant data from a small area of evaluation in the outlet.

In order to determine the average of the velocity values of the RBCs at the entrance and at the outlet of each contraction, the sequence of frames was analyzed using the PIVLab image analysis toolbox, integrated in MATLAB. First, the pre-treated images were imported into the software and calibrated (relatively to their dimensions and time between frames), and a ROI mask was applied to remove the areas where there are no RBCs. Following, the motion of the particles between the frames was analyzed and the instantaneous velocities were calculated by the variation of the distance traveled by the RBCs between each time step. Then, the average velocity vectors (U_x and U_y) were calculated in the x and y directions and the velocity field of each sample (U_{xy}) was determined based on the equation: $|U_{xy}| = \text{sqrt}\,(U_x^2 + U_y^2)$. Finally, a filter was applied to smooth the images and remove the high frequencies, which could indicate spikes of velocity without physical significance. Figure 2d presents an example of the velocity field distribution at the entrance of the contraction. It is possible to observe that the velocity of the RBCs is significantly higher in the zone of the narrowing entrance, reasoning that the abrupt transition causes an increase of the velocity of the RBCs. Note that, due to limitations of the available equipment, it was not possible to acquire frames with RBCs moving at high velocity in the interior of the microchannel contraction. As a result, almost no cells were registered in that region, explaining the 0 velocity in the interior of the contraction in the PIVLab image (Figure 2d), this way the results section will approach and compare the DI and velocity of the RBCs at the entrance and outlet of the contractions, neglecting the study of cells inside the contraction regions. Note that both RBC deformability and velocity are measured in the same area (as defined in Figure 2c, left and right) in order to establish a relation between the RBCs' deformability and their velocity. After obtaining the velocity distribution immediately before the entrance and after the outlet of the contraction, a criterion for determining the RBCs' velocity was defined (as presented in the Results Section 3): From the region of interest (Figure 2c, left and right), where the velocities are higher, the 100 pixels with highest velocity (obtained in PIVLab) were selected and those velocities were averaged, neglecting the surrounding areas with lowest velocities.

Additional details on the ImageJ and PIVLab procedures for the determination of RBC deformability and velocity can be found in [25].

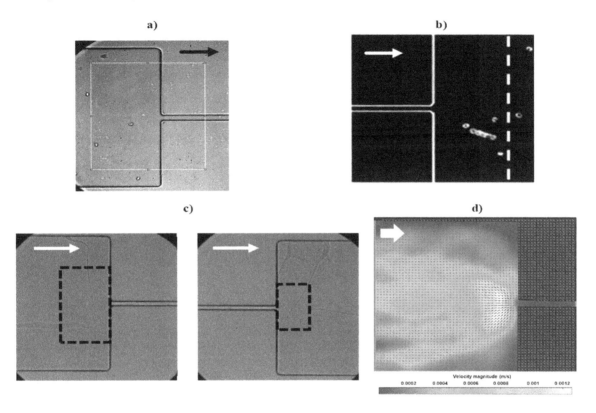

Figure 2. (**a**) Example of a cut-off of a transfer zone (308 μm × 332 μm) in the entrance of the microchannel contraction, using the crop function of ImageJ; (**b**) Example of a tracked red blood cell (RBC) at the outlet of the microchannel contraction, using ImageJ, where the dashed line represents a region where the RBCs expand after the outlet (relaxation area); (**c**) Definition of the areas (inside the dashed lines) for measuring the RBCs' deformability and velocity at the entrance (left—121 μm × 237 μm region) and at the outlet (right—86 μm × 142 μm region) of the microchannel contraction (Magnification: 40×); (**d**) Example of the velocity distribution, obtained with PIVLab, of healthy RBCs (non-modified) at the entrance of the microchannel contraction (the arrows indicate the flow direction in each frame). Note that, due to limitations of the available equipment (frame rate acquisition), it was not possible to acquire frames with RBCs moving at high velocity in the interior of the microchannel contraction and, as a result, no cells were registered in that region, explaining the 0 velocity in the image.

3. Results and Discussion

This section presents the deformability and velocity results (obtained as in Section 2.4) of the comparison between healthy and chemically modified RBCs with glucose, glutaraldehyde, and diamide. All the presented results are an average of three assays. For each assay, a sequence of 10,000 frames was considered and around 10 RBCs were followed to measure their DI. Figure 3 shows examples of RBCs from different assays at the entrance and at the outlet of the contraction in the PDMS microchannel, for different percentages of glucose, considering a 5 μL/min flow rate, and for a healthy RBC sample (for control—0% glucose). From Figure 3a, it is possible to detect a difference between RBC deformability as the glucose percentage increases, i.e., the RBCs change from a deformed/stretched shape to a non-deformed shape, as the cells have more difficulties to deform and tend to keep their original shape.

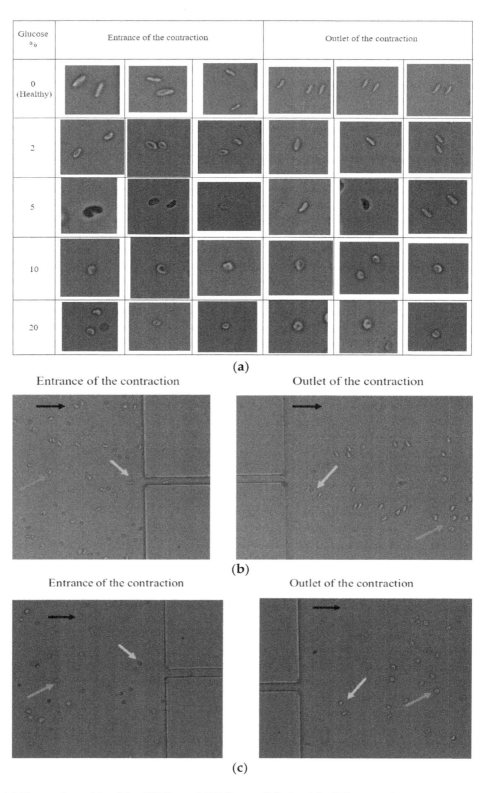

(a)

Entrance of the contraction   Outlet of the contraction

(b)

Entrance of the contraction   Outlet of the contraction

(c)

Figure 3. (**a**) Examples of healthy RBCs and RBCs modified with different glucose percentages at the entrance and at the outlet of the microchannel contraction, extracted from three assays; (**b**) Healthy RBCs (red arrow, left) deforming at the entrance of the contraction (green arrow, left), leaving the contraction still deformed (green arrow, right), and recovering their original shape following the outlet on an expansion area (red arrow, right); (**c**) 10% glucose-modified RBCs (red arrow, left) with almost no deformation at the entrance of the contraction (green arrow, left) and leaving the contraction (green arrow, right), recovering their original shape on an expansion area (red arrow, right). The black arrows indicate the flow direction.

These results suggest that the glucose concentration affects the RBCs' deformability, in agreement with several past studies regarding the influence of glucose over RBC deformability [31,32]. The increase of glucose (hyperglycemia) in RBCs causes damage in the RBCs' membranes and increases the blood viscosity, also increasing the cells' aggregation, which leads to a significant decrease on the RBCs' DI. When the RBCs were modified with glutaraldehyde or diamide, the results were similar to the ones observed for glucose (shown in Figure 3), and, therefore, only the glucose images are presented. Following the outlet of the microchannel contraction, the RBCs start to recover their shape, again decreasing their deformation index, as shown in Figure 3b,c, for an assay with healthy RBCs and one assay with 10% glucose-modified RBCs.

Figure 4 presents the DI for healthy and modified RBCs (with glucose, glutaraldehyde, and diamide), at the entrance and at the outlet of the microchannel 8 μm contraction, as well as at the relaxation area (see Figure 2b), for the 5 μL/min flow rate.

The results show that, as the percentage of glucose, glutaraldehyde, or diamide increases, the cells tend to become more rigid, decreasing their DI [29]. While the healthy cells deformed at the entrance of the contraction to pass throughout the contraction and then recovered their initial shape after reaching the microchannel expansion area, the modified RBCs did not deform and some aggregation of the cells was observed, increasing the difficulty to cross the contraction. At the outlet of the contraction, where the deformability was measured, the RBCs tend to start to recover their original shape, which is verified in Figure 4: The RBCs at the outlet have lower DI than at the entrance of the contraction. As the rigidity of the cells increases, the difference between the DI at entrance and at the outlet of the contraction decreases. Since the evaluation regions at entrance and at the outlet have a different total area (as defined in Figure 2c), it may also help to explain the hysteresis in the results between entrance and outlet (the entrance evaluation area is larger than the outlet evaluation area).

Table 1 presents the differences between the averaged RBC deformability at the entrance of the contraction and at the relaxation area, for all the tested conditions. This allows us to observe the cells' maximum deformability, passing from their deformed shape entering the contraction, until their recovered shape after relaxation. The results show that, as the rigidity of the cells increases, the difference in the deformability between the entrance and the relaxation area (ΔDI) decreases, and this behavior is similar for the three chemicals tested: Glucose, glutaraldehyde, and diamide.

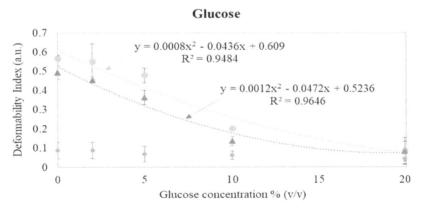

(a)

Figure 4. *Cont.*

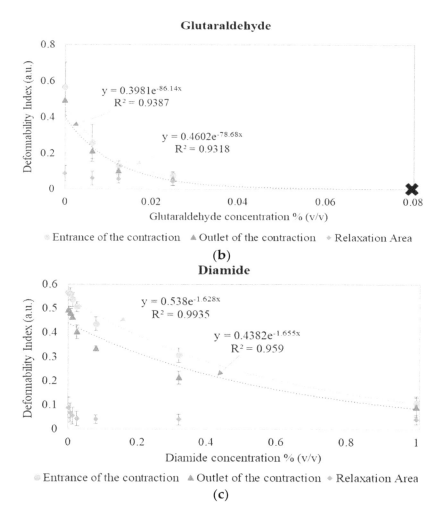

Figure 4. Deformation index (DI) and error bars for healthy and (**a**) glucose-, (**b**) glutaraldehyde-, and (**c**) diamide-modified RBCs, at the entrance (blue series), at the outlet (orange series) and at the relaxation area (green series) of the microchannel contraction and trend lines. In (b), the X represents the clogging of the microchannel, with no deformability or velocity data. Each point of the plots is the average of 30 RBCs (three assays for each condition and 10 RBCs followed in each assay).

Table 1. Difference of the deformation index (ΔDI) between red blood cell (RBC) deformability at the entrance of the contraction (Figure 2c, left) and at the relaxation area (Figure 2b) for all the tested conditions, obtained from the data presented in Figure 4.

Sample	Concentration (%)	ΔDI
Healthy RBCs	0	0.479
RBCs + Glucose	2	0.463
	5	0.410
	10	0.139
	20	0.041
RBCs + Glutaraldehyde	0.00625	0.196
	0.0125	0.074
	0.025	0.034
	0.08	X
RBCs + Diamide	0.00625	0.493
	0.0125	0.482
	0.025	0.464
	0.08	0.396
	0.32	0.267
	1	0.068

It was also observed that, for 0.08% (v/v) glutaraldehyde-modified RBCs, the rigidified cells clogged the entrance of the contraction and no deformability or velocity data could be extracted (this is represented by X in Figure 4b). Therefore, for a high concentration of glutaraldehyde, it was unable to measure the transiting velocity of the cells. Figure 5 presents an example of clogging at the entrance of the contraction, when the RBCs were modified with a 0.08% (v/v) concentration of glutaraldehyde.

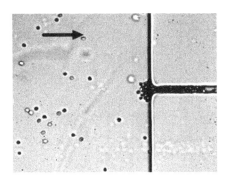

Figure 5. Detail of clogging at the entrance of the 8 μm contraction when the RBCs were modified with a 0.08% (v/v) concentration of glutaraldehyde.

Elevated blood glucose in the RBCs alters RBC membrane proteins through glycosylation and oxidation. Glutaraldehyde penetrates into cell membranes and non-specifically cross-links the cytosol, the cytoskeletal, and the transmembrane proteins, acting on all components of the cell and increasing the effective viscosity of the cytoplasm and lipid membrane. Diamide is a spectrin-specific cross-linker, oxidizing thiol groups while forming disulfide bonds within the structural region [30]. The obtained results indicate that viscous effects in the cytoplasm and/or lipid membrane are a dominant factor when dictating dynamic responses of RBCs in pressure-driven flows, explaining the higher effect of the glutaraldehyde in damaging the RBCs and the microchannel clogging, when compared to diamide and glucose [30].

Figure 6 presents the average cell velocity for healthy and modified RBCs (with glucose, glutaraldehyde, and diamide), at the entrance and at the outlet of the microchannel 8 μm contraction, for the 5 μL/min flow rate.

Overall, the results agree with those of deformability. When the average velocity at the high velocity regions was evaluated, it was found that the impaired RBCs (by adding glucose, glutaraldehyde, or diamide) presented lower velocities than healthy RBCs, indicating that the increase of the RBCs' rigidity causes the non-deformed cells to follow streamlines that on average have lower velocity, while the stretched and healthy RBCs follow streamlines that on average have higher velocity. Supplementary material videos show how the cells gain velocity when entering the contraction, explaining the higher velocity immediately at the outlet of the contraction (when compared to the velocity at the entrance), before starting to relax and recover their original shape. Similarly to the deformability results, for 0.08% (v/v) glutaraldehyde-modified RBCs, the rigidified cells clogged at the entrance of the contraction and, as a result, no velocity data could be extracted (this is represented by X in Figure 6b).

Additionally, it would be interesting to quantitatively study the relation between deformation index and velocity inside the microchannel contraction, besides the data presented at entrance and outlet (Figures 4 and 6). However, due to technical limitations of the high speed acquisition system, it was not possible to acquire an enough number of RBCs with high quality contrast to perform the measurements of RBC deformability and velocity with the software tools referred in Section 2. Despite that limitation, some RBCs could still be observed within the contraction. Examples of RBCs (healthy, with 0.025% diamide, and with 10% glucose) flowing within the contraction are shown in Figure 7.

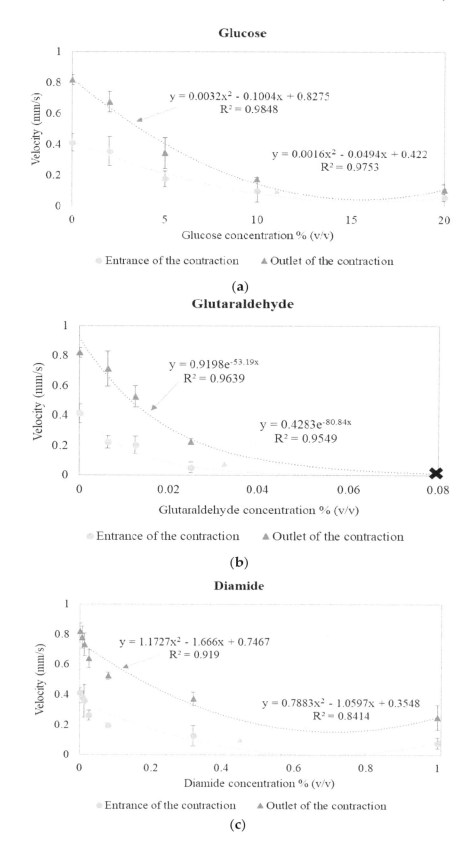

Figure 6. Velocity (mm/s) and error bars for healthy and (**a**) glucose-, (**b**) glutaraldehyde-, and (**c**) diamide-modified RBCs, at the entrance (blue series) and at the outlet (orange series) of the microchannel contraction and trend lines. In (b), the *X* represents the clogging of the microchannel, with no deformability or velocity data.

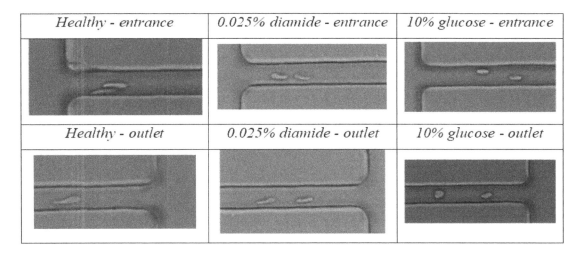

Figure 7. Examples of healthy RBCs, RBCs modified with 0.025% diamide, and RBCs modified with 10% glucose inside the 8 μm width microchannel contraction, at different areas (entrance and outlet of the contraction).

A qualitative analysis of the presented results shows that healthy RBCs cross the microchannel contraction in a more deformed shape than the 0.025% diamide and 10% glucose samples, and the 10% glucose samples are less deformable than the 0.025% diamide ones, which corroborates the quantitative results (before the entrance and after the outlet) presented in Figure 6. Supplementary material presents videos of healthy and modified RBCs flowing at the entrance and at the outlet of the contraction, allowing a better observation of the RBCs' behavior at the different regions of the microchannel contraction.

Since one of the main objectives of this work was to establish a relation between the RBCs' deformability and their velocity, Figure 8 presents the velocity vs DI calibration curves for glucose-, glutaraldehyde-, and diamide-modified RBCs at the entrance and at the outlet of the microchannel contraction. This figure purpose is to show the dispersion that occurs between the cells. Therefore, instead of presenting all RBCs averaged together (as in Figures 4 and 6), it is intended to evaluate how each small group of cells fits the deformability vs velocity curve, in order to understand their individualized behavior. Therefore, from the performed assays, the RBCs were gathered in groups of three cells measured under the same conditions and their average was calculated (each blue dot of the plots). Consequently, each plot of Figure 8 gathers data from a high number of RBCs (three RBCs × number of dots in each plot, leading to a range of RBCs between $3 \times 16 = 48$ in Figure 8d and $3 \times 28 = 84$ in Figure 8e), measured in the areas defined in Figure 2.

Based on the results, it is observed that, overall and as expected, for all synthetically modified RBCs, an increase of cell deformation index leads to an increase of the cells' velocity, both at the entrance and at the outlet of a microchannel contraction. When comparing the velocity with the deformability correlation at entrance and at outlet, it is clear, for all the tested methods, that the results at the outlet present a better fitting to the linear tendency curve than at the entrance (based on the R^2 values). Therefore, in the future, when advancing for a diagnostic tool, the analysis must be performed at the outlet of the contraction (the place to integrate a sensor), where the RBCs' behavior is more reliable. Additionally, our results indicate that diamide is the most interesting approach for mimicking the malaria effects on RBCs with the intention of exploring sensor applications, as the velocity vs DI results show a better fitting to the linear tendency curve ($R^2 = 0.89$) and, consequently, it is easier to control the velocity vs deformability curve. These results are a promising step to help the development of integrated sensors in microfluidic devices that allow the design of an autonomous malaria detection system of high sensitivity, precise, low-cost, portable, and with low energy consumption.

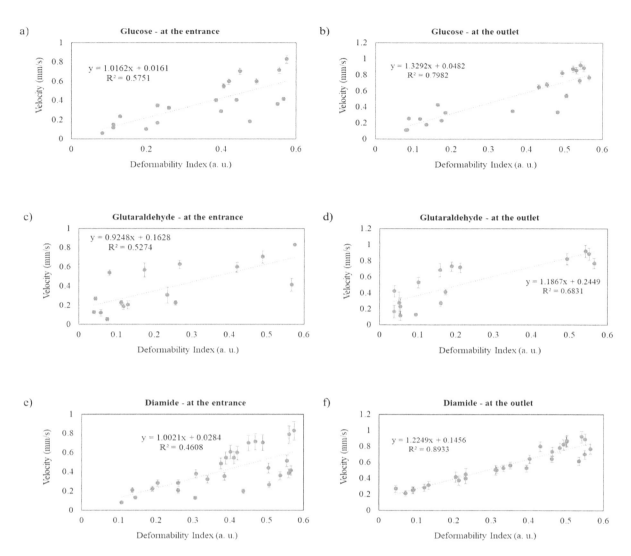

Figure 8. Velocity (mm/s) vs. deformability (a.u.) curve, measured at the entrance and at the outlet of the 8 μm contraction, for the RBC samples modified with (**a**) at entrance; glucose, (**b**) at outlet; glucose (**c**) at entrance; glutaraldehyde; (**d**) at outlet; glutaraldehyde, (**e**) at entrance; diamide, and (**f**) at outlet; diamide.

4. Future Perspectives

Future works will include an increase in cell quantity in order to define the average property of the entire cell population with higher accuracy, since the physical properties of individual RBCs within the same RBC population can vary significantly [38]. Additionally, since the ultimate goal is to develop a clinical tool, more blood samples from different donors will be assessed to increase the RBCs' variability and to include more independent data. It is also planned to improve our high speed video microsystem, allowing the capture of good enough quality images to quantitatively measure both velocity and deformability of the RBCs flowing across the microchannel contraction. This improvement will allow to develop an improved association between RBC deformability and transiting velocity through the narrow constrictions. Finally, after obtaining an improved correlation with synthetically modified samples, it is intended to test real parasite-affected RBC samples [39] to measure their deformability and velocity, compare disease and artificially impaired RBCs, establish target values, and fully validate the proposed approach. This improved correlation will be used to relate the RBCs' behavior according to the various stages of malaria and to develop integrated sensors in microfluidic devices for RBC velocity measurements.

5. Conclusions

This work has investigated the deformability and the velocity of healthy and chemically modified RBCs, attempting to mimic the effect of malaria in RBCs and to establish a relation between RBCs' velocity and deformability. The glucose, glutaraldehyde, and diamide effect in the RBCs was compared using PDMS microchannels with 8 μm narrow contractions that forced the RBCs to undergo deformation when they passed through them. It was concluded that, by adding glucose, glutaraldehyde, or diamide, the RBC membrane tends to become stiffer, decreasing the cell's deformability and, consequently, decreasing the cell shape recovery capacity. Additionally, when the RBCs' rigidity increased, the RBCs' velocity decreased.

When the relation between deformability and velocity was evaluated, it was concluded that, for all synthetically modified RBCs, an increase of the cells' deformation index led to an increase of the cells' velocity. It was also verified that diamide was the most interesting approach to impair the cells and mimic the malaria effects on RBCs, as the velocity vs deformation index results have showed the best fitting to the linear tendency curve and, consequently, it would be easier to control the deformability and velocity of the cells based on this method.

Despite still being a challenge, this work will be a valuable contribution to help establishing the development of simple, reagent-free, inexpensive, and accurate new malaria diagnostic systems towards point-of-care devices.

Video S1: 10% glucose RBCs at the entrance of the contraction, Video S2: 10% glucose RBCs at the outlet of the contraction, Video S3: Healthy RBCs at the entrance of the contraction, Video S4: Healthy RBCs at the outlet of the contraction.

Author Contributions: Conceptualization, R.L. and S.O.C.; Methodology, R.L. and S.O.C.; Validation, R.L., J.M.M., C.S.V.F. and G.M.; Investigation, L.V.B. and V.F.; Data Analysis, L.V.B. and V.F.; Writing-Original Draft Preparation, S.O.C.; Writing-Review & Editing, S.O.C., R.L., J.M.M., C.S.V.F. and G.M.; Supervision, C.S.V.F. and S.O.C.

Acknowledgments: The authors would like to thank Diana Pinho from the IP Bragança for providing the blood samples and for the support in the experimental tests.

References

1. WHO. *Malaria World Report*; World Health Organization: Geneva, Switzerland, 2016.
2. WHO. *Malaria Rapid Diagnostic Test Performance: Results of WHO Product Testing of Malaria RDTs*; World Health Organization: Geneva, Switzerland, 2017.
3. Wongsrichanalai, C.; Barcus, M.J.; Muth, S.; Sutamihardja, A.; Wernsdorfer, W.H. A review of malaria diagnostic tools: Microscopy and rapid diagnostic test (RDT). *Am. J. Trop. Med. Hyg.* **2007**, *77*, 119–127. [PubMed]
4. Lucchi, N.; Ljolje, D.; Silva-Flannery, L.; Udhayakumar, V. Use of malachite green-loop mediated isothermal amplification for detection of *Plasmodium* spp. parasites. *PLoS ONE* **2016**, *11*, e0151437. [CrossRef] [PubMed]
5. QuantuMDx. Available online: http://quantumdx.com/applications/malaria (accessed on 1 March 2018).
6. Saha, R.; Karmakar, S.; Roy, M. Computational investigation on the photoacoustics of malaria infected red blood cells. *PLoS ONE* **2012**, *7*, e51774. [CrossRef] [PubMed]
7. Diez-Silva, M.; Dao, M.; Han, J.; Lim, C.T.; Suresh, S. Shape and biomechanical characteristics of human red blood cells in health and disease. *MRS Bull.* **2010**, *35*, 382–388. [CrossRef] [PubMed]
8. Handayani, S.; Chiu, D.T.; Tjitra, E.; Kuo, J.S.; Lampah, D.; Kenangalem, E.; Russell, B. High deformability of *Plasmodium vivax*-infected red blood cells under microfluidic conditions. *J. Infectious Dis.* **2009**, *199*, 445–450. [CrossRef] [PubMed]
9. Shelby, J.P.; White, J.; Ganesan, K.; Rathod, P.K.; Chiu, D.T. A microfluidic model for single-cell capillary obstruction by *Plasmodium falciparum*-infected erythrocytes. *Proc. Natl. Acad. Sci. USA* **2003**, *100*, 14618–14622. [CrossRef] [PubMed]
10. How, T.V.; Black, R.; Hughes, P. Hemodynamics of vascular prostheses. In *Advances in Hemodynamics and Hemorheology*; How, T.V., Ed.; Elsevier: Amsterdam, The Netherlands, 1996; Volume 1, pp. 373–423.

11. Tomaiuolo, G. Biomechanical properties of red blood cells in health and disease towards microfluidics. *Biomicrofluidics* **2014**, *8*, 051501. [CrossRef] [PubMed]

12. Johnson, R.M. Ektacytometry of red blood cells. *Methods Enzymol.* **1989**, *173*, 35–54. [PubMed]

13. Lim, C.; Dao, M.; Suresh, S.; Sow, C.; Chew, K. Large deformation of living cells using laser traps. *Acta Mater.* **2004**, *52*, 1837–1845. [CrossRef]

14. Grier, D.G. A revolution in optical manipulation. *Nature* **2003**, *424*, 810–816. [CrossRef] [PubMed]

15. Hochmuth, R. Micropipette aspiration of living cells. *J. Biomech.* **2000**, *33*, 15–22. [CrossRef]

16. Rodrigues, R.O.; Pinho, D.; Faustino, V.; Lima, R. A simple microfluidic device for the deformability assessment of blood cells in a continuous flow. *Biomed. Microdevices* **2015**, *17*, 108. [CrossRef] [PubMed]

17. Zhao, R.; Antaki, J.F.; Naik, T.; Bachman, T.N.; Kameneva, M.V.; Wu, Z.J. Microscopic investigation of erythrocyte deformation dynamics. *Biorheology* **2006**, *43*, 747–765. [PubMed]

18. Yaginuma, T.; Oliveira, M.S.N.; Lima, R.; Ishikawa, T.; Yamaguchi, T. Human red blood cell behavior under homogeneous extensional flow in a hyperbolic shaped microchannel. *Biomicrofluidics* **2013**, *7*, 054110. [CrossRef] [PubMed]

19. Faustino, V.; Pinho, D.; Yaginuma, T.; Calhelha, R.C.; Ferreira, I.C.; Lima, R. Extensional flow-based microfluidic device: Deformability assessment of red blood cells in contact with tumor cells. *BioChip J.* **2014**, *8*, 42–47. [CrossRef]

20. Lee, S.S.; Yim, Y.; Ahn, K.H.; Lee, S.J. Extensional flow-based assessment of red blood cell deformability using hyperbolic converging microchannel. *Biomed. Microdevices* **2009**, *11*, 1021–1027. [CrossRef] [PubMed]

21. Bento, D.; Rodrigues, R.O.; Faustino, V.; Pinho, D.; Fernandes, C.S.; Pereira, A.I.; Garcia, V.; Miranda, J.M.; Lima, R. Deformation of red blood cells, air bubbles, and droplets in microfluidic devices: Flow visualizations and measurements. *Micromachines* **2018**, *9*, 151. [CrossRef]

22. Hou, H.; Hou, H.W.; Bhagat, A.A.S.; Chong, A.G.L.; Mao, P.; Tan, K.S.W.; Han, J.; Lim, C.T. Deformability based cell margination—A simple microfluidic design for malaria-infected erythrocyte separation. *Lab Chip* **2010**, *10*, 2605–2613. [CrossRef] [PubMed]

23. Passos, A.; Sherwood, J.; Agrawal, R.; Pavesio, C.; Balabani, S. The effect of RBC stiffness on microhaemodynamics. In Proceedings of the 5th Micro and Nano Flows Conference, Milan, Italy, 11–14 September 2016.

24. Chien, S. Red blood cell deformability and its relevance to blood flow. *Ann. Rev. Physiol.* **1987**, *49*, 177–192. [CrossRef] [PubMed]

25. Vilas Boas, L.; Lima, R.; Minas, G.; Fernandes, C.S.; Catarino, S.O. Imaging of healthy and malaria-mimicked red blood cells in polydimethylsiloxane microchannels for determination of cells deformability and flow velocity. In *VipIMAGE—ECCOMAS 2017. Lecture Notes in Comp. Vision and Biomechanics*; Tavares, J., Natal Jorge, R., Eds.; Springer: New York, NY, USA, 2018; pp. 915–922.

26. Kaneko, M.; Ishida, T.; Tsai, C.D.; Ito, H.; Chimura, M.; Taniguchi, T.; Ohtani, T.; Sakata, Y. On-Chip RBC Deformability Checker Embedded with Vision Analyzer. In Proceedings of the 2015 IEEE International Conference on Mechatronics and Automation, Takamatsu, Japan, 6–9 August 2017; pp. 2005–2010.

27. Tsai, C.D.; Tanaka, J.; Kaneko, M.; Horade, M.; Ito, H.; Taniguchi, T.; Ohtani, T.; Sakata, Y. An On-Chip RBC Deformability Checker Significantly Improves Velocity-Deformation Correlation. *Micromachines* **2016**, *7*, 176. [CrossRef]

28. Jeong, J.H.; Sugii, Y.; Minamiyama, M.; Okamoto, K. Measurement of RBC deformation and velocity in capillaries in vivo. *Microvasc. Res.* **2006**, *71*, 212–217. [CrossRef] [PubMed]

29. Rodrigues, R.O.; Faustino, V.; Pinto, E.; Pinho, D.; Lima, R. Red Blood Cells deformability index assessment in a hyperbolic microchannel: The diamide and glutaraldehyde effect. *Webmed Cent. Biomed. Eng.* **2013**, *4*, WMC004375.

30. Forsyth, A.M.; Wan, J.; Ristenpart, W.D.; Stone, H.A. The dynamic behavior of chemically "stiffened" red blood cells in microchannel flows. *Microvasc. Res.* **2010**, *80*, 37–43. [CrossRef] [PubMed]

31. Babu, N.; Singh, M. Influence of hyperglycemia on aggregation, deformability and shape parameters of erythrocytes. *Clin. Hemorheol. Microcirc.* **2004**, *31*, 273–280. [PubMed]

32. Shin, S.; Ku, Y.H.; Suh, J.S.; Singh, M. Rheological characteristics of erythrocytes incubated in glucose media. *Clin. Hemorheol. Microcirc.* **2008**, *38*, 153–161. [PubMed]

33. Pinto, V.C.; Sousa, P.J.; Cardoso, V.F.; Minas, G. Optimized SU-8 Processing for Low-Cost Microstructures Fabrication without Cleanroom Facilities. *Micromachines* **2014**, *5*, 738–755. [CrossRef]

34. Faustino, V.; Catarino, S.O.; Lima, R.; Minas, G. Biomedical microfluidic devices by using low-cost fabrication techniques: A review. *J. Biomech.* **2016**, *49*, 2280–2292. [CrossRef] [PubMed]

35. Abramoff, M.; Magalhães, P.; Ram, S. Image processing with ImageJ. *Biophotonics Int.* **2004**, *11*, 36–42.

36. Thielicke, W.; Stamhuis, E.J. PIVlab—Towards User-friendly, Affordable and Accurate Digital Particle Image Velocimetry in MATLAB. *J. Open Res. Softw.* **2014**, *2*, e30. [CrossRef]

37. Thielicke, W.; Stamhuis, E.J. PIVlab—Time-Resolved Digital Particle Image Velocimetry Tool for MATLAB. Available online: https://figshare.com/articles/PIVlab_version_1_35/1092508 (accessed on July 2017).

38. Picot, J.; Ndour, P.A.; Lefevre, S.D.; El Nemer, W.; Tawfik, H.; Galimand, J.; Costa, L.D.; Ribeil, J.-A.; Montalembert, M.d.; Brousse, V.; et al. A biomimetic microfluidic chip to study the circulation and mechanical retention of red blood cells in the spleen. *Am. J. Hematol.* **2015**, *90*, 339–345. [CrossRef] [PubMed]

39. Barber, B.E.; Russell, B.; Grigg, M.J.; Zhang, R.; William, T.; Amir, A.; Lau, Y.L.; Chatfield, M.D.; Dondorp, A.M.; Anstey, N.M.; et al. Reduced red blood cell deformability in *Plasmodium knowlesi malaria*. *Blood Adv.* **2018**, *2*, 433–443. [CrossRef] [PubMed]

14

Microfluidic-Based Biosensor for Blood Viscosity and Erythrocyte Sedimentation Rate Using Disposable Fluid Delivery System

Yang Jun Kang 🄾

Department of Mechanical Engineering, Chosun University, 309 Pilmun-daero, Dong-gu, Gwangju 61452, Korea; yjkang2011@chosun.ac.kr

Abstract: To quantify the variation of red blood cells (RBCs) or plasma proteins in blood samples effectively, it is necessary to measure blood viscosity and erythrocyte sedimentation rate (ESR) simultaneously. Conventional microfluidic measurement methods require two syringe pumps to control flow rates of both fluids. In this study, instead of two syringe pumps, two air-compressed syringes (ACSs) are newly adopted for delivering blood samples and reference fluid into a T-shaped microfluidic channel. Under fluid delivery with two ACS, the flow rate of each fluid is not specified over time. To obtain velocity fields of reference fluid consistently, RBCs suspended in 40% glycerin solution (hematocrit = 7%) as the reference fluid is newly selected for avoiding RBCs sedimentation in ACS. A calibration curve is obtained by evaluating the relationship between averaged velocity obtained with micro-particle image velocimetry (μPIV) and flow rate of a syringe pump with respect to blood samples and reference fluid. By installing the ACSs horizontally, ESR is obtained by monitoring the image intensity of the blood sample. The averaged velocities of the blood sample and reference fluid ($<U_B>$, $<U_R>$) and the interfacial location in both fluids (α_B) are obtained with μPIV and digital image processing, respectively. Blood viscosity is then measured by using a parallel co-flowing method with a correction factor. The ESR is quantified as two indices (t_{ESR}, I_{ESR}) from image intensity of blood sample ($<I_B>$) over time. As a demonstration, the proposed method is employed to quantify contributions of hematocrit (Hct = 30%, 40%, and 50%), base solution (1× phosphate-buffered saline [PBS], plasma, and dextran solution), and hardened RBCs to blood viscosity and ESR, respectively. Experimental Results of the present method were comparable with those of the previous method. In conclusion, the proposed method has the ability to measure blood viscosity and ESR consistently, under fluid delivery of two ACSs.

Keywords: blood viscosity; Erythrocyte sedimentation rate (ESR); T-shaped microfluidic channel; air-compressed syringe (ACS); micro-particle image velocimetry

1. Introduction

Microcirculation plays a substantial role in regulating blood flows and exchanging substances (gases, nutrients, and waste) between blood samples and peripheral tissues. Impaired microcirculation commonly leads to organ failures or mortality [1]. There is a need for comprehensive research that offers an insight that intrinsic properties and flow characteristics of blood samples share with microcirculatory disorders such as hypertension, sickle cell anemia, and diabetes [2]. The previous study has reported that biophysical properties of blood samples (hematocrit (Hct), viscosity, and erythrocyte sedimentation rate (ESR)) are strongly correlated with coronary heart diseases [3]. Thereafter, the biophysical properties of the blood sample have been studied extensively for the effective monitoring of circulatory disorders [4–9].

Under normal physiological conditions, red blood cells (RBCs) occupy 40–50% of blood volume. As RBCs are the most abundant cells in the blood sample, the biophysical properties of the blood sample are determined dominantly by properties of RBCs. The characteristics of RBCs, including morphology, membrane viscoelasticity, and RBCs count, are evaluated by quantifying several biophysical properties of blood samples, including viscoelasticity (or viscosity), deformability, and hematocrit. In that regard, plasma proteins in blood samples induce RBC aggregation, which occurs at an extremely low shear rate (i.e., $\dot{\gamma} = 1{\sim}10\ \mathrm{s}^{-1}$) [10] or stasis. Among the biophysical properties of blood samples, blood viscosity is determined by several factors, including hematocrit, plasma viscosity, RBCs deformability, and RBCs aggregation. Thus, their properties of blood samples are employed to monitor variations in the characteristics of blood samples. At lower shear rates, RBC aggregation causes to increase blood viscosity. At high shear rates, the deformation and alignment of RBCs lead to a decrease in blood viscosity. In other words, blood viscosity provides information on aggregation and deformability simultaneously. However, at extremely low shear rates, a syringe pump (SP) exhibits fluidic instability and RBC sedimentation continuously occurs. A microfluidics-based viscometer does not provide consistent values of blood viscosity. Conventionally, blood viscosity has been measured at sufficiently high shear rates (i.e., $\dot{\gamma} > 10\ \mathrm{s}^{-1}$ [11,12] or $\dot{\gamma} > 50{-}100\ \mathrm{s}^{-1}$ [13,14]), especially in microfluidic environments. For the reason, blood viscosity obtained with a microfluidic device does not give sufficient information on the contributions of plasma proteins to RBC aggregation. To evaluate variations in plasma proteins consistently, it is additionally necessary to quantify RBCs aggregation or ESR.

A microfluidic device has several advantages, including small volume consumption, fast measurement, easy sample handling, high sensitivity, and disposability. Thus, it has been widely used to measure various biophysical properties of blood samples (i.e., blood viscosity [15], RBCs aggregation [16], RBCs deformability [17,18], and hematocrit [19]).

The previous methods for measuring blood viscosity are conveniently divided into three categories (i.e., driving sources, devices, and quantification techniques). First, extrinsic driving sources such as SPs [20], pressure sources, and hand-held pipettes [13] have been suggested for delivering a blood sample into a specific device. Additionally, intrinsic driving sources such as capillary force (or surface tension) [21,22] and gravity force [23] have been applied to supply blood samples into a device. Second, various devices such as a microelectromechanical system (MEMS)-based microfluidic device, a 3D-printed microfluidic device [13,24], and a paper-based device [25] have been suggested for inducing blood flow in a specifically constrained direction. Third, quantification techniques such as advancing meniscus (i.e., variations of a blood column over time) [15,22,26,27], the falling time of a metal sphere in a tube [28], electric impedances (i.e., resistance, capacitance) [29,30], droplet length [31], digital flow compartment with a microfluidic channel array [11,12], interface detection in co-flowing streams [32,33], and reversal flow switching in a Wheatstone bridge analog of a fluidic circuit [14] have been suggested to measure blood viscosity.

To measure RBCs aggregation in microfluidic environments, a blood sample is placed into a microfluidic channel. By applying shear stress to the blood sample with external driving systems (i.e., an SP [34], pinch valve [16], or stirring motor [35]), the RBCs in the blood sample are aggregated or disaggregated, depending on the shear rate. Several quantification methods, such as light intensity (i.e., transmission, and back-scattering) [16], electrical conductivity [36,37], microscopic RBC images [38–40], ultrasonic images [41], and optical tweezers [42] have been suggested for obtaining temporal variations of RBCs aggregation. As another approach, RBC aggregation can be quantified by measuring the sedimentation distances of RBCs in a blood sample during a specific duration (i.e., ESR). Unlike the conventional Westergren ESR method, a microfluidic-based ESR measurement is quantified by measuring the conductivity of the blood sample in a PDMS chamber with a square cross-section (i.e., each side = 4 mm, depth = 5 mm) [43]. Owing to the continuous ESR in the driving syringe, RBC-free regions (or depleted regions) expand from the top layer with an elapse of time. The blood sample is supplied into a microfluidic device from the top layer of the driving syringe. To monitor blood flows in the microfluidic channel, microscopic images are sequentially captured with a high speed camera. Image intensity of each microscopic image is calculated over time by conducting digital image processing. The ESR is then evaluated by quantifying temporal variations of the image intensity [44].

To measure blood viscosity and RBC aggregation inexpensively, two SPs should be replaced with an inexpensive and disposable delivery system. To remove the syringe pump, single ACS is suggested to infuse the blood sample into a microfluidic device for measuring pressure and RBCs aggregation over continuously varying flow rates [45]. In this study, the ultimate goal of this study is to measure blood viscosity and RBC aggregation (or ESR), without two SPs.

In this study, a simple method for measuring blood viscosity and ESR is proposed. It involves the quantification of the interfacial location in a co-flowing channel and microscopic image intensity of blood sample flowing in a microfluidic device. Two air-compressed syringes (ACSs) are employed to simultaneously deliver the blood sample and reference fluid. Based on an ACS for delivering blood samples as suggested in previous studies [46,47], two ACSs are suggested to deliver blood samples and reference fluid simultaneously. Since the flow rates of both fluids are not specified under fluid delivery with the ACSs, it is necessary to quantify them with a time-resolved micro-particle image velocimetry (µ-PIV) technique. Based on a parallel co-flowing method with a correction factor [32], the blood viscosity is measured by monitoring the interfacial location in a co-flowing channel. Unlike the previous studies [46,47], two ACSs are installed horizontally to measure ESR effectively. Continuous sedimentation in the ACS causes an expansion of an RBC-free layer from the top layer. When blood samples are delivered to the blood channel from the ACS, the populations of RBCs (or hematocrit) are reduced over time. Since a continuous ESR contributes to increasing microscopic image intensity of blood flows, the ESR can be quantified by monitoring the image intensity of the blood sample.

When compared to previous methods that have the ability to measure blood viscosity under fluid delivery with syringe pumps, two syringe pumps are replaced by two ACSs as a novelty of this method. Here, a 40% glycerin solution is newly selected as the reference fluid. RBCs as fluid tracers are added into reference fluid. Velocity fields of both fluids are obtained consistently over time by conducting a time-resolved micro-PIV technique.

By installing the ACSs horizontally, the continuous ESR inside the ACS is filled with the blood sample causing it to expand RBC-free regions. As RBCs aggregation tends to increase substantially at lower hematocrit or lower velocity, it contributes to increasing the image intensity of blood samples. Thus, it is possible to evaluate the ESR by monitoring the microscopic image intensity of the blood sample.

2. Materials and Methods

2.1. Fabrication of Microfluidic Device and Experimental Procedure

A microfluidic device for measuring blood viscosity and ESR consisted of two inlets (a, b), one outlet (a), and a T-shaped channel (width = 250 µm, depth = 20 µm), as shown in Figure 1A-a. The T-shaped channel was composed of a blood channel, a reference channel, and a co-flowing channel. When analyzing the velocity fields of each fluid, the T-shaped channel does not require to align each microscopic image in the horizontal direction. Conventional micro-electromechanical-system techniques, such as photolithography and deep reactive ion etching (DRIE), were employed to fabricate 4-inch silicon mold. To peel off PDMS block from the master mold easily, plasma surface treatment was conducted after the DRIE process [48]. PDMS elastomer (Sylgard 184, Dow Corning, Midland, MI, USA) was mixed with a curing agent at a ratio of 10:1. After positioning the mold on a petri dish, the PDMS mixture was poured into the mold. Air bubbles dissolved in the PDMS were removed by operating a vacuum pump (WOB-L Pump, Welch, Gardner Denver, Milwaukee, WI, and USA) for 1 h. After curing the PDMS in a convective oven at 70 °C for 1 h, a PDMS block was peeled off from the mold. It cut with a razor blade. Two inlets and outlets were punched with a biopsy punch (outer diameter = 1.0 mm). After treating the surfaces of the PDMS block and a glass slide with an oxygen plasma system (CUTE-MPR, Femto Science Co., Gyeonggi-do, Korea), the PDMS block was bonded on a glass substrate. A microfluidic device was finally prepared by placing it on a hotplate at 120 °C for 10 min.

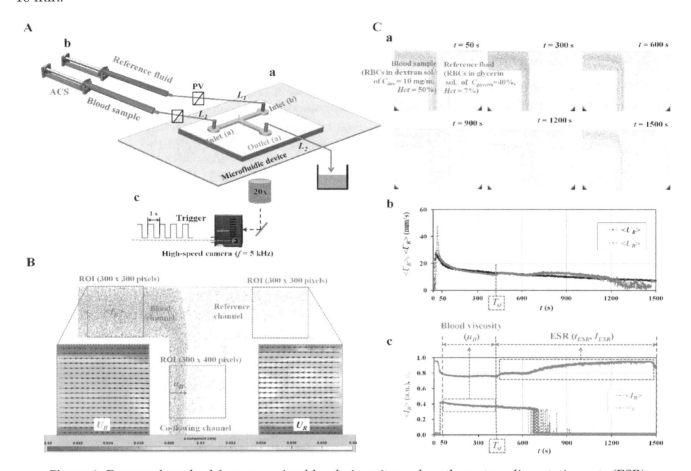

Figure 1. Proposed method for measuring blood viscosity and erythrocyte sedimentation rate (ESR) under fluid delivery of two air-compressed syringes (ACSs). (**A**) Schematic diagram of the proposed technique, including a microfluidic device, two ACSs, and an image acquisition system. (**a**) A microfluidic device consisting of two inlets (**a,b**), one outlet (**a**), and a T-shaped channel (i.e., blood channel, reference channel, and co-flowing channel). (**b**) Two ACSs for delivering blood samples and reference fluid. Each ACS was composed of a disposable syringe (~1 mL), a fixture, and a pinch valve. (**c**) The microfluidic device is located in an optical image acquisition system composed of optical microscopy with a 20× objective lens (NA = 0.4), and a high-speed camera. The camera had a frame rate of 5 kHz and captured sequential snapshots at an interval of 1 s. (**B**) Three regions-of-interest (ROIs) were selected for evaluating four parameters ($<I_B>$, U_B, U_R, and α_B). $<I_B>$ and α_B were obtained by conducting digital image processing. U_B and U_R were obtained by conducting a micro-particle image velocimetry (PIV) technique. (**C**) As a preliminary demonstration, blood sample (normal RBCs in 10 mg/mL dextran solution (Hct = 50%)) and reference fluid (RBCs in 40% glycerin solution (Hct = 7%)) were delivered to each inlet with two ACSs. (**a**) Microscopic images captured at a specific time (t) (t = 50, 300, 600, 900, 1200, and 1500 s). (**b**) Temporal variations of $<U_B>$ and $<U_R>$. (**c**) Temporal variations of $<I_B>$ and α_B. Separation time (T_{st}) was obtained as the time when $<I_B>$ started to increase. First, blood viscosity was evaluated from three parameters (U_B, U_R, and α_B) obtained within T_{st}. Second, the ESR of the blood sample was evaluated from $<I_B>$ obtained above T_{st}.

As shown in Figure 1A-b, two polyethylene tubes (L_1) (length = 300 mm, inner diameter = 500 μm, and thickness = 500 μm) were tightly fitted into two inlets (a, b). The end of each tube was connected to the individual syringe needle of the ACS. The outlet of each ACS was clamped with a pinch valve. The other tube (L_2) (length = 200 mm, inner diameter = 500 μm, and thickness = 500 μm) was tightly fitted into outlet (a). The end of the tube (L_2) was connected to a waste dish. To remove air bubbles and avoid non-specific binding of plasma proteins to the inner surface of the channels, the channel was filled with bovine serum albumin (BSA) solution (C_{BSA} = 2 mg/mL) through outlet (a). After an elapse of 10 min, the microfluidic channel was newly filled with 1× PBS.

Based on the concept of ACS as reported in a previous study [45], two ACSs were employed to deliver the blood sample and reference fluid into the microfluidic device. Figure A1A (Appendix A) showed two ACSs filled with the blood sample (Hct = 50%) and reference fluid (RBCs suspended in 40% glycerin solution (Hct = 7%)). Each ACS was composed of a disposable syringe (~ 1 mL), a fixture, and a pinch valve. Two pinch valves were used to stop or allow the fluid flow of each fluid. Each ACS was placed horizontally on the stage of the optical microscope and fixed with an adhesive tape. Here, an angle of inclination of the ACS only depended on an individual fixture. It was certain that the installation angle of the ACS remained identical because the same fixture of the ACS was used for all experiments.

As shown in Figure A1B (Appendix A), the operation of each ACS was classified into five steps: (1) piston movement at the lowest position forward at $t = t_1$, (2) air suction by moving the piston to 0.7 mL backward at $t = t_2$, (3) blood suction by moving the piston to 0.3 mL backward at $t = t_3$, (4) air compression by moving the piston to 0.3 mL forward at $t = t_4$, and (5) blood delivery by removing the pinch valve at $t = t_5$. As the air cavity inside the ACS was compressed to 0.3 mL, internal pressure increased substantially above atmospheric pressure. Similarly, the reference fluid was sucked into the syringe. The remainder of the procedure was the same as blood delivery. By removing two pinch valves, blood sample and reference fluid were delivered to the corresponding inlets because pressure difference increased inside the ACS.

The microfluidic device was positioned on an optical microscope (BX51, Olympus, Tokyo, Japan) equipped with a 20× objective lens (NA = 0.4). As shown in Figure 1A-c, a high-speed camera (FASTCAM MINI, Photron, Tokyo, Japan) was used to obtain sequential microscopic images of the blood sample and reference fluid flowing in the microfluidic channels. The camera offered a spatial resolution of 1280 × 1000 pixels. Each pixel corresponded to 10 μm physically. A function generator (WF1944B, NF Corporation, Yokohama, Japan) triggered the high-speed camera at an interval of 1 s. Then, two microscopic images were captured at a frame rate of 5 kHz.

To minimize the effect of temperature on blood viscosity, all experiments were conducted at a room temperature of 25 °C. Contributions of two factors (i.e., humidity, and atmospheric pressure) to the present method were neglected. After the blood sample was injected into an ACS, the blood sample did not contact with environment air. Additionally, the ACS was operated by pressure difference (ΔP) between pressure inside ACS (P_{ACS}) and atmosphere pressure (P_{atm}) (i.e., $\Delta P = P_{ACS} - P_{atm}$) [47]. The pressure difference depended on air volume inside the ACS (i.e., gauge pressure), rather than atmospheric pressure.

2.2. Quantification of Microscopic Image Intensity, Blood Velocity Fields, and Interfacial Location

First, blood viscosity was obtained by quantifying the velocity fields of blood sample flowing in the blood channel, the velocity fields of reference fluid flowing in the reference channel, and the interface location between two fluids flowing in the co-flowing channel.

RBCs as fluid tracers were added into reference fluid to obtain the velocity fields of the reference fluid. To measure velocity fields of reference fluid consistently, RBCs should be distributed uniformly in reference fluid during experiments. According to previous studies [1,2], when reference fluid was prepared by adding RBCs into 1× PBS and filled into the ACS, sedimentation of RBCs in ACS occurred continuously over time. RBCs in reference fluid did not flow uniformly over time. After a certain lapse of time, there were no fluid tracers in reference fluid. It was then impossible to obtain the velocity fields of the reference fluid. To resolve the critical issue, a 40% glycerin solution was carefully selected as a base solution in reference fluid. Additionally, to minimize contributions of RBCs to velocity fields and viscosity, hematocrit of RBCs added into reference fluid was fixed at Hct = 7%.

As shown in Figure 1B, an ROI (300 × 300 pixels) was selected to obtain the velocity fields of the blood sample flowing in the blood channel. Another ROI with 300 x 300 pixels was selected to obtain the velocity fields of the reference fluid flowing in the reference channel. By conducting a time-resolved μPIV technique, the velocity fields of the blood sample (U_B) across the blood channel width were obtained over time. Additionally, velocity fields of the reference fluid flow (U_R) across the reference channel width were obtained over time. The size of the interrogation window was selected as 64 × 64 pixels. The window overlap was set to 75%. The velocity fields were validated and corrected with a median filter. The averaged velocities ($<U_B>$, $<U_R>$) of both fluids were calculated as an arithmetic average over the specific ROI. To obtain the interface (i.e., blood sample-filled width) in the co-flowing channel (α_B), an ROI with 300 × 400 pixels was selected in the co-flowing channel. A gray-scale microscopic image was converted into a binary image by adopting Otsu's method [49]. By conducting an arithmetic average over the ROI, variations of the interfacial location in the co-flowing channel (α_B) were obtained over a period of time.

Second, the ESR was evaluated by quantifying the microscopic image intensity of the blood sample flowing in the blood channel. To evaluate the microscopic image intensity of blood flows, and ROI with 300 x 300 pixels was selected in the blood channel. The image intensity of the blood sample flowing in the blood channel was obtained by conducting digital image processing with a commercial software package (Matlab 2019, Mathworks, Natick, MA, USA). An averaged value of microscopic image intensity ($<I_B>$) was obtained by performing an arithmetic average of image intensity over the specific ROI.

2.3. Quantification of Blood Viscosity and ESR

As a preliminary demonstration, blood samples (normal RBCs suspended in specific dextran solution (10 mg/mL), Hct = 50%) and reference fluid were delivered to the corresponding inlets (a, b) under the fluid delivery with two ACSs. To visualize the velocity fields of the reference fluid flowing in the reference channel, the reference fluid was prepared by adding normal RBCs (Hct = 7%) into a 40% glycerin solution.

Figure 1C-a showed microscopic images captured at specific times (t) (t = 50, 300, 600, 900, 1200, and 1500 s). Above t = 600 s, the populations of RBCs flowing in the blood channel decreased substantially over time. As shown in Figure 1C-b, temporal variations of U_B and U_R were obtained by conducting the μPIV technique. As the pressure difference between the inner pressure and atmospheric pressure tended to decrease over time in the ACS, the averaged velocity of the reference fluid ($<U_R>$) tended to decrease stably over time. However, owing to the continuous ESR inside the ACS, an RBC-free liquid was observed in a tube, as shown in Figure A1C (Appendix A). The averaged velocity of the blood sample ($<U_B>$) varied unstably above t = 400 s. Figure 1C-c showed the temporal variations in the image intensity of the blood sample flowing in the blood channel ($<I_B>$), and the interface between the two fluids in the co-flowing channel (α_B). Similar to U_B, the continuous ESR inside the ACS led to unstable behaviors in $<I_B>$ and α_B. In this study, the separation time when unstable behavior began was denoted as T_{st}. At $t < T_{st}$, three factors ($<U_B>$, $<U_R>$, and $<\alpha_B>$) exhibited stable variations over time. Thus, the blood viscosity was quantified from the three factors ($<U_B>$, $<U_R>$, and α_B). For a rectangular channel with an extremely low aspect ratio, an approximate formula of fluidic resistance was derived approximately as $R = \frac{12\,\mu_B\,L}{w\,h^3}$. A co-flowing channel was filled with a blood sample and reference fluid, respectively. For simple mathematical representation, both streams were represented as two fluidic resistances connected in parallel. The corresponding fluidic resistance for each fluid was derived as $R_B = \frac{12\,\mu_B\,L}{W\alpha_B h^3}$ for a blood sample, and $R_R = \frac{12\,\mu_R\,L}{W(1-\alpha_B)\,h^3}$ for reference fluid. Here, μ_R meant the viscosity of the reference fluid. As both fluids had the same pressure drop (i.e., $\Delta P = R_B \cdot Q_B = R_R \cdot Q_R$), blood viscosity formula (μ_B) was derived as $\mu_B = \mu_R \times \left(\frac{\alpha_B}{1-\alpha_B}\right) \times \left(\frac{Q_R}{Q_B}\right)$. Here, Q_B and Q_R represented the flow rate of the blood sample and reference fluid, respectively. The simple mathematical model did not account for real boundary conditions in co-flowing flows. Thus, to compensate for the deviation from the real boundary condition, the previous study included a correction factor in the analytical formula of blood viscosity. According to the blood viscosity formula reported in a parallel co-flowing method with a correction factor [32], the blood viscosity formula (μ_B) was modified as $\mu_B = C_f \times \mu_R \times \left(\frac{\alpha_B}{1-\alpha_B}\right) \times \left(\frac{Q_R}{Q_B}\right)$.

Since the correction factor (C_f) was varied depending on the channel size, a numerical simulation was conducted to determine the correction factor. Based on a procedure discussed in a previous study [32], a numerical simulation using commercial computational fluid dynamics (CFD) software (CFD ACE+, ESI Group, Paris, France) for a rectangular channel (width = 250 μm, depth = 20 μm) was conducted to obtain the viscosity of the test fluid with respect to the interface. For convenience, it was assumed that the reference fluid and test fluid behaved as Newtonian fluids. Both fluids had the same value, as $\mu_{ref} = \mu_{test} = 1$ cP. The interface between both fluids was relocated by varying the flow rate ratio of the reference fluid to test fluid. As shown in Figure A2A (Appendix A), when the interface moved from center line ($\alpha_x = 0.5$) to each wall (i.e., $\alpha_x = 0$ or 1), the blood viscosity without the correction factor (i.e., μ_n) showed a large deviation when compared with the viscosity of the test fluid ($\mu_{test} = 1$ cP). Considering that the viscosity of the test fluid should have a constant value of $\mu_{test} = 1$ cP with respect to the interface, the correction factor (C_f) could be obtained by reciprocating μ_n with respect to α_x (i.e., $C_f = 1/\mu_n$). By conducting a regression analysis, the variations of the correction factor with respect to the interface were obtained as $C_f = 9.7212\alpha_x^4 - 19.442\alpha_x^3 + 15.687\alpha_x^2 - 5.9659\alpha_x + 1.8992$ ($R^2 = 0.9968$). As shown in Figure A2B (Appendix A), to validate C_f, the viscosities of the test fluid were given as (a) $\mu_{test} = 1$ cP and (b) $\mu_{test} = 4.08$ cP. The flow rates of both fluids were the same, at 1 mL/h (i.e., $Q_{ref} = Q_{test} = 1$ mL/h). By applying the correction factor, the viscosities of the test fluids were determined as 1 cP and 4.14 cP, respectively. From the results, it was found that the parallel co-flowing method with the correction factor had the ability to measure the viscosity of a test fluid within 1.4% of a normalized difference. However, at $t > T_{st}$, the continuous ESR inside the ACS caused unstable behaviors in blood flows. To quantify the ESR, two indices (i.e., I_{ESR}, T_{ESR}) were suggested from $<I_B>$ and T_{st}, as shown in Figure 5. Based on previous studies [45,50], one ESR index (I_{ESR}) was suggested simply by integrating $<I_B>$ from $t = T_{st}$ to $t = T_{end}$ (i.e., $I_{ESR} = \int_{t=T_{st}}^{t=T_{end}} <I_B>dt$). Here, T_{end} represented the end time of each experiment. Additionally, $T_{ESR} = T_{st} - T_i$. T_i indicated the initial time when the blood sample started to fill the blood channel.

From the preliminary demonstration, four factors ($<U_B>$, $<U_R>$, α_B, and $<I_B>$) could be effectively employed to obtain the blood viscosity and ESR when two ACSs were employed to deliver the blood sample and reference fluid into a microfluidic device.

2.4. Selection of Base Solution in Reference Fluid

To visualize the velocity fields of the reference fluid, RBCs were added into the reference fluid as fluid tracers. Glycerin solution was suggested as a reference fluid to minimize the sedimentation of RBCs inside the ACS. According to a previous study [51], the density (ρ) and viscosity (μ) increased at higher concentrations of glycerin solution as shown in Figure A3A (Appendix A). To evaluate the sedimentation rate of the RBCs added into the reference fluid, a simple ESR tester was prepared by using a disposable syringe (~1 mL) as shown in Figure A3C (Appendix A). The disposable syringe was fitted vertically into a hole (outer diameter = 4 mm) of the PDMS block. The outlet of the hole was closed with 3M adhesive tape. The syringe was filled with a specific concentration of glycerin solution (~0.5 mL). A 50 μL RBCs droplet was dropped into a specific concentration of glycerin solution. To monitor the sedimentation rate of the RBCs droplet in the simple ESR tester, snapshots were captured at an interval of 1 s with a smartphone camera (Galaxy A5, Samsung, Korea). As shown in Figure A3B (Appendix A), temporal variations of sedimentation height (H) were obtained by varying the concentration of the glycerin solution ($C_{glycerin}$) ($C_{glycerin}$ = 5%, 10%, 20%, 30%, and 40%). Figure A3C (Appendix A) showed sedimentation of the RBCs droplet in 30% glycerin solution over time (t) (t = 0, 156, 192, 249, 259, 270, and 275 s). From the results, the RBCs droplet in the 40% glycerin solution remained nearly identical at the upper position, even without sedimentation. Furthermore, considering that the densities of normal RBCs range from 1090 kg/m³ to 1106 kg/m³ [52], the reference fluid was selected as a 40% glycerin solution ($C_{glycerin}$ = 40%), because its density was greater than that of the RBCs.

2.5. Statistical Analysis

The statistical significance was evaluated by conducting statistical analyses with a commercial software package (Statistical Package for the Social Sciences (SPSS) Statistics version 24, IBM Corp., Armonk, NY, USA). Two ESR indices (I_{ESR}, T_{ESR}) and blood viscosity ($<\mu_B>$) obtained by the present method were compared with results reported in a previous study (i.e., blood viscosity: μ_B, ESR index: S_{EAI}). An analysis of variance (ANOVA) test was applied to verify significant differences between comparative results. A linear regression analysis was conducted to verify the correlations between two parameters. All experimental results were expressed as mean ± standard deviation. If the p-value was less than 0.05, the experimental results exhibited significant differences within a 95% confidence interval.

3. Results and Discussion

3.1. Contribution of RBCs Added into Reference Fluid to Viscosity and Velocity Fields

To evaluate the effects of the RBCs added into the reference fluid on fluid viscosity, the viscosity of the reference fluid was measured by varying the volume of the RBCs added to the reference fluid (i.e., hematocrit [Hct]). In that regard, a 1× PBS was delivered to the blood channel (i.e., left-side channel) at a constant flow rate of Q_{PBS} = 1 mL/h with a syringe pump (SP) (neMESYS, Centoni Gmbh, Germany). The hematocrit (Hct) of the reference fluid was adjusted to Hct = 3%, 5%, 7%, and 9% by adding normal RBCs into the 40% glycerin solution. The reference fluid was delivered to the reference channel (i.e., right-side channel) at a constant flow rate of $Q_{glycerin}$ = 1 mL/h with an SP. Figure 2A showed microscopic images for evaluating the interfacial location in the co-flowing channel with respect to Hct ((a) Hct = 0%, (b) Hct = 3%, (c) Hct = 5%, (d) Hct = 7%, and (e) Hct = 9%). To verify the contribution of the hematocrit in the reference fluid to the velocity fields (U_R), the velocity fields of the reference fluid were obtained across the reference channel width with respect to Hct. As shown in Figure 2B-a, a variation of the velocity profile (U_R) was obtained across the reference channel width with respect to Hct. The inset showed the microscopic image and velocity profile of the reference fluid with Hct = 3%. From the results, the velocity profile did not show a distinctive difference depending on the hematocrit. Figure 2B-b showed variations of the averaged velocity of the reference fluid ($<U_R>$) with respect to Hct. The hematocrit in the reference fluid did not contribute to varying $<U_R>$ significantly. As shown in Figure 2C-a, the variations of the interface in the co-flowing channel (α_R) and the viscosity (μ_R) were obtained with respect to Hct. The interface and viscosity remained constant as α_R = 0.771 ± 0.003 and μ_R = 3.868 ± 0.068 cP for the reference fluid, with up to 9% hematocrit. From the results, it could be observed that providing up to a 9% hematocrit in the reference fluid did not significantly contribute to increasing the viscosity of the reference fluid. In addition, as shown in Figure A3A (Appendix A), an empirical formula [51] indicated that a 40% glycerin solution without any RBCs had a viscosity value of 4.07 cP. Based on the parallel co-flowing method with the correction factor [32], the viscosity of the reference fluid was measured consistently within a 5% difference when compared with the empirical formula. Furthermore, a previous flow-switching method [14] was employed to measure the viscosity of the reference fluid with respect to hematocrit. The inset of Figure 2C-b showed reversal flow-switching in the junction channel for the reference fluid with Hct = 7%. By increasing the flow rate of the 1× PBS (Q_{PBS}) from Q_{PBS} = 1 mL/h to Q_{PBS} = 3.1 mL/h, the hydrodynamic balancing in both side channels caused to reverse flow direction from left direction to right direction (i.e., reversal flow-switching phenomena) [14]. In other words, the junction channel was filled with blood at Q_{PBS} = 1 mL/h. However, it was filled with 1× PBS at Q_{PBS} = 3.1 mL/h. Based on the viscosity formula suggested in the flow-switching method, the viscosity of the reference fluid was quantified as μ_R = 3.1 ± 0.05 cP. As shown in Figure 2C-b, the viscosity obtained by both methods remained stable, with respect to hematocrit. Similar to the case in the parallel co-flowing method with the correction factor, the results of the flow-switching method indicated that the RBCs added into the reference fluid did not contribute to varying the viscosity within 9% hematocrit. The viscosity obtained by the flow-switching method was underestimated by approximately 20% when compared with that obtained by the parallel co-flowing method with the correction factor. From these results, in this study, the reference fluid was prepared by adding normal RBCs (*Hct* = 7%) into a 40% glycerin solution throughout all experiments.

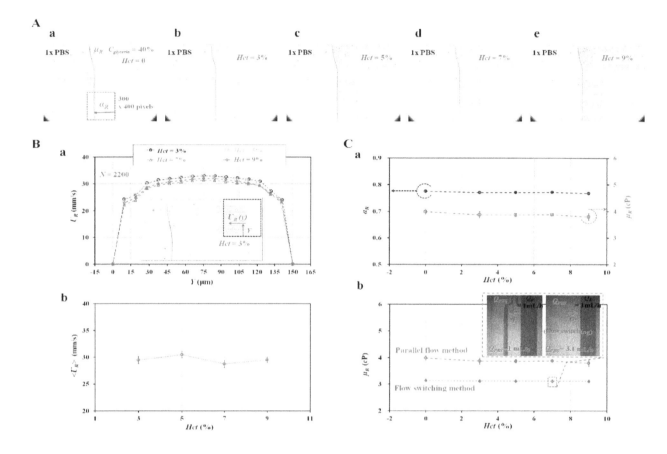

Figure 2. Contributions of RBCs added into the reference fluid to viscosity. 1× PBS was delivered to the blood channel at a constant flow rate of 1 mL/h with a syringe pump (SP). The hematocrit (*Hct*) of reference fluid was adjusted by adding normal RBCs into 40% glycerin solution (*Hct* = 0, 3%, 5%, 7%, and 9%). The reference fluid was delivered to the reference channel at a constant flow rate of 1 mL/h with an SP. (**A**) Microscopic images for obtaining interface (α_R) in co-flowing channel with respect to *Hct* ((**a**) *Hct* = 0, (**b**) *Hct* = 3%, (**c**) *Hct* = 5%, (**d**) *Hct* = 7%, and (**e**) *Hct* = 9%). (**B**) Contributions of hematocrit in reference fluid to velocity fields (U_R). (**a**) Variation of velocity fields (U_R) across reference channel width with respect to *Hct*. The inset showed a microscopic image and a velocity profile of the reference fluid with *Hct* = 3%. (**b**) Variations of <U_R> averaged over a region of interest (ROI) with respect to *Hct*. (**C**) Effect of *Hct* in reference to fluid on viscosity (μ_R). (**a**) Variations of α_R and μ_R with respect to *Hct*. (**b**) Comparison between the proposed method (i.e., the parallel-flow method with correction factor) and previous method (i.e., flow-switching method) with respect to *Hct*.

3.2. Relationship between Flow Rate of Syringe Pump and Averaged Velocity Obtained by μPIV

To obtain blood viscosity, the flow rates of the blood sample and reference fluid should be measured from the averaged velocity obtained by conducting the μPIV technique. In other words, there was a need to obtain the relationship between the flow rate delivered by the SP (Q_{sp}) and the averaged velocity obtained by conducting the μPIV technique (<U>).

The hematocrit of the blood sample was adjusted to Hct = 30%, 40%, and 50% by adding normal RBCs into the base solution (1× PBS, plasma). Using two SPs, the flow rate of each fluid decreased stepwise from Q_{sp} = 1.5 mL/h to Q_{sp} = 0.1 mL/h, at an interval of 0.2 mL/h. With respect to each flow rate, the SP had been operated for 8 min. The blood sample was prepared by adding normal RBCs into plasma. As shown in Figure 3A-a, temporal variations of the averaged velocity ($<U_B>$) and the flow rate of the SP (Q_{sp}) were obtained by varying the hematocrit. At a higher flow rate of Q_{sp}, the hematocrit contributed to decreasing $<U_B>$. At a lower flow rate of Q_{sp}, $<U_B>$ remained constant, without contribution from the hematocrit. By changing the base solution from plasma to a 1× PBS, temporal variations of $<U_B>$ and Q_{sp} were obtained with respect to Hct. As shown in Figure 3A-b, the variations of $<U_B>$, with respect to hematocrit, were very similar to those of a blood sample composed of plasma. By averaging $<U_B>$ with respect to Q_{sp}, $<U_B>$ was quantified as mean ± standard deviation with respect to Q_{sp}. To determine the relationship between $<U_B>$ and Q_{sp}, a scatter plot was used to plot $<U_B>$ on a vertical axis and Q_{sp} on a horizontal axis. Figure 3A-c showed variations of $<U_B>$ with respect to Q_{sp} and Hct in a blood sample composed of plasma. For example, $<U_B>$ was estimated as about 30 mm/s for Q_{sp} =1.3 mL/h. Based on formula of flow rate (i.e., $Q_{\mu P} = <U_B>A_c$, A_c = w x h), flow rate obtained by μPIV was estimated as $Q_{\mu PIV}$ = 0.54 mL/h. When compared with Q_{sp} =1.3 mL/h, the normalized difference between Q_{sp} and $Q_{\mu PIV}$ was estimated as 59%. In this study, instead of the flow rate formula, the flow rate of the blood sample or reference fluid was estimated from the calibration formula obtained in advance. Thus, it was necessary to determine the relationship between velocity ($<U_B>$) and Q_{sp}. A regression analysis was conducted by assuming the regression formula as a quadratic model. Regression formulas between $<U_B>$ and Q_{sp} with respect to Hct were obtained, as shown inside of Figure 3A-c. The regression formulas for each hematocrit were obtained as $<U_B>$ = −5.027 Q_{sp}^2 + 30.279 Q_{sp} (R^2 = 0.998) for Hct = 30%, $<U_B>$ = −6.262 Q_{sp}^2 + 30.660 Q_{sp} (R^2 = 0.999) for Hct = 40%, and $<U_B>$ = −5.916 Q_{sp}^2 + 29.137 Q_{sp} (R^2 = 0.999) for Hct = 50%. Figure 3A-d showed variations of $<U_B>$ with respect to the Q_{sp} and Hct in a blood sample composed of 1× PBS. From the regression analysis, as shown inside Figure 3A-d, the regression formulas for each hematocrit were obtained as $<U_B>$ = −4.850 Q_{sp}^2 + 30.791 Q_{sp} (R^2 = 0.998) for Hct = 30%, $<U_B>$ = −7.897 Q_{sp}^2 + 33.519 Q_{sp} (R^2 = 1.000) for Hct = 40%, and $<U_B>$ = −5.717 Q_{sp}^2 + 29.286 Q_{sp} (R^2 = 0.999) for Hct = 50%. For the same hematocrit, the base solution (i.e., plasma or 1× PBS) did not contribute to varying the coefficients of the quadratic formula (i.e., normalized difference < 4% except Hct = 40%). However, for the same base solution, the coefficients of a quadratic model varied significantly with respect to hematocrit.

A regression formula between Q_{sp} and $<U_R>$ for the reference fluid (i.e., 40% glycerin solution) with RBCs (Hct = 7%) was obtained by using a similar procedure to that used for the blood sample. Figure 3B-a showed the temporal variations of Q_{sp} and $<U_R>$ for the reference fluid. $<U_R>$ was obtained as a mean ± standard deviation for a corresponding Q_{sp}. When compared with the blood sample, $<U_R>$ increased substantially, owing to the lower value of the hematocrit. As shown in Figure 3B-b, variations of $<U_R>$ with respect to Q_{sp} were represented by a scatter plot. From a regression analysis, the regression formula between $<U_R>$ and Q_{sp} was obtained as $<U_R>$ = −7.770 Q_{sp}^2 + 37.127 Q_{sp} (R^2 = 0.9875).

From the results, the coefficients of the quadratic formula were varied significantly with respect to hematocrit. However, the base solution (i.e., 1× PBS, or plasma) did not contribute to changing the coefficients of the regression formula. Using regression formulae between Q_{sp} and $<U_R>$ (or $<U_B>$) obtained in advance, the $<U_R>$ or $<U_B>$ obtained by conducting the μPIV technique was converted into a flow rate (i.e., Q_B, Q_R, respectively).

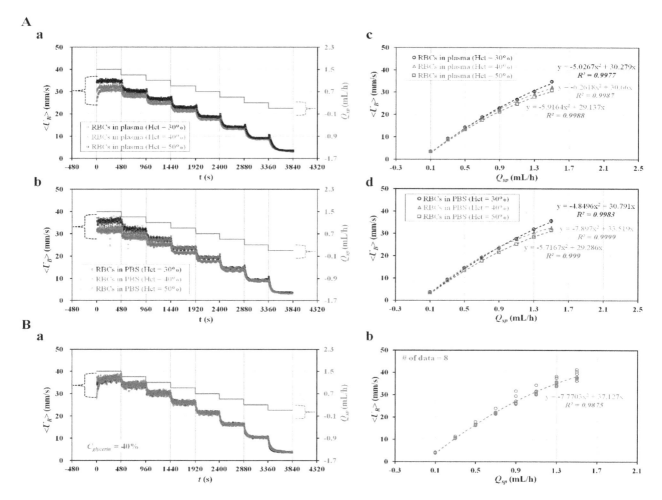

Figure 3. Calibration formula for the relationship between flow rate controlled by SP (Q_{sp}) and averaged velocity obtained by μPIV technique ($<U>$). Hematocrit (*Hct*) of blood was adjusted to *Hct* = 30%, 40%, and 50% by adding normal RBCs into a base solution (1× PBS or plasma). With two syringe pumps, the flow rate of each fluid decreased stepwise from Q_{sp} = 1.5 mL/h to Q_{sp} = 0.1 mL/h at an interval of 0.2 mL/h. Each flow rate was maintained for 8 min. (**A**) Relationship between Q_{sp} and $<U_B>$ with respect to hematocrit and base solution. (**a**) Temporal variations in $<U_B>$ and Q_{sp} of blood sample (normal RBCs in plasma) with respect to *Hct*. (**b**) Temporal variations in $<U_B>$ and Q_{sp} of blood sample (normal RBCs in 1× PBS) with respect to *Hct*. (**c**) Regression formula between $<U_B>$ and Q_{sp} of blood sample (normal RBCs in plasma) with respect to *Hct*. (**d**) Regression formula between $<U_B>$ and Q_{sp} of blood sample (normal RBCs in 1× PBS) with respect to *Hct*. (**B**) Calibration formula of relationship between Q_{sp} and $<U_R>$ of reference fluid (40% glycerin solution with RBCs (*Hct* = 7%). (**a**) Temporal variations of Q_{sp} and $<U_R>$. (**b**) Regression formula between $<U_B>$ and Q_{sp}.

3.3. Quantitative Comparison of Blood Viscosity with Respect to Fluid Delivery System (ACS, SP)

Since the $<U_R>$ and $<U_B>$ obtained from the μPIV technique were converted into flow rates (Q_R and Q_B) from regression formulae obtained in advance, the blood viscosity could be measured by monitoring the interface (α_B) in the co-flowing channel, under fluid delivery with an ACS. The blood viscosity obtained by the ACS was quantitatively compared with one obtained by an SP. Blood samples (*Hct* = 30%, 40%, and 50%) were prepared by adding normal RBCs into the base solution (1× PBS, plasma).

Figure 4A-a showed the temporal variations of Q_R, Q_B, and α_B for the blood sample (normal RBCs in 1× PBS, *Hct* = 50%). In addition, Figure 4A-b depicted the temporal variations of Q_R, Q_B, and α_B for the blood sample (normal RBCs in plasma, *Hct* = 50%). Using the blood viscosity formula, the blood viscosity was obtained by using the temporal variations of Q_R, Q_B, and α_B. Here, the viscosity of the reference fluid was given as μ_R = 4.08 cP by using measurement results reported in previous studies [14,51]. For a rectangular channel (width = w, depth = h) with a lower aspect ratio [32], the formula of shear rate ($\dot{\gamma}$) was given as approximately $\dot{\gamma} = \frac{6Q_B}{wh^2}$. The corresponding shear rate of the blood viscosity obtained at a specific blood flow rate (Q_B) was estimated by using the shear rate formula. A scatter plot was employed to plot μ_B on a vertical axis, and $\dot{\gamma}$ on a horizontal axis. As shown in Figure 4B-a, variations of μ_B were obtained with respect to the shear rate under fluid delivery with the two ACSs. Here, the blood sample ($Hct = 50\%$) was prepared by adding normal RBCs into plasma or 1× PBS. The blood sample has behaved as a Newtonian fluid at sufficiently higher shear rates ($\dot{\gamma} > 10^3 \ s^{-1}$). From the experimental results, μ_B remained constant with respect to the shear rate. By conducting an arithmetic average of μ_B over specific shear rates, the blood viscosity was expressed as $<\mu_B>$ = mean ± standard deviation. The viscosity of the blood sample composed of plasma ($<\mu_{B, plasma}>$ = 2.381 ± 0.042 cP) was significantly higher than that of the blood sample composed of 1× PBS ($<\mu_{B, PBS}>$ = 1.845 ± 0.0573 cP). To compare with the blood viscosity obtained under fluid delivery with two ACSs, the same blood samples were employed to measure the blood viscosity under fluid delivery with two SPs. Two fluids (blood sample, reference fluid) were delivered to each inlet of the microfluidic device, at the same flow rate ($Q_B = Q_R$).

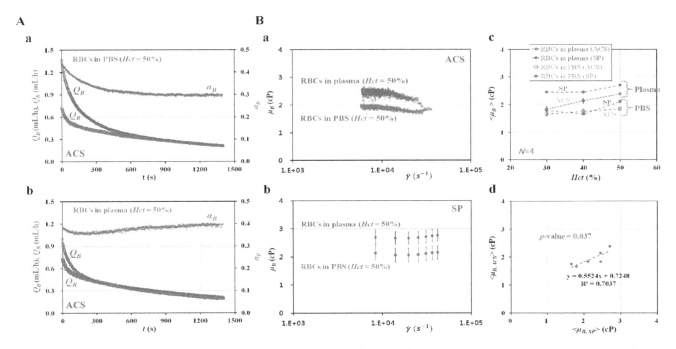

Figure 4. Quantitative comparison of blood viscosity for blood samples (normal RBCs in plasma and PBS, $Hct = 50\%$) with respect to the fluid delivery system (ACS, SP). (**A**) Variations of flow rates (Q_B, Q_R) and interface (α_B) with respect to the base solution (1× PBS, plasma). (**a**) Temporal variations of Q_B, Q_R, and α_B for a blood sample (normal RBCs in 1× PBS, and $Hct = 50\%$). (**b**) Temporal variations of Q_B, Q_R, and α_B for a blood sample (normal RBCs in plasma, and $Hct = 50\%$). (**B**) Variation of blood viscosity depending on the base solution, hematocrit, and fluid delivery system (ACS and SP). (**a**) Variations of blood viscosity (μ_B) of blood samples with respect to the base solution (1× PBS, plasma) and shear rate under fluid delivery of ACS. (**b**) Variations of μ_B with respect to the base solution (1× PBS, plasma) and shear rate under fluid delivery of two SPs. (**c**) Variations of $<\mu_B>$ with respect to base solution (1× PBS, plasma), hematocrit ($Hct = 30\%$, 40%, and 50%), and fluid delivery system (ACS, SP). $<\mu_B>$ was quantified as $<\mu_B>$ = mean ± standard deviation by conducting an arithmetic average of μ_B obtained over shear rates. (**d**) Correlation between blood viscosity obtained under ACS ($<\mu_{B, ACS}>$) and blood viscosity obtained under SP ($<\mu_{B, SP}>$).

As represented in Figure 3A-a and Figure 3A-b, the flow rate of the SP (Q_{sp}) decreased stepwise from Q_{sp} = 1.5 mL/h to Q_{sp} = 0.1 mL/h at an interval of 0.2 mL/h. Each flow rate had been maintained for 8 min. As shown in Figure 4B-b, variations in μ_B of the blood samples (normal RBCs in plasma and 1× PBS, $Hct = 50\%$) were obtained with respect to the shear rate. The blood viscosity remained constant with respect to the shear rate. The viscosity of the blood sample composed of plasma ($<\mu_{B, plasma}> = 2.728 \pm 0.0918$ cP) was higher than that of the blood sample composed of 1× PBS ($<\mu_{B, PBS}> = 2.109 \pm 0.0429$ cP). When compared with the blood viscosity obtained by the ACS, blood viscosity obtained by the SP increased by approximately 12.5%. To determine the effects of hematocrit on blood viscosity, variations of blood viscosity were obtained by varying the hematocrit ($Hct = 30\%$, 40%, and 50%), base solution (1× PBS, plasma), and fluid delivery system (ACS, SP). Figure 4B-c showed the variations of $<\mu_B>$ with respect to Hct, base solution, and the fluid delivery system. Under fluid delivery with an ACS, $<\mu_B>$ tended to increase with respect to Hct. Under fluid delivery with an SP, there was no significant difference between $Hct = 30\%$ and $Hct = 40\%$. The blood viscosity increased at $Hct = 50\%$ when compared with $Hct = 30\%$ or 40%. To determine the correlation between the blood viscosity obtained by the ACS ($<\mu_{B, ACS}>$) and the blood viscosity obtained by the SP ($<\mu_{B, SP}>$), a scatterplot was used to plot $<\mu_{B, ACS}>$ on a vertical axis, and $<\mu_{B, SP}>$ on a horizontal axis, as shown in Figure 4B-d. According to a linear regression analysis, $<\mu_{B, ACS}>$ was expressed as $<\mu_{B, ACS}> = 0.5524 <\mu_{B, SP}> + 0.7248$ ($R^2 = 0.7037$, p-value = 0.037). Here, p-value = 0.037 indicated that a linear regression showed sufficient relationship between two viscosity values (i.e., $<\mu_{B, ACS}>$ vs. $<\mu_{B, SP}>$). In addition, R^2 was obtained as a high value of $R^2 = 0.7037$. Although two SPs were effectively used to deliver two fluids during measurement of blood viscosity, the arrangement included challenges, such as a bulky size and a high cost. From the correlation between $<\mu_{B, ACS}>$ and $<\mu_{B, SP}>$, it was found that the ACS can be effectively employed to deliver two fluids in the measurement of blood viscosity. Thus, the blood viscosity can be measured consistently under fluid delivery with two ACSs.

3.4. Quantitative Measurement of ESR with Respect to base Solution and Hematocrit

The ESR of the blood sample was evaluated by quantifying the microscopic image intensity of the blood sample ($<I_B>$) flowing in the blood channel. Two ESR indices (t_{ESR}, I_{ESR}) were suggested by quantifying the temporal variations of $<I_B>$. The blood samples ($Hct = 30\%$, 40%, and 50%) were prepared by adding normal RBCs into a base solution (1× PBS, plasma).

As shown in Figure 5A-a, variations of $<I_B>$ for the blood sample (normal RBCs in plasma) were obtained with respect to Hct. $<I_B>$ tended to decrease at higher values of Hct. In addition, T_{st} tended to be shorter at lower values of the hematocrit. To exclude the contribution of plasma protein to the ESR, the plasma was replaced with the 1× PBS. As shown in Figure 5A-b, temporal variations of $<I_B>$ for the blood sample (normal RBCs in 1× PBS) were obtained by varying Hct. $<I_B>$ tended to decrease at higher values of Hct. With a certain elapse of time, $<I_B>$ remained constant. There was no existence of separation time within 2000 s (i.e., $T_{st} > 2000$ s). The results indicated that the 1× PBS did not sufficiently contribute to enhancing ESR when compared with plasma.

To quantify the ESR of the blood sample (normal RBCs in plasma) from $<I_B>$ as shown in Figure 5A-a, two ESR indices (t_{ESR}, I_{ESR}) were obtained with respect to the hematocrit. Figure 5B-a showed variations of t_{ESR} and I_{ESR} with respect to Hct. According to the results, t_{ESR} tended to increase significantly with respect to hematocrit (p-value = 0.0004). I_{ESR} tended to decrease substantially with respect to hematocrit (p-value = 0.001). Under blood delivery with the ACS, the RBCs tended to fall down continuously inside the ACS, which was installed horizontally. Owing to the continuous ESR inside the ACS, the populations of RBCs delivered to the blood channel decreased over time. Thus, $<I_B>$ increased gradually over time, as shown in Figure 5A-a. However, when the plasma was replaced with the 1× PBS, the blood sample did not exhibit an ESR inside the ACS. For this reason, after a certain period of time, $<I_B>$ remained constant over time, as shown in Figure 5A-b. To quantitatively compare with results reported in a previous study, two indices (t_{ESR}, I_{ESR}) and S_{EAI} (previous ESR index) [45] were plotted on a vertical axis and horizontal axis, respectively. S_{EAI} exhibited larger scatters than t_{ESR} or I_{ESR}. From the regression analysis, the linear regression exhibited higher values of $R^2 = 0.7474 \sim 0.7755$. The results indicated that the two ESR indices exhibited consistent variations with respect to hematocrit when compared with S_{EAI}. Thus, the two ESR indices (t_{ESR}, I_{ESR}) can be effectively used to evaluate the variation of ESR with respect to hematocrit.

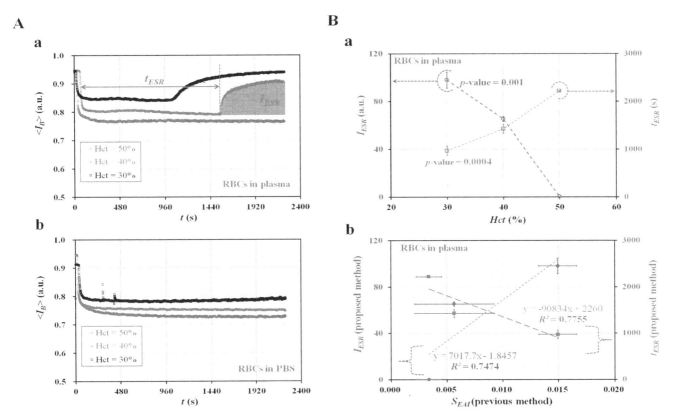

Figure 5. Evaluation of ESR for blood samples with respect to base solutions (1× PBS, and plasma) and hematocrit (*Hct* = 30%, 40%, and 50%). (**A**) Variations of <I_B> with respect to base solution and hematocrit. (**a**) Temporal variations of <I_B> of blood sample (normal RBCs in plasma) with respect to *Hct*. (**b**) Temporal variations of <I_B> of blood sample (normal RBCs in 1× PBS) with respect to *Hct*. (**B**) Variations of two ESR indices (t_{ESR}, I_{ESR}) for blood sample (normal RBCs in plasma) with respect to *Hct*. (**a**) Variations of t_{ESR} and I_{ESR} with respect to *Hct*. (**b**) Correlation between proposed ESR indices (t_{ESR}, I_{ESR}) and previous ESR index (S_{EAI}).

3.5. Variations of Blood Viscosity and ESR for Blood Samples Composed of Specific Dextran Solutions

A specific dextran solution as a base solution was prepared to enhance the ESR of the blood sample. To exclude the contributions of hematocrit to ESR, the hematocrit of the blood sample was adjusted to *Hct* = 50%. The blood samples were prepared by adding normal RBCs into specific concentrations of dextran solution (i.e., C_{dex} = 0, 5, 10, 15, and 20 mg/mL). C_{dex} = 0 meant 1× PBS as control. As shown in Figure 6A-a, temporal variations of Q_B were obtained with respect to C_{dex}. From the results, the blood sample composed of dextran solution (C_{dex} <= 5 mg/mL) exhibited stable variations of Q_B over time. However, above C_{dex} >= 10 mg/mL, the separation time (T_{st}) tended to reduce at higher concentrations of the dextran solution. Figure 6A-b showed temporal variations of α_B with respect to C_{dex}. Similar to the case with Q_B, α_B varied unstably above C_{dex} >= 10 mg/mL. T_{st} tended to be shorter at higher concentrations of the dextran solution. By using stable variations of Q_B and α_B obtained at t < T_{st}, variations of μ_B were obtained with respect to the shear rate. As shown in Figure 6A-c, blood viscosities were obtained at sufficiently higher shear rates ($\dot{\gamma} > 10^3\ s^{-1}$). They remained constant with respect to the shear rate. Additionally, the blood viscosity tended to increase at higher concentrations of the dextran solution. By averaging the μ_B values obtained at shear rates, the blood viscosity was expressed as <μ_B> = mean ± standard deviation. Figure 6A-d showed variations of <μ_B> with respect to C_{dex} and the fluid delivery system (ACS, SP). When compared with the results reported in a previous study [45], the present results exhibited sufficiently consistent variations of <μ_B> with respect to C_{dex}.

In addition, there was no significant difference between the ACS and SP. As shown in Figure 6A-e, to determine the correlation between $<\mu_B>$ obtained by the proposed method (two ACSs) and μ_B obtained by the previous method (two SPs) [45], a scatter plot was used to plot $<\mu_B>$ (proposed method) on a vertical axis and μ_B (previous method) on a horizontal axis. According to linear regression analysis, the high value of $R^2 = 0.9767$ indicated that the proposed method could give comparable results when compared with the previous method. Thus, ACSs could be effectively employed to deliver fluid samples. After measuring the blood viscosity with respect to C_{dex}, the contributions of the dextran solution to the ESR were evaluated by quantifying the image intensity of the blood sample flowing in the blood channel ($<I_B>$). As shown in Figure 6B-a, temporal variations of $<I_B>$ were obtained with respect to C_{dex}. As a result, T_{st} was reduced at higher concentrations of the dextran solution. Using $<I_B>$ with respect to C_{dex}, two ESR indices (t_{ESR}, I_{ESR}) were obtained with respect to C_{dex}. As shown in Figure 6B-b, the ESR indices remained constant up to $C_{dex} = 5$ mg/mL. Above $C_{dex} >= 10$ mg/mL, t_{ESR} tended to decrease substantially with respect to C_{dex} (p-value = 0.0001). I_{ESR} increased largely at higher concentrations of dextran solution (p-value = 0.0001). To compare with the results reported in a previous study [45], a scatterplot was used to plot t_{ESR} and I_{ESR} (i.e., proposed method) on a vertical axis, and S_{EAI} (i.e., previous method: periodic on-off control with an SP) on a horizontal axis. As shown in Figure 6B-c, a linear regression analysis was conducted to determine the correlation between the proposed method and the previous method. The higher value of $R^2 = 0.8202$–0.8548 indicated that the two ESR indices (t_{ESR}, I_{ESR}) gave comparable results when compared with the previous method. Thus, the ESR indices can be effectively used to quantify the ESRs of blood samples.

3.6. Variations of Blood Viscosity and ESR for Blood Samples Composed of Hardened RBCs

As the last demonstration, the proposed method was applied to evaluate the contribution of hardened RBCs to the ESR. As shown in Figure 5A-a, a blood sample ($Hct = 50\%$) composed of plasma did not contribute to variations in the ESR. To stimulate the ESR of a blood sample with a high value of $Hct = 50\%$, the plasma as a base solution was replaced with a specific concentration of dextran solution (i.e., $C_{dex} = 15$ mg/mL). Hardened RBCs were prepared by sufficiently exposing normal RBCs to specific concentrations of GA solution (C_{GA}) (i.e., $C_{GA} = 0, 5, 10$, and 15 µL/mL). $C_{GA} = 0$ indicated normal RBCs as control. The blood samples ($Hct = 50\%$) were then prepared by adding hardened RBCs into the specific dextran solutions.

Figure 7A showed the temporal variations of Q_B with respect to C_{GA}. T_{st} tended to increase at higher concentrations of the GA solution. At $C_{GA} = 15$ µL/mL, Q_B tended to decrease stably over time. Figure 7B showed the temporal variations of α_B with respect to C_{GA}. The variations of α_B were very similar to those of Q_B. At $C_{GA} = 15$ µL/mL, α_B remained constant after a certain period of time. Figure 7C showed the temporal variations of $<I_B>$ with respect to C_{GA}. Except for at $C_{GA} = 15$ µL/mL, $<I_B>$ tended to increase stably over time. Additionally, T_{st} tended to increase at higher concentrations of the GA solution. By measuring three factors (Q_B, α_B, and $<I_B>$) simultaneously, the hardened blood sample composed of hardened RBCs fixed with $C_{GA} = 15$ µL/mL did not exhibit an ESR inside the ACS. Thus, there were no significant variations of Q_B and α_B. As shown in Figure 7D, variations of $<\mu_B>$ were obtained with respect to C_{GA}. $<\mu_B>$ tended to increase considerably with respect to C_{GA}. As the GA solution contributed to stiffening the RBCs' membranes, it was reasonable that the blood viscosity increased at higher concentrations of the GA solution. Figure 7E showed variations of the two ESR indices (t_{ESR}, I_{ESR}) with respect to C_{GA}. t_{ESR} tended to increase with respect to C_{GA}. I_{ESR} tended to decrease with respect to C_{GA}.

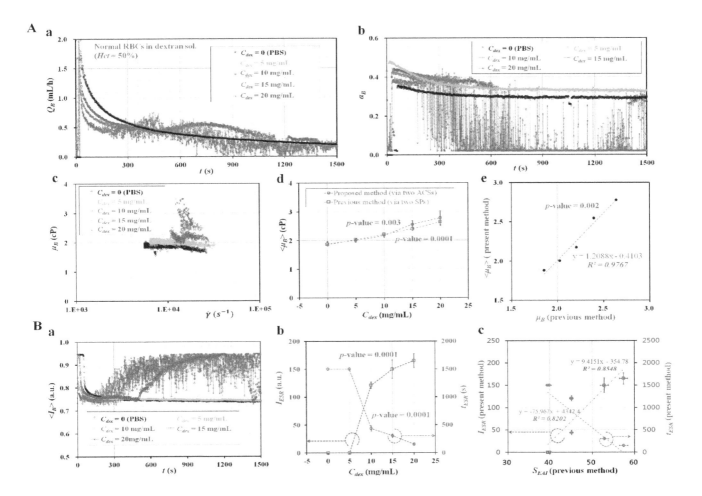

Figure 6. Measurement of blood viscosity and ESR for blood samples composed of specific concentrations of dextran solution. Blood samples ($Hct = 50\%$) were prepared by adding normal RBCs into various concentration of dextran solution (C_{dex}) (i.e., $C_{dex} = 0$, 5, 10, 15, and 20 mg/mL). $C_{dex} = 0$ meant 1× PBS as control. (**A**) Variations of blood viscosity with respect to C_{dex}. (**a**) Temporal variations of Q_B with respect to C_{dex}. (**b**) Temporal variations of α_B with respect to C_{dex}. (**c**) Variations of μ_B with respect to shear rate and C_{dex}. (**d**) Variations of $<\mu_B>$ with respect to the C_{dex} and fluid delivery system (ACS, SP). (**e**) Correlation between blood viscosity obtained by the proposed method and blood viscosity obtained by the previous method. (**B**) Variations of ESR with respect to C_{dex}. (**a**) Temporal variations of $<I_B>$ with respect to C_{dex}. (**b**) Variations of two ESR indices (t_{ESR}, I_{ESR}) with respect to C_{dex}. (**c**) Quantitative comparison between the proposed method (t_{ESR}, I_{ESR}) and previous method (S_{EAI}).

From the experimental results, it was found that the GA solution caused an increase in blood viscosity. Furthermore, the proposed method had the ability to consistently measure blood viscosity and ESR, under simultaneously fluid delivery from two ACSs.

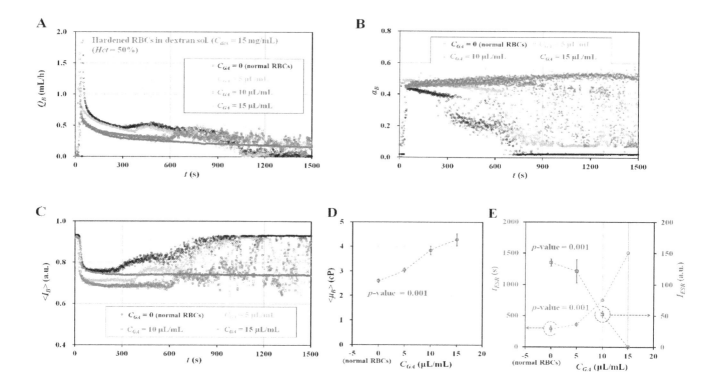

Figure 7. Measurement of blood viscosity and ESR and blood viscosity for blood samples composed of hardened RBCs with glutaraldehyde (GA) solution. To prepare hardened RBCs from normal RBCs, normal RBCs were sufficiently exposed to specific concentrations of GA solution (C_{GA}) ($C_{GA} = 0$, 5, 10, and 15 µL/mL). $C_{GA} = 0$ meant normal RBCs as control. Blood sample ($Hct = 50\%$) was prepared by adding hardened RBCs into the dextran solution ($C_{dex} = 15$ mg/mL). (**A**) Temporal variations of Q_B with respect to C_{GA}. (**B**) Temporal variations of α_B with respect to C_{GA}. (**C**) Temporal variations of $<I_B>$ with respect to C_{GA}. (**D**) Variations of $<\mu_B>$ with respect to C_{GA}. (**E**) Variations of two ESR indices (t_{ESR}, I_{ESR}) with respect to C_{GA}.

4. Conclusions

In this study, a simple method of measuring blood viscosity and ESR was demonstrated by quantifying averaged velocities of a blood sample and reference fluid, where the blood sample and reference fluid were delivered to a microfluidic device with two ACSs. According to the experimental results, a 40% glycerin solution with RBCs ($Hct = 7\%$) was selected as the reference fluid to obtain velocity fields and avoid sedimentation of RBCs in the ACS. Using a calibration formulae between the flow rate of an SP (Q_{sp}) and the averaged velocity obtained by the µPIV technique ($<U_B>$) in advance, $<U_B>$ or $<U_R>$ was converted into Q_B or Q_R, respectively. As a demonstration, the proposed method was employed to evaluate the contributions of the hematocrit ($Hct = 30\%$, 40%, and 50%), base solution (1× PBS, plasma, dextran solution), and hardened RBCs to the blood viscosity and ESR, respectively. The results of the proposed method were comparable with those reported in previous studies that used two SPs. From the experimental results, it could be concluded that the proposed method had the ability to consistently measure blood viscosity and ESR under simultaneous fluid delivery with two ACSs. However, image acquisition for quantifying blood flows in microfluidic channels was demonstrated from the optical microscope and a high-speed camera. To resolve the issue, the proposed method should be improved substantially by adopting a portable image acquisition system in the near future.

Appendix A.

Appendix A.1. Figure A1

A

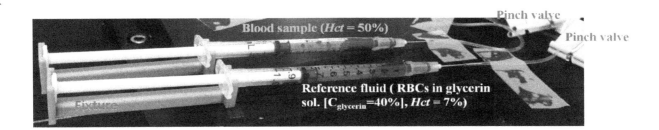

B   **C**

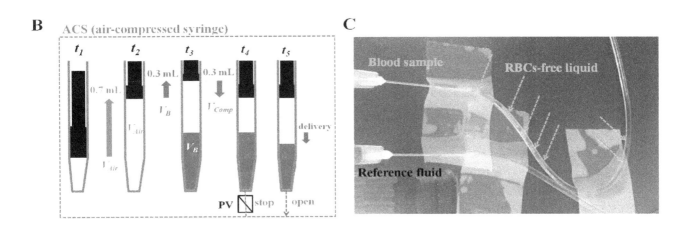

Figure A1. Fabrication and operation of the air-compressed syringe. (**A**) Two air-compressed syringes (ACSs) filled with blood sample (Hct = 50%) and reference fluid (RBCs in 40% glycerin sol. [Hct = 7%]). Each ACS was composed of a disposable syringe (~ 1mL), a fixture, and a pinch valve. (**B**) Operation of ACS: piston movement at the lowest position forward at $t = t_1$, air suction (V_{Air} = 0.7 mL) by moving piston to 0.7 mL backward at $t = t_2$, blood suction by moving piston to 0.3 mL backward (V_B = 0.3 mL) at $t = t_3$, air compression by moving piston to 0.3 mL forward (V_{comp} = 0.3 mL) at $t = t_4$, and blood delivery by removing pinch valve at $t = t_5$. Similarly, the reference fluid was sucked into the syringe instead of blood. The remaining procedure was the same as blood delivery with the ACS. The blood sample and reference fluid were then delivered into the corresponding inlets with two ACSs. (**C**) Snapshots for showing RBC-free liquid in a tube under blood delivery using an ACS. Owing to the continuous erythrocyte sedimentation rate (ESR) inside the ACS, a red blood cell (RBC)-free liquid was observed in the microfluidic channel after a certain lapse of time.

Appendix A.2. Figure A2

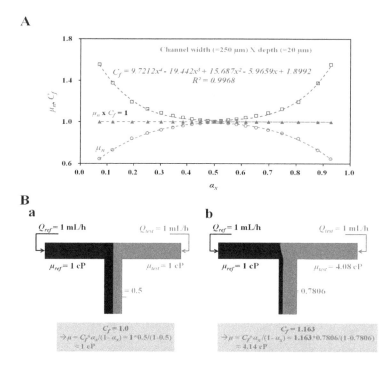

Figure A2. A correction factor of the parallel flow method estimated by conducting a numerical simulation. (**A**) The polynomial formula of a correction factor (C_f) estimated from a numerical simulation. (**B**) Numerical simulation results for showing interfacial location depending on the viscosity of test fluid. (**a**) $\alpha_x = 0.5$ for $\mu_{test} = 1$ cP. Viscosity of test fluid was estimated as 1 cP by considering correction factor of $C_f = 1$. (**b**) $\alpha_x = 0.7806$ for $\mu_{test} = 4.08$ cP. The viscosity of test fluid was estimated as 4.14 cP by considering the correction factor of $C_f = 1.163$.

Appendix A.3. Figure A3

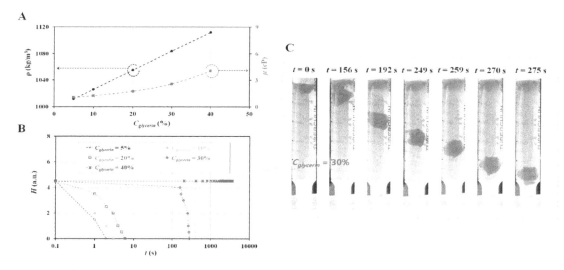

Figure A3. Selection of proper reference fluid by quantifying density (ρ) and sedimentation of RBCs droplet with respect to $C_{glycerin} = 5\%$, 10%, 20%, 30%, and 40%. (**A**) Variations of ρ and viscosity (μ) with respect to $C_{glycerin}$. (**B**) Temporal variation of sedimentation height (H) with respect to $C_{glycerin}$. (**C**) Snapshots for showing sedimentations of RBCs droplet with elapsed time (t) ($t = 0$, 156, 192, 249, 259, 270, and 275 s). Here, the syringe was filled with a 30% glycerin solution.

Appendix A.4. Blood Sample Preparation

According to the protocol approved by the Ethics Committee of Chosun University Hospital (CUH) (CHOSUN 2018-05-11), all experimental procedures were conducted after confirming that the procedures involved were appropriate and humane.

Human concentrated RBCs and fresh frozen plasma (FFP) were purchased from the Gwangju-Chonnam blood bank (Gwangju, Korea). The concentrated RBCs and FFP were kept at 4 °C and −20 °C, respectively. The concentrated RBCs were preserved in an anticoagulant solution (i.e., citrate phosphate dextrose adenine [CPDA]). To remove the CPDA from the concentrated RBCs, washing procedures were performed twice. The concentrated RBCs (~20 mL) were mixed with phosphate-buffered saline (PBS) (1×, pH 7.4, Gibco, Life Technologies, New York, NY, USA) (~20 mL) in a 40 mL tube. After inserting the tube in a centrifuge (Allegra X-30R benchtop, Beckman Coulter, Brea, CA, USA), the centrifuge was set to 4000 rpm and was operated for 10 min. Owing to differences in density, the blood sample was distinctively separated into two layers (i.e., upper layer: liquid, and lower layer: RBCs) in the tube. Normal RBCs were collected after removing the liquid positioned in the upper layer. To completely remove the anticoagulant solution, a washing procedure was repeated twice. The FFP was thawed under a room temperature of 25 °C. For removing debris existing in the FFP, pure plasma was collected by passing the FFP through a syringe filter (mesh size = 5 μm, Minisart, Sartorius, and Germany). Finally, the normal RBCs and plasma were stored at 4 °C in a refrigerator before the experiment. Various blood samples were prepared by adding normal or hardened RBCs into a specific base solution. Except for experiments to determine the contributions of hematocrit to blood viscosity or ESR, the hematocrit of the blood sample was fixed at $Hct = 50\%$ for consistent measurement.

First, to evaluate the contributions of hematocrit to blood viscosity and ESR, the hematocrit of the blood sample was adjusted to $Hct = 30\%$, 40%, and 50% by adding normal RBCs into base solution (i.e., 1× PBS, and plasma). Second, to enhance the ESR in ACS, five different concentrations of dextran solution (i.e., $C_{dex} = 0$, 5, 10, 15, and 20 mg/mL) were prepared by adding dextran powder (*Leuconostoc* spp., MW = 450–650 kDa, Sigma-Aldrich, USA) into 1× PBS. Then, blood samples ($Hct = 50\%$) were prepared by adding normal RBCs into specific concentrations of the dextran solution. Third, four concentrations of glutaraldehyde (GA) solution (i.e., $C_{GA} = 0$, 5, 10, and 15 μL/mL) were diluted by mixing the GA solution (Grade II, 25% in H_2O, Sigma-Aldrich, USA) with 1× PBS. Homogeneous hardened RBCs were prepared by exposing normal RBCs to each concentration of the GA solution for 10 min. To enhance ESR in blood sample ($Hct = 50\%$) significantly, plasma was replaced with a specific concentration of dextran solution ($C_{dex} = 15$ mg/mL). A hardened blood sample ($Hct = 50\%$) was then prepared by adding homogeneous hardened RBCs into the specific dextran solution.

Appendix A.5. Variation of Velocity, Interface, and Viscosity with Respect to Relocation of Object Plane

Variations of velocity, interface, and viscosity were evaluated by moving an object plane (Z_f) in the depth direction. The object plane (Z_f) relocated from $Z_f = -60$ μm to $Z_f = 60$ μm at intervals of 15 μm. $Z_f = 0$ represented that the microscopic images were captured at the focus plane (i.e., the best conditions for focus). $Z_f > 0$ meant that the microfluidic device moved vertically and that the microscopic images were captured at an out-of-focus plane. $Z_f < 0$ meant that the microfluidic device moved in a gravitational direction and that the microscopic images were captured at the out-of-focus plane. The blood sample ($Hct = 50\%$) was prepared by adding normal RBCs in a 1× PBS. The reference fluid with RBCs ($Hct = 7\%$) was prepared by adding normal RBCs into a 40% glycerin solution. Using two SPs, the reference fluid or blood sample was delivered to the reference channel (i.e., right-side channel). Simultaneously, the 1× PBS was delivered to the blood channel (i.e., left-side channel). The flow rate of each fluid remained at a constant flow rate of 1 mL/h.

First, with respect to the blood sample, the contribution of the object plane to velocity fields and viscosity was evaluated with respect to the relocation of the object plane. As shown in Figure A4-(A-a), variations of the velocity profile of the blood sample (U_B) across the reference channel width were obtained with respect to $Z_f = -60, -30, 0, 30,$ and 60 μm. Using data sets of $n = 180$, each velocity was averaged and expressed as a mean ± standard deviation. The inset of Figure A4-(A-a) depicted the velocity profile of blood flow (U_B) estimated from sequential microscopic images captured at the focal plane ($Z_f = 0$). When Z_f increased from $Z_f = 0$ to an out-of-focus plane, U_B tended to decrease. In other words, the velocity fields varied depending on the object plane.

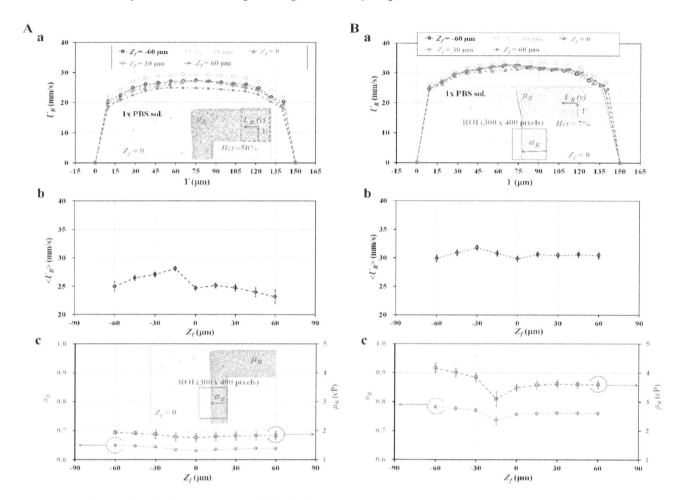

Figure A4. Effect of the relocation of object plane (Z_f) on velocity, interface, and viscosity with respect to the blood sample and reference fluid. A blood sample ($Hct = 50\%$) was prepared by adding normal RBCs into a 1× PBS. A reference fluid with RBCs ($Hct = 7\%$) was prepared by adding normal RBCs into a 40% glycerin solution. Both fluids were delivered to inlets at a constant flow rate of 1 mL/h with two SPs. (**A**) Effects of the relocation of object plane on velocity, interface, and viscosity for the blood sample. (**a**) Variations of U_B across reference channel width with respect to $Z_f = -60, -30, 0,$ 30, and 60 μm. The inset depicted the velocity profile of the blood sample flowing in the reference channel at $Z_f = 0$. (**b**) Variations of $<U_B>$ with respect to Z_f. (**c**) Variations of α_B and μ_B with respect to Z_f. The inset showed interfacial location (α_B) at $Z_f = 0$. (**B**) Effect of the relocation of object plane on velocity, interface, and viscosity for reference fluid with RBCs ($Hct = 7\%$). (**a**) Variations of U_R across reference channel width with respect to $Z_f = --60, -30, 0, 30,$ and 60 μm. The inset represented U_R and α_R at $Z_f = 0$. (**b**) Variations of $<U_R>$ with respect to Z_f. (**c**) Variations of α_R and μ_R with respect to Z_f.

Based on an analytical formula for a depth of correlation (DOC) suggested in a previous study [53], the DOC was estimated as 33.9 μm. Since the DOC was sufficiently higher than the channel depth of 20 μm (i.e., DOC > depth), all RBCs in the microfluidic channel could contribute to calculating the velocity fields uniformly. According to the estimated DOC, the μPIV technique measured averaged velocity fields in the depth direction at the focal plane ($Z_f = 0$). The averaged velocities of the blood sample and reference fluid ($<U_R>$, and $<U_B>$) were calculated as an arithmetic average over the specific ROI.

Figure A4-(A-b) showed variations of $<U_B>$ with respect to Z_f. When Z_f increased from the focal plane ($Z_f = 0$) to an out-of-focus plane, $<U_B>$ tended to gradually decrease. The averaged blood velocity ($<U_B>$) remained constant from $Z_f = 0$ to $Z_f = 30$ µm. From the results, $<U_B>$ remained constant until the microfluidic device moved vertically with regard to DOC. In that regard, when Z_f decreased from $Z_f = -15$ µm, $<U_B>$ tended to gradually decrease.

Figure A4-(A-c) showed variations of α_B and μ_B with respect to Z_f. The inset of Figure A4 (A-c) showed the interfacial location of blood flow (α_B) in a microscopic image captured at the focal plane ($Z_f = 0$). The blood viscosity (μ_B) was obtained by inserting α_B into the viscosity formula as reported in previous studies [32,33]. As α_B and μ_B remained constant with respect to Z_f, the relocation of the object plane did not contribute to varying the blood viscosity.

Second, with respect to the reference fluid with RBCs ($Hct = 7\%$), the effects of the object plane on velocity and viscosity were evaluated by quantifying variations of the velocity fields and viscosity when the object plane moved vertically. As shown in Figure A4-(B-a), variations of velocity profile (U_R) were obtained with respect to $Z_f = -60, -30, 0, 30$, and 60 µm. The inset of Figure A4-(B-a) represented U_R at the focal plane ($Z_f = 0$). Except for $Z_f = -30$ µm, the relocation of the object plane did not contribute to varying significant variations of $<U_R>$. Figure A4-(B-b) showed variations of $<U_R>$ with respect to Z_f. When Z_f relocated vertically from the focal plane ($Z_f = 0$), $<U_R>$ remained constant with respect to Z_f. From the results, $<U_R>$ remained constant, even though the object plane relocated vertically outside the DOC. However, when Z_f relocated in a gravitational direction from the focal plane ($Z_f = 0$), $<U_R>$ fluctuated along the object plane. As shown in Figure A4-(B-c), variations of α_R and μ_R were obtained with respect to Z_f. Similar to $<U_R>$, α_R and μ_R remained constant when Z_f relocated in the vertical depth direction. However, α_R and μ_R exhibited large fluctuations and increased when relocating Z_f in a gravitational direction.

From these experimental results, it was found that the averaged velocities of the blood sample and reference fluid ($<U_B>$, and $<U_R>$) remained constant throughout the relocation of the object plane outside the DOC. In other words, when a microfluidic device moved up to the DOC vertically, the averaged velocity and interface remained constant. However, when a microfluidic device moved in the gravitational direction, it contributed to fluctuations of velocity, interface, and viscosity. For consistent measurement of velocity fields and the interfacial location, a microfluidic device was positioned at $Z_f = 0$–30 µm. In other words, a microscopic image was then captured at the focus plane or at a slightly out-of-focus plane.

References

1.   Popel, A.S.; Johnson, P.C. Microcirculation and hemorheology. *Annu. Rev. Fluid Mech.* **2005**, *37*, 43–69. [CrossRef] [PubMed]
2.   Lipowsky, H.H. Microvascular Rheology and Hemodynamics. *Microcirculation* **2005**, *12*, 5–15. [CrossRef]
3.   Danesh, J.; Collins, R.; Peto, R.; Lowe, G.D.O. Haematocrit, viscosity, erythrocyte sedimentation rate: Meta-analyses of prospective studies of coronary heart disease. *Eur. Heart J.* **2000**, *21*, 515–520. [CrossRef] [PubMed]
4.   Jones, C.M.; Baker-Groberg, S.M.; Cianchetti, F.A.; Glynn, J.J.; Healy, L.D.; Lam, W.Y.; Nelson, J.W.; Parrish, D.C.; Phillips, K.G.; Scott-Drechsel, D.E.; et al. Measurement science in the circulatory system. *Cell Mol. Bioeng.* **2014**, *7*, 1–14. [CrossRef] [PubMed]
5.   Oore-ofe, O.; Soma, P.; Buys, A.V.; Debusho, L.K.; Pretorius, E. Characterizing pathology in erythrocytes using morphological and biophysical membrane properties: Relation to impaired hemorheology and cardiovascular function in rheumatoid arthritis. *Biochim. Biophys. Acta-Biomembr.* **2017**, *1859*, 2381–2391.
6.   Kang, Y.J.; Lee, S.-J. In vitro and ex vivo measurement of the biophysical properties of blood using microfluidic platforms and animal models. *Analyst* **2018**, *143*, 2723–2749. [CrossRef]

7.   Yeom, E.; Kim, H.M.; Park, J.H.; Choi, W.; Doh, J.; Lee, S.-J. Microfluidic system for monitoring temporal variations of hemorheological properties and platelet adhesion in LPS-injected rats. *Sci. Rep.* **2017**, *7*, 1801. [CrossRef]

8.   Kang, Y.J.; Yeom, E.; Lee, S.-J. Microfluidic biosensor for monitoring tmporal variations of hemorheological and hemodynamic properties using an extracorporeal rat bypass loop. *Anal. Chem.* **2013**, *85*, 10503–10511. [CrossRef]

9.   Kang, Y.J.; Lee, S.-J. Blood viscoelasticity measurement using steady and transient flow controls of blood in a microfluidic analogue of Wheastone-bridge channel. *Biomicrofluidics* **2013**, *7*, 054122. [CrossRef]

10. Schmid-Schonbein, H.; Gaehtgens, P.; Hirsch, H. On the shear rate dependence of red cell aggregation in vitro. *J. Clin. Investig.* **1968**, *47*, 1447–1454. [CrossRef]

11. Kim, B.J.; Lee, S.Y.; Jee, S.; Atajanov, A.; Yang, S. Micro-viscometer for measuring shear-varying blood viscosity over a wide-ranging shear rate. *Sensors* **2017**, *17*, 1442. [CrossRef] [PubMed]

12. Kang, Y.J.; Yang, S. Integrated microfluidic viscometer equipped with fluid temperature controller for measurement of viscosity in complex fluids. *Microfluid. Nanofluidics* **2013**, *14*, 657–668. [CrossRef]

13. Oh, S.; Kim, B.; Lee, J.K.; Choi, S. 3D-printed capillary circuits for rapid, low-cost, portable analysis ofblood viscosity. *Sens. Actuator B Chem.* **2018**, *259*, 106–113. [CrossRef]

14. Kang, Y.J.; Ryu, J.; Lee, S.-J. Label-free viscosity measurement of complex fluids using reversal flow switching manipulation in a microfluidic channel. *Biomicrofluidics* **2013**, *7*, 044106. [CrossRef]

15. Khnouf, R.; Karasneh, D.; Abdulhay, E.; Abdelhay, A.; Sheng, W.; Fan, Z.H. Microfluidics-based device for the measurement of blood viscosity and its modeling based on shear rate, temperature, and heparin concentration. *Biomedical Microdevices* **2019**, *21*, 80. [CrossRef]

16. Isiksacan, Z.; Erel, O.; Elbuken, C. A portable microfluidic system for rapid measurement of the erythrocyte sedimentation rate. *Lab Chip* **2016**, *16*, 4682–4690. [CrossRef]

17. Zeng, N.F.; Mancuso, J.E.; Zivkovic, A.M.; Smilowitz, J.T.; Ristenpart, W.D. Red blood cells from individuals with abdominal obesity or metabolic abnormalities exhibit less deformability upon entering a constriction. *PLoS ONE* **2016**, *11*, e0156070. [CrossRef]

18. Guo, Q.; Duffy, S.P.; Matthews, K.; Deng, X.; Santoso, A.T.; Islamzada, E.; Ma, H. Deformability based sorting of red blood cells improves diagnostic sensitivity for malaria caused by Plasmodium falciparum. *Lab Chip* **2016**, *16*, 645–654. [CrossRef]

19. Berry, S.B.; Fernandes, S.C.; Rajaratnam, A.; DeChiara, N.S.; Mace, C.R. Measurement of the hematocrit using paper-based microfluidic devices. *Lab Chip* **2016**, *16*, 3689–3694. [CrossRef]

20. Kim, B.J.; Lee, Y.S.; Zhbanov, A.; Yang, S. A physiometer for simultaneous measurement of whole blood viscosity and its determinants: Hematocrit and red blood cell deformability. *Analyst* **2019**, *144*, 3144–3157. [CrossRef]

21. Han, Z.; Tang, X.; Zheng, B. A PDMS viscometer for microliter Newtonian fluid. *J. Micromech. Microeng.* **2007**, *17*, 1828–1834. [CrossRef]

22. Srivastava, N.; Davenport, R.D.; Burns, M.A. Nanoliter Viscometer for Analyzing Blood Plasma and Other Liquid Samples. *Anal. Chem.* **2005**, *77*, 383–392. [CrossRef] [PubMed]

23. Kim, H.; Cho, Y.I.; Lee, D.-H.; Park, C.-M.; Moon, H.-W.; Hur, M.; Kim, J.Q.; Yun, Y.-M. Analycal performance evaluation of the scanning tube viscometer for measurement of whole blood viscosity. *Clin. Biochem.* **2013**, *46*, 139–142. [CrossRef] [PubMed]

24. Hong, H.; Song, J.M.; Yeom, E. 3D printed microfluidic viscometer based on the co-flowing stream. *Biomicrofluidics* **2019**, *13*, 014104. [CrossRef] [PubMed]

25. Kang, H.; Jang, I.; Song, S.; Bae, S.-C. Development of a paper-based viscometer for blood plasma using colorimetric analysis. *Anal. Chem.* **2019**, *91*, 4868–4875. [CrossRef]

26. Marinakis, G.N.; Barbenel, J.C.; Tsangaris, S.G. A new capillary viscometer for small samples of whole blood. *Proc. Inst. Mech. Eng.* **2002**, *216*, H1502. [CrossRef]

27. Solomon, D.E.; Abdel-Raziq, A.; Vanapalli, S.A. A stress-controlled microfluidic shear viscometer based on smartphone imaging. *Rheol. Acta* **2016**, *55*, 727–738. [CrossRef]

28. Kim, W.-J.; Kim, S.; Huh, C.; Kim, B.K.; Kim, Y.J. A novel hand-held viscometer applicable for point-of-care. *Sens. Actuator B Chem.* **2016**, *234*, 239–246. [CrossRef]

29. Pop, G.A.M.; Sisschops, L.L.A.; Iliev, B.; Struijk, P.C.; van der Heven, J.G.; Hoedemaekers, C.W.E. On-line blood viscosity monitoring in vivo with a central venous catheter using electrical impedance technique. *Biosens. Bioelectron.* **2013**, *41*, 595–601. [CrossRef]

30. Zeng, H.; Zhao, Y. Rheological analysis of non-Newtonian blood flow using a microfluidic device. *Sens. Actuator A Phys.* **2011**, *166*, 207–213. [CrossRef]

31. Li, Y.; Ward, K.R.; Burns, M.A. Viscosity measurements using microfluidic droplet length. *Anal. Chem.* **2017**, *89*, 3996–4006. [CrossRef] [PubMed]

32. Kang, Y.J. Periodic and simultaneous quantification of blood viscosity and red blood cell aggregation using a microfluidic platform under in-vitro closed-loop circulation. *Biomicrofluidics* **2018**, *12*, 024116. [CrossRef] [PubMed]

33. Kang, Y.J. Microfluidic-based technique for measuring RBC aggregation and blood viscosity in a continuous and simultaneous fashion. *Micromachines* **2018**, *9*, 467. [CrossRef] [PubMed]

34. Kang, Y.J.; Kim, B.J. Multiple and periodic measurement of RBC aggregation and ESR in parallel microfluidic channels under on-off blood flow control. *Micromachines* **2018**, *9*, 318. [CrossRef] [PubMed]

35. Nam, J.-H.; Yang, Y.; Chung, S.; Shin, S. Comparison of light-transmission and -backscattering methods in the measurement of red blood cell aggregation. *J. Biomed. Opt.* **2010**, *15*, 027003. [CrossRef]

36. Baskurt, O.K.; Uyuklu, M.; Meiselman, H.J. Time Course of Electrical Impedance During Red Blood Cell Aggregation in a Glass Tube: Comparison with Light Transmittance. *IEEE Trans. Biomed. Eng.* **2010**, *57*, 969–978. [CrossRef]

37. Antonova, N.; Riha, P.; Ivanov, I. Time dependent variation of human blood conductivity as a method for an estimation of RBC aggregation. *Clin. Hemorheolo. Microcir.* **2008**, *39*, 69–78. [CrossRef]

38. Brust, M.; Aouane, O.; Thie'baud, M.; Flormann, D.; Verdier, C.; Kaestner, L.; Laschke, M.W.; Selmi, H.; Benyoussef, A.; Podgorski, T.; et al. The plasma protein fibrinogen stabilizes clusters of red blood cells in microcapillary flows. *Sci. Rep.* **2014**, *4*, 4348. [CrossRef]

39. Kaliviotis, E.; Sherwood, M.; Balabani, S. Partitioning of red blood cell aggregates in bifurcating microscale flows. *Sci. Rep.* **2017**, *7*, 44563. [CrossRef]

40. Tomaiuolo, G.; Lanotte, L.; Ghigliotti, G.; Misbah, C.; Guido, S. Red blood cell clustering in Poiseuille microcapillary flow. *Phys. Fluids* **2012**, *24*, 051903. [CrossRef]

41. Yeom, E.; Lee, S.-J. Microfluidic-based speckle analysis for sensitive measurement of erythrocyte aggregation: A comparison of four methods for detection of elevated erythrocyte aggregation in diabetic rat blood. *Biomicrofluidics* **2015**, *9*, 024110. [CrossRef]

42. Lee, K.; Kinnunen, M.; Khokhlova, M.D.; Lyubin, E.V.; Priezzhev, A.V.; Meglinski, I.; Fedyanin, A.A. Optical tweezers study of red blood cell aggregation and disaggregation in plasma and protein solutions. *J. Biomed. Opt.* **2016**, *21*, 035001. [CrossRef]

43. Zhbanov, A.; Yang, S. Effects of aggregation on blood sedimentation and conductivity. *PLoS ONE* **2015**, *10*, e0129337. [CrossRef]

44. Kang, Y.J.; Ha, Y.-R.; Lee, S.-J. Microfluidic-based measurement of erythrocyte sedimentation rate for biophysical assessment of blood in an in vivo malaria-infected mouse. *Biomicrofluidics* **2014**, *8*, 044114. [CrossRef]

45. Kang, Y.J. Microfluidic-based biosensor for sequential measurement of blood pressure and RBC aggregation over continuously varying blood flows. *Micromachines* **2019**, *10*, 577. [CrossRef]

46. Kang, Y.J. Simultaneous measurement of blood pressure and RBC aggregation by monitoring on–off blood flows supplied from a disposable air-compressed pump. *Analyst* **2019**, *144*, 3556–3566. [CrossRef]

47. Kang, Y.J. RBC deformability measurement based on variations of pressure in multiple micropillar channels during blood delivery using a disposable air-compressed pump. *Anal. Methods* **2018**, *10*, 4549–4561. [CrossRef]

48. Gao, J.X.; Yeo, L.P.; Chan-Park, M.B.; Miao, J.M.; Yan, Y.H.; Sun, J.B.; Lam, Y.C.; Yue, C.Y. Antistick postpassivation of high-aspect ratio silicon molds fabricated by deep-reactive ion etching. *J. Microelectromech. Syst.* **2006**, *15*, 84–93. [CrossRef]

49. Otsu, N. A threshold selection method from gray-level histograms. *IEEE Trans. Syst. Man. Cybern.* **1979**, *9*, 62–66. [CrossRef]

50. Kang, Y.J. Continuous and simultaneous measurement of the biophysical properties of blood in a microfluidic environment. *Analyst* **2016**, *141*, 6583–6597. [CrossRef]

51.   Cheng, N.-S. Formula for the viscosity of a glycerol-water mixture. *Ind. Eng. Chem. Res.* **2008**, *47*, 3285–3288. [CrossRef]

52.   Linderkamp, O.; Friederichs, E.; Boehler, T.; Ludwig, A. Age dependency of red blood cell deformability and density: Studies in transient erythroblastopenia of childhood. *Br. J. Haematol.* **1993**, *83*, 125–129. [CrossRef]

53.   Bourdon, C.J.; Olsen, M.G.; Gorby, A.D. The depth of corretion in miciro-PIV for high numerical aperature and immersion objectives. *J. Fluid Eng. Trans. ASME* **2006**, *128*, 883–886. [CrossRef]

Permissions

The contributors of this book come from diverse backgrounds, making this book a truly international effort. This book will bring forth new frontiers with its revolutionizing research information and detailed analysis of the nascent developments around the world.

We would like to thank all the contributing authors for lending their expertise to make the book truly unique. They have played a crucial role in the development of this book. Without their invaluable contributions this book wouldn't have been possible. They have made vital efforts to compile up to date information on the varied aspects of this subject to make this book a valuable addition to the collection of many professionals and students.

This book was conceptualized with the vision of imparting up-to-date information and advanced data in this field. To ensure the same, a matchless editorial board was set up. Every individual on the board went through rigorous rounds of assessment to prove their worth. After which they invested a large part of their time researching and compiling the most relevant data for our readers.

The editorial board has been involved in producing this book since its inception. They have spent rigorous hours researching and exploring the diverse topics which have resulted in the successful publishing of this book. They have passed on their knowledge of decades through this book. To expedite this challenging task, the publisher supported the team at every step. A small team of assistant editors was also appointed to further simplify the editing procedure and attain best results for the readers.

Apart from the editorial board, the designing team has also invested a significant amount of their time in understanding the subject and creating the most relevant covers. They scrutinized every image to scout for the most suitable representation of the subject and create an appropriate cover for the book.

The publishing team has been an ardent support to the editorial, designing and production team. Their endless efforts to recruit the best for this project, has resulted in the accomplishment of this book. They are a veteran in the field of academics and their pool of knowledge is as vast as their experience in printing. Their expertise and guidance has proved useful at every step. Their uncompromising quality standards have made this book an exceptional effort. Their encouragement from time to time has been an inspiration for everyone.

The publisher and the editorial board hope that this book will prove to be a valuable piece of knowledge for researchers, students, practitioners and scholars across the globe.

List of Contributors

Ezekiel O. Adekanmbi, Anthony T. Giduthuri and Soumya K. Srivastava
Department of Chemical and Materials Engineering, University of Idaho, Moscow, ID 83844-1021, USA

Risa Munechika
Department of Engineering, Nagoya Institute of Technology, Nagoya 466-8555, Japan

Shukei Sugita
Department of Engineering, Nagoya Institute of Technology, Nagoya 466-8555, Japan
Department of Electrical and Mechanical Engineering, Nagoya Institute of Technology, Nagoya 466-8555, Japan

Zhigang Gao, Weijie Zhao, Jiu Deng, Xiaorui Li, Yueyang Qu, Lingling Xu and Yong Luo
School of Pharmaceutical Science and Technology, Dalian University of Technology, Dalian 116024, China

Zongzheng Chen
Integrated Chinese and Western Medicine Postdoctoral research station, Jinan University, Guangzhou 510632, China

Yao Lu
Dalian Institute of Chemical Physics, Chinese Academy of Sciences, Dalian 116023, China

Tingjiao Li
College of Stomatology, Dalian Medical University, Dalian 116024, China

Bingcheng Lin
School of Pharmaceutical Science and Technology, Dalian University of Technology, Dalian 116024, China
Dalian Institute of Chemical Physics, Chinese Academy of Sciences, Dalian 116023, China

Masanori Nakamura and Daichi Ono
Department of Electrical and Mechanical Engineering, Nagoya Institute of Technology, Nagoya 466-8555, Japan

Yuan Fang
School of Automation and Information Engineering, Xi'an University of Technology, Xi'an 710048, China
School of Electrical and Electronic Engineering, Baoji University of Arts and Sciences, Baoji 721016, China

Ningmei Yu, Yuquan Jiang and Chaoliang Dang
School of Automation and Information Engineering, Xi'an University of Technology, Xi'an 710048, China

Vera Faustino
Center for Micro Electromechanical Systems (CMEMS-UMinho), University of Minho, Campus de Azurém, 4800-058 Guimarães, Portugal
MEtRICs, Mechanical Engineering Department, University of Minho, Campus de Azurém, 4800-058 Guimarães, Portugal

Raquel O. Rodrigues
Center for Micro Electromechanical Systems (CMEMS-UMinho), University of Minho, Campus de Azurém, 4800-058 Guimarães, Portugal

Elísio Costa and Alice Santos-Silva
UCIBIO-REQUINTE, Faculty of Pharmacy of University of Porto, Rua de Jorge Viterbo Ferreira, 4150-755 Porto, Portugal

Vasco Miranda
Dialysis Clinic of Gondomar, Rua 5 de Outubro, 4420-086 Gondomar, Portugal

Joana S. Amaral
CIMO, Centro de Investigação de Montanha, Instituto Politécnico de Bragança, Campus de Sta. Apolónia, 5300-253 Bragança, Portugal
REQUIMTE-LAQV, Pharmacy Faculty, University of Porto, 4099-002 Porto, Portugal

Rui Lima
CEFT, Faculdade de Engenharia da Universidade do Porto (FEUP), Rua Roberto Frias, 4200-465 Porto, Portugal
MEtRICs, Mechanical Engineering Department, University of Minho, Campus de Azurém, 4800-058 Guimarães, Portugal

Yang Jun Kang
Department of Mechanical Engineering, Chosun University, 309 Pilmun-daero, Dong-gu, Gwangju 61452, Korea

J. Ponmozhi, J. B. L. M. Campos and J. M. Miranda
Transport Phenomena Research Center (CEFT), Department of Chemical Engineering, Faculty of Engineering, University of Porto, Rua Dr. Roberto Frias s/n, 4200-465 Porto, Portugal

J. M. R. Moreira and F. J. Mergulhão
Laboratory for Process Engineering, Environment (LEPABE), Biotechnology and Energy, Department of Chemical Engineering, Faculty of Engineering, University of Porto, Rua Dr. Roberto Frias s/n, 4200-465 Porto, Portugal

Susana O. Catarino and Raquel O. Rodrigues
Center for Micro Electromechanical Systems (CMEMS-UMinho), University of Minho, Campus de Azurém, 4800-058 Guimarães, Portugal

Diana Pinho
Research Centre in Digitalization and Intelligent Robotics (CeDRI), Instituto Politécnico de Bragança, Campus de Santa Apolónia, 5300-253 Bragança, Portugal
CEFT, Faculdade de Engenharia da Universidade do Porto (FEUP), Rua Roberto Frias, 4200-465 Porto, Portugal
Center for Micro Electromechanical Systems (CMEMS-UMinho), University of Minho, Campus de Azurém, 4800-058 Guimarães, Portugal
MEtRICs, Mechanical Engineering Department, University of Minho, Campus de Azurém, 4800-058 Guimarães, Portugal

João M. Miranda
CEFT, Faculdade de Engenharia da Universidade do Porto (FEUP), Rua Roberto Frias, 4200-465 Porto, Portugal

Naoki Takeishi and Shigeo Wada
Graduate School of Engineering Science, Osaka University, 1-3 Machikaneyama, Toyonaka, Osaka 560-8531, Japan

Hiroaki Ito
Department of Mechanical Engineering, Osaka University, Suita, Osaka 565-0871, Japan

Department of Physics, Graduate School of Science, Chiba University, Chiba 263-8522, Japan

Makoto Kaneko
Department of Mechanical Engineering, Osaka University, Suita, Osaka 565-0871, Japan

Byung Jun Kim
Department of Biomedical Science and Engineering, Gwangju Institute of Science and Technology (GIST), Gwangju 61005, Korea

Liliana Vilas Boas
Microelectromechanical Systems Research Unit (CMEMS-UMinho), University of Minho, 4800-058 Guimarães, Portugal
Instituto Politécnico de Bragança, ESTiG, C. Sta. Apolónia, 5300-253 Bragança, Portugal

Vera Faustino
Microelectromechanical Systems Research Unit (CMEMS-UMinho), University of Minho, 4800-058 Guimarães, Portugal
MEtRICs, DEM, University of Minho, 4800-058 Guimarães, Portugal

João Mário Miranda
CEFT, University of Porto, 4000-008 Porto, Portugal

Graça Minas and Susana Oliveira Catarino
Microelectromechanical Systems Research Unit (CMEMS-UMinho), University of Minho, 4800-058 Guimarães, Portugal

Carla Sofia Veiga Fernandes
Instituto Politécnico de Bragança, ESTiG, C. Sta. Apolónia, 5300-253 Bragança, Portugal

Index